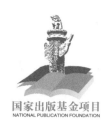

国家出版基金项目
NATIONAL PUBLICATION FOUNDATION

National Key Book Publishing Planning Project of the 13th Five-Year Plan

"十三五"国家重点图书出版规划项目

International Clinical Medicine Series Based on the Belt and Road Initiative

"一带一路"背景下国际化临床医学丛书

Preventive Medicine

预防医学

Chief Editor Lyu Quanjun

主编 吕全军

U0339679

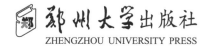

郑州大学出版社

ZHENGZHOU UNIVERSITY PRESS

图书在版编目(CIP)数据

预防医学 = Preventive Medicine：英文／吕全军主编. — 郑州：郑州大学出版社，2020. 12

("一带一路"背景下国际化临床医学丛书)

ISBN 978-7-5645-6652-4

Ⅰ. ①预… Ⅱ. ①吕… Ⅲ. ①预防医学 – 英文 Ⅳ. ①R1

中国版本图书馆 CIP 数据核字(2019)第 167946 号

预防医学 = Preventive Medicine：英文

项目负责人	孙保营 杨秦予		策 划 编 辑	孙保营
责 任 编 辑	陈文静		装 帧 设 计	苏永生
责 任 校 对	张彦勤		责 任 监 制	凌 青 李瑞卿

出 版 发 行	郑州大学出版社有限公司		地 址	郑州市大学路 40 号(450052)
出 版 人	孙保营		网 址	http://www.zzup.cn
经 销	全国新华书店		发行电话	0371-66966070
印 刷	河南文华印务有限公司			
开 本	850 mm×1 168 mm 1 / 16			
印 张	23.75		字 数	912 千字
版 次	2020 年 12 月第 1 版		印 次	2020 年 12 月第 1 次印刷

书 号	ISBN 978-7-5645-6652-4		定 价	129.00 元

Staff of Expert Steering Committee

Chairmen

Zhong Shizhen Li Sijin Lü Chuanzhu

Vice Chairmen

Bai Yuting Chen Xu Cui Wen Huang Gang Huang Yuanhua

Jiang Zhisheng Li Yumin Liu Zhangsuo Luo Baojun Lü Yi

Tang Shiying

Committee Member

An Dongping	Bai Xiaochun	Cao Shanying	Chen Jun	Chen Yijiu
Chen Zhesheng	Chen Zhihong	Chen Zhiqiao	Ding Yueming	Du Hua
Duan Zhongping	Guan Chengnong	Huang Xufeng	Jian Jie	Jiang Yaochuan
Jiao Xiaomin	Li Cairui	Li Guoxin	Li Guoming	Li Jiabin
Li Ling	Li Zhijie	Liu Hongmin	Liu Huifan	Liu Kangdong
Song Weiqun	Tang Chunzhi	Wang Huamin	Wang Huixin	Wang Jiahong
Wang Jiangang	Wang Wenjun	Wang Yuan	Wei Jia	Wen Xiaojun
Wu Jun	Wu Weidong	Wu Xuedong	Xie Xieju	Xue Qing
Yan Wenhai	Yan Xinming	Yang Donghua	Yu Feng	Yu Xiyong
Zhang Lirong	Zhang Mao	Zhang Ming	Zhang Yu'an	Zhang Junjian
Zhao Song	Zhao Yumin	Zheng Weiyang	Zhu Lin	

专家指导委员会

主 任 委 员

钟世镇　李思进　吕传柱

副主任委员（以姓氏汉语拼音为序）

白育庭　陈　旭　崔　文　黄　钢　黄元华　姜志胜

李玉民　刘章锁　雒保军　吕　毅　唐世英

委　　员（以姓氏汉语拼音为序）

安东平　白晓春　曹山鹰　陈　君　陈忆九　陈哲生

陈志宏　陈志桥　丁跃明　杜　华　段钟平　官成浓

黄旭枫　简　洁　蒋尧传　焦小民　李才锐　李国新

李果明　李家斌　李　玲　李志杰　刘宏民　刘会范

刘康栋　宋为群　唐纯志　王华民　王慧欣　王家宏

王建刚　王文军　王　渊　韦　嘉　温小军　吴　军

吴卫东　吴学东　谢协驹　薛　青　鄢文海　闫新明

杨冬华　余　峰　余细勇　张莉蓉　张　茂　张　明

张玉安　章军建　赵　松　赵玉敏　郑维扬　朱　林

编审委员会

Editorial Staff

作者名单

主　审
　　吴卫东　　新乡医学院
　　王惠欣　　瑞典斯德哥尔摩大学
主　编
　　吕全军　　郑州大学
副主编
　　孟晓静　　南方医科大学
　　马玉霞　　河北医科大学
　　王美林　　南京医科大学
　　许雅君　　北京大学
　　姚三巧　　新乡医学院
　　于　燕　　西安交通大学
编　委　（以姓氏汉语拼音为序）
　　程　悦　　西安交通大学
　　韩　蓓　　西安交通大学
　　黄　波　　南华大学
　　黄　辉　　郑州大学
　　姜碧杰　　新乡医学院
　　罗小琴　　西安交通大学
　　王百齐　　天津医科大学
　　王　玲　　澳门科技大学
　　吴　媚　　四川大学
　　燕　贞　　海南医学院
　　杨　瑾　　山西医科大学
　　曾怀才　　南华大学
　　张　勤　　四川大学
　　赵奇红　　安徽医科大学
　　赵　茜　　厦门大学
　　朱静媛　　郑州大学

Preface

At the Second Belt and Road Summit Forum on International Cooperation in 2019 and the Seventy-third World Health Assembly in 2020, General Secretary Xi Jinping stated the importance for promoting the construction of the "Belt and Road" and jointly build a community for human health. Countries and regions along the "Belt and Road" have a large number of overseas Chinese communities, and shared close geographic proximity, similarities in culture, disease profiles and medical habits. They also shared a profound mass base with ample space for cooperation and exchange in Clinical Medicine. The publication of the International Clinical Medicine series for clinical researchers, medical teachers and students in countries along the "Belt and Road" is a concrete measure to promote the exchange of Chinese and foreign medical science and technology with mutual appreciation and reciprocity.

Zhengzhou University Press coordinated more than 600 medical experts from over 160 renowned medical research institutes, medical schools and clinical hospitals across China. It produced this set of medical tools in English to serve the needs for the construction of the "Belt and Road". It comprehensively coversaspects in the theoretical framework and clinical practicesin Clinical Medicine, including basic science, multiple clinical specialities and social medicine. It reflects the latest academic and technological developments, and the international frontiers of academic advancements in Clinical Medicine. It shared with the world China's latest diagnosis and therapeutic approaches, clinical techniques, and experiences in prescription and medication. It has an important role in disseminating contemporary Chinese medical science and technology innovations, demonstrating the achievements of modern China's economic and social development, and promoting the unique charm of Chinese culture to the world.

The series is the first set of medical tools written in English by Chinese medical experts to serve the needs of the "Belt and Road" construction. It systematically and comprehensively reflects the Chinese characteristics in Clinical Medicine. Also, it presents a landmark achievement in the implementation of the "Belt and Road" initiative in promoting exchanges in medical science and technology. This series is theoretical in nature, with each volume built on the mainlines in traditional disciplines but at the same time introducing contemporary theories that guide clinical practices, diagnosis and treatment methods, echoing the latest research findings in Clinical Medicine.

As the disciplines in Clinical Medicine rapidly advances, different views on knowledge, inclusiveness, and medical ethics may arise. We hope this work will facilitate the exchange of ideas, build common ground while allowing differences, and contribute to the building of a community for human health in a broad spectrum of disciplines and research focuses.

Nick Lemoine

Foreign Academician of the Chinese Academy of Engineering
Dean, Academy of Medical Sciences of Zhengzhou University
Director, Barts Cancer Institute, London, UK
6th August, 2020

Foreword

The book reviews national health achievements in recent decades, but also examines the hidden vulnerabilities. The concept of health as a public good is discussed, as it is the fundamental duty of government to promote and protect the health of the public.

This book provides a complete guide to common occupational and environmental injuries and illnesses, their diagnosis and treatment, and preventive measures in the workplace and community. Our aim is to help health care professionals understand the complexities of occupational and environmental health issues and provide useful clinical information on common illnesses and injuries. The book contains three sections.

Part 1 is living Environment and Health. This part povides a comprehensive discussion of environmental medicine and some of the complex societal issues that accompany industrialization and technologic advances throughout the world. Environmental health is the field of science that studies how the environment influences human health and disease. Environmental health addresses all the physical, chemical, and biological factors external to a person, and all the related factors impacting behaviors. It encompasses the assessment and control of those environmental factors that can potentially affect health. It is targeted towards preventing disease and creating health–supportive environments.

Promoting health remains an arduous task and nothing short of concerted international efforts is required for truly delivering the goal of "health for all". The systems and entities that protect and promote the public's health, already have been challenged by problems like obesity, toxic environments, a large uninsured population, and health disparities and must also confront emerging threats, such as antimicrobial resistance and bioterrorism and the new era. The social, cultural, and global contexts of the nation's health are also undergoing rapid and dramatic change. Scientific and technological advances, such as genomics and informatics, extend the limits of knowledge and human potential more rapidly than their implications can be absorbed and acted upon. At the same time, people, products, and germs migrate and the nation's demographics are shifting in ways that challenge public and private resources. So a framework for assuring the public's health in the new century should be described.

Part 2 is Diet, Nutrition and Health. This part comprises six chapters, each considering a particular aspect of nutrition. It introduces the nutrition basics, comprehensive consideration of community nutrition, nutrition in life circle, nutrition–related diseases, clinical nutrition, food safety and foodborne diseases.

Part 3 is Occupational Environment and Health. This part defines the practice of occupational and environmental medicine and introduce the health care provider to the diagnosis of occupational injuries and illnesses. These chapters offer guidance for identifying workplace and community exposures to toxic material—putting this information to immediate clinical use and applying it toward better health and safety practices in the workplace. This section presents a comprehensive discussion of disability prevention and management and considers the important issues in the international practice of occupational and environmental medicine.

We hope this book is very helpful for the international students to study public health and preventive medicine.

Authors

Contents

Part 1   Living Environment and Health

Part 2　Diet, Nutrition and Health

Part 3　Occupational Environment and Health

Chapter 1

Introduction

1.1 Basic concepts

1.1.1 Health is more difficult to define than disease

Perhaps the best-known definition of health comes from the preamble to the constitution of the World Health Organization: "Health is a state of complete physical, mental, and social well-being and not merely the absence of disease or infirmity." This definition has the strengths of recognizing that any meaningful concept of health must include all the dimensions of human life, and that such a definition must be positive (i. e. , "not merely the absence of disease or infirmity"). Nevertheless, the definition has been criticized for two weaknesses. It is too idealistic in its expectations for complete well-being, and it is too static in viewing health as a state rather than as a dynamic process that requires constant effort and activity to maintain. Better health is central to human happiness and well-being. It also makes an important contribution to economic progress, as healthy populations live longer, are more productive, and save more. Many factors influence health status and a country's ability to provide quality health services for its people. "The biggest enemy of health in the developing world is poverty. " (Kofi Annan). Health promotion is the process of enabling people to increase control over, and to improve their health. It moves beyond a focus on individual behavior and towards a wide range of social and environmental interventions.

1.1.2 Public health

1.1.2.1 Definitions of public health

The term of "public health" has two meanings. The first one refers to the health status of the public, for a defined population. The second meaning refers to the organized social efforts made to preserve and improve the health of a defined population. The best-known definition of public health in terms of this second meaning was written in 1920 by C. E. A. Winslow and it is still remarkably current significance.

Public health is the science and art of preventing disease, prolonging life, and promoting physical health and efficiency through organized community efforts for the sanitation of the environment, the control of community infections, the education of the individual in principles of personal hygiene, the organization of medical and nursing service for the early diagnosis and treatment of disease, and the development of the social machinery which will ensure to every individual in the community a standard of living adequate for the maintenance of health.

This definition is profound in many ways. First, it states the central emphasis of all public health work, that is, promoting health and preventing disease. Second, it emphasizes the diverse strategies that are required to bring this about, including environmental sanitation, specific disease control efforts, health education, medical care, and an adequate standard of living. Third, it clarifies that for these goals to be achieved, organized social action is required. This action is largely expressed in the policies of the federal, state, and local governments and in the activities of the agencies designed to promote and protect the health of the public. As the Institute of Medicine (IOM) indicated in its 1988 report entitled *The Future of Public Health*, Public health is what we, as a society, do collectively to ensure the conditions in which people can be healthy.

1.1.2.2 Missions, functions and services of public health

There are two missions of public health: Promote physical and mental health. Prevent disease, injury, and disability.

The three core public health functions are assessment, assurance and policy development. These three functions revolve in a continuous motion. Because the scope of these three functions is so broad, the 10 essential public health services have been developed to further differentiate the stages of the public health process.

There are ten essential public health services namely: ①Monitor health status to identify and solve community problems; ②Diagnose and investigate health problems and health hazards in the community; ③Inform, educate, and empower people about health issues; ④Mobilize community partnerships and action to identify and solve health problems; ⑤Develop policies and plans that support individual and community health efforts; ⑥Enforce laws and regulations that protect health and ensure safety; ⑦Link people to needed personal health services; ⑧Ensure a competent public and personal health care workforce; ⑨Evaluate effectiveness, accessibility, and quality of personal and population-based health services; ⑩Research for new insights and innovative solutions to health problems.

Public health surveillance is the continuous, systematic collection, analysis and interpretation of health-related data needed for the planning, implementation, and evaluation of public health practice. Such surveillance can: ①Serve as an early warning system for impending public health emergencies; ②Document the impact of an intervention, or track progress towards specified goals; ③And monitor and clarify the epidemiology of health problems, to allow priorities to be set and to develop public health policy and strategies.

1.1.2.3 Preventive medicine

The preventive medicine is the science about environment and health. It refers to the relationship between environment and population health by use of the theory and methods of basic medicine, clinical medicine, environmental medicine and social medicine. It demonstrates useful and harmful factors that influence health and environment-related diseases and their genesis, development and epidemic.

The fields of preventive medicine and public health share the goals of promoting general health, preventing specific diseases, and applying the concepts and techniques of epidemiology toward these goals. Preventive medicine seeks to enhance the lives of individuals by helping them improve their own health, whereas public health attempts to promote health in populations through the application of organized community efforts. Although preventive medicine and public health are discussed separately here, there should be a seamless continuum between the practice of preventive medicine by clinicians, the attempts of individuals and families to promote their own and their neighbors' health, and the efforts of governments and voluntary agencies to achieve the same health goals for populations.

1.2   Natural history of public health

1.2.1   Natural history of public health in the United States

In the United States, Lemuel Shattuck's "Report of the Sanitary Commission of Massachusetts" in 1850 outlined existing and future public health needs for that state and became America's blueprint for development of a public health system. Shattuck called for the establishment of state and local health departments to organize public efforts aimed at sanitary inspections, communicable disease control, food sanitation, vital statistics, and services for infants and children. These local health departments developed rapidly in the seaports and other industrial urban centers, beginning with a health department in Baltimore in 1798, because these were the settings where the problems were reaching unacceptable levels.

This sketch of the development of public health in the United State would be incomplete without a brief introduction to the roles and powers of the federal government. Federal health powers, at least as enumerated in the U. S. Constitution, are minimal. It is surprising to some to learn that the word health does not even appear in the Constitution. As a result of not being a power granted to the federal government (such as defense, foreign diplomacy, international and interstate commerce, or printing money), health became a power to be exercised by states or reserved to the people themselves.

Although the complete history of public health is a fascinating saga in its own right, this section presents only selected highlights. When ancient cultures perceived illness as the manifestation of supernatural forces, they also felt that little in the way of either personal or collective action was possible. For many centuries, disease was synonymous with epidemic. Diseases including horrific epidemics of infectious diseases such as the Black Death (plague), leprosy, and cholera, were phenomena to be accepted. It was not until the so-called Age of Reason and the Enlightenment that scholarly inquiry began to challenge the "givens" or accepted realities of society. Eventually, the expansion of the science and knowledge base would reap substantial rewards.

With the advent of industrialism and imperialism, the stage was set for epidemic diseases to increase their terrible toll. As populations shifted to urban centers for purpose of commerce and industry, public health conditions worsened: The mixing of dense populations living in unsanitary conditions and working long hours in unsafe and exploitative industries with wave after wave of cholera, smallpox, typhoid, tuberculosis, yellow fever, and other diseases was a formula for disaster. Such disaster struck again and again across the globe, but most seriously and most often at the industrialized seaport cities that provided the portal of entry for diseases transported as stowaways alongside commercial cargo. The experience and subsequent susceptibilty of different cultures to these diseases partly explain how relatively small bands of Europeans were able to overcome and subjugate vast Native American cultures. Seeing the Europeans unaffected by scourges such as smallpox served to reinforce beliefs that these light-skinned visitors were supernatural figures unaffected by natural forces.

The British colonies in North America and the fledgling United States certainly bore their share of the burden. American diaries of the 17th and 18th centuries chronicle one infectious disease onslaught after another. These epidemics left their mark on families, communities, and even history. For example, the national capital had to be moved out of Philadelphia because of a devastating yellow fever epidemic in 1793. This epidemic also prompted the city to develop its first board of health in that same year.

The formation of local boards of distinguished citizens, the first boards of health, was one of the earliest organized responses to epidemics. This response was revealing in that it represented an attempt to confront disease collectively.

Because science had not yet determined that specific microorganisms were the causes of epidemics, avoidance had long been the primary tactic used. Avoidance meant evacuating the general location of the epidemic until it subsided or isolating diseased individuals or those recently exposed to diseases on the basis of a mix of fear, tradition, and scientific speculation. Several developments, however, were swinging the pendulum ever closer to more effective counteractions.

The public health pioneers such as Edward Jenner, John Snow and Edwin Chadwick illustrated the value of public health, even when its methods are applied amid scientific uncertainty. Long before Koch's postulates established scientific methods for linking bacteria with specific diseases and before Pasteur's experiments helped to establish the germ theory, both Jenner and Snow used deductive logic and common sense to do battle with smallpox and cholera, respectively. In 1796, Jenner successfully used vaccination for a disease that ran rampant through communities across the globe. This was the initial shot in a long and arduous campaign that by the year 1977 had totally eradicated smallpox from all of its human hiding places in every country in the world.

Snow's accomplishments even further advanced the art and science of public health. In 1854, Snow traced an outbreak of cholera to the well water drawn from the pump at Broad Street and helped to prevent hundreds, perhaps thousands, of cholera cases. In that same year, he demonstrated that another large outbreak could be traced to one particular water company that drew its water from the Thames River, downstream from London, and that another company that drew its water upstream from London was not linked with cholera cases. In both efforts, Snow's ability to collect and analyze data allowed him to determine causation, which in turn allowed him to implement corrective actions that prevented additional cases. All of this occurred without the benefit of the knowledge that there was an odd-shaped little bacterium that was carried in water and spread from person to person by hand-to-mouth contact.

England's General Board of Health conducted its own investigations of these outbreaks and concluded that air, rather than contaminated water, was the cause. Its approach, however, was one of collecting a vast amount of information and accepting only that which supported its view of disease causation. Snow, on the other hand, systematically tested his hypothesis by exploring evidence that ran in contrast to his initial expectations.

Chadwick was a more official leader of what has become known as the sanitary movement of the latter half of the 19th century. In a variety of official capacities, he played a major part in structuring government's role and responsibilities for protecting the public's health. Because of the growing concern over the social and sanitary conditions in England, the National Vaccination Board was established in 1837. Shortly thereafter, Chadwick's "Report on an Inquiry into the Sanitary Conditions of the Laboring Population of Great Britain" articulated a framework for broad public actions that served as a blueprint for the growing sanitary movement. One result was the establishment in 1848 of the General Board of Health. Interestingly, Chadwick's interest in public health had its roots in Jeremy Bentham's utilitarian movement. For Chadwick, disease was viewed as cause of poverty, and poverty was responsible the great social ills of the time, including societal disorder and high taxation to provide the general welfare. Public health efforts are necessary to reduce poverty and its wider social effects. This view recognizes a link between poverty and health that differs somewhat from current views. Today, it is more common to consider poor health as a result of poverty, rather than as its cause.

Chadwick was also a key participant in the partly scientific, partly political debate that took place in British government as to whether deaths should be attributed to clinical conditions or to their underlying factors, such as hunger and poverty. It was Chadwick's view that pathologic, as opposed to less proximal social and behavioral, factors should be the basis for classifying deaths. Chadwick's arguments prevailed, although aspects of this debate continue to this day. William Farr, sometimes called the father of modern vital statistics, championed the opposing view.

In the latter half of the 19th century, as sanitation and environmental engineering methods evolved, more effective interventions became available against epidemic diseases. Furthermore, the scientific advances of this period paved the way for modern disease control efforts targeting specific microorganisms.

1.2.2   Natural history of public health in China

When the People's Republic of China was founded in 1949, China had a weak medical and health system due to low levels of development in its economy and society. The nation had only 3,670 medical and health institutions, 541,000 health workers and 85,000 beds at health institutions. The average life expectancy was 35 years. To change this situation, the government devoted great efforts to developing the medical and health services, and implemented guidelines which stipulated that the health services were to serve vast majority of the people, that prevention should be stressed, that both Western medicine and Traditional Chinese Medicine (TCM) should be utilized, and that health promotion and people's involvement should be incorporated. The people were mobilized to carry out health promotion programs, and basic knowledge about healthcare was widely spread. All of this greatly enhanced the people's health, and major breakthroughs were made in medical sciences. Chlamydia rachomatis was identified for the first time by Chinese scientists; Chinese doctors performed the world's first replantation of a severed limb; and artemisinin, an effective cure for malaria, was extracted in a Chinese laboratory.

Following the introduction of the reform and opening-up drive in 1978, to address problems such as a severe shortage of medical and health resources and a lack of service capability and low efficiency, the government allowed multichannel financing for the medical industry, and encouraged medical development in various forms, by increasing resource supply, opening up the pharmaceuticals manufacturing and circulation market, developing the pharmaceutical industry, and promoting TCM. Economic incentives were adopted to encourage medical personnel to enhance their performance. At the First National Health Service Meeting in 1996, a decision was made on implementing the guiding principles for health services in the new era, namely, "focusing on the rural areas, prioritizing prevention, equal emphasis on Western medicine and TCM, relying on science and education, encouraging public participation, promoting public health, and serving socialist modernization. " In 1998, China began to form a social medical insurance system to cover the basic medical needs of workers. In 2000, it set the goal of establishing an urban medical and healthcare system in line with the socialist market economy, so that the people could enjoy reasonably priced, high-quality medical services, and thus become healthier. In 2002, the government released the Decision on Further Enhancing Health Services in Rural Areas. Taking into consideration the levels of economic and social development in rural areas, the government decided to drive health services reform to a deeper level, and put in more funding to rural areas, to provide different levels of medical services to rural residents.

In 2003, under the firm leadership of the Communist Party and the government, the Chinese people, united as one, won a decisive victory in their combat against the severe acute respiratory syndrome pandemic.

Learning a lesson from this experience, the government took comprehensive measures to improve public health services, and the prevention and control of serious diseases. Marked progress was made in the prevention and control system for serious diseases, in the response mechanism for public health emergencies, in the development of community healthcare services in rural and urban areas, and in the new-type rural cooperative medical care and basic medical insurance for urban residents.

In 2009, China launched a new round of reform of the medical and healthcare system. With the release of the Opinions on Deepening Reform of the Medical and Healthcare System, the government delivered a message that the basic medical and healthcare system should be available to all citizens as a public product. The nonprofit nature of public medical and healthcare was made clearly. In the document, it was proposed that China would develop the "four systems" of public health, medical services, medical security and drug supply and the "eight supporting mechanisms" of medical and healthcare management, operation, investment, pricing, supervision, technology and personnel, information, and law-based development, in an effort to form a basic medical and healthcare system and promote the all-around, balanced, and sustainable development of the health sector. Soon after that, China issued the Plan for Reforming Key Areas of the Medical and Healthcare System (2009—2011) and Plan for Deepening Reform of the Medical and Healthcare System during the 12th Five-Year Plan Period (2011—2015). In these two documents, the government set the goals of the reform, which were accelerating the basic medical security system, improving community-level medical and healthcare services, and promoting equal access to basic public health services.

Since 2012 China has redoubled its effort to reform the medical and healthcare system; it has accelerated the comprehensive reform of public hospitals and the price reform of drugs and medical service; it has also implemented serious illness insurance policies covering both urban and rural residents, adopted a multi-layer diagnosis and treatment mechanism, and improved the policies regarding the production, distribution and use of drugs. In 2015, enhancing public health and fitness was formally introduced in the government. In 2016, at the National Health and Fitness Conference, it was stated that the government will "follow the correct guidelines for promoting health and fitness services, focus on lower-level medical institutions, strive to reform and make innovations in the medical sector, prioritize disease prevention, lay equal emphasis on Western medicine and TCM, incorporate health promotion in all policies, and involve all citizens in promoting public health and thereby bring health benefits to all". The state issued "Healthy China 2030" Planning Outline, a guiding document on promoting public health and fitness, with plans to make the Chinese people healthier.

1.3   The subjects and missions of hygiene and preventive medicine

The subjects investigated in hygiene and preventive medicine are environmental factors such as natural and social environment. Public concern about the environment today tends to focus on hazards such as chemical toxins (e. g. , dioxin), radiation (including electromagnetic, ionizing, and solar ultraviolet radiation), radon, "sick" buildings, and other relatively new and "high-tech" environmental and occupational hazards.

The missions of the preventive medicine include: ①Prevent epidemics and the spread of disease; ②Protect against environmental hazards; ③Prevent injuries; ④Promote and encourage healthy behaviors; ⑤Respond to disasters and assist communities in recovery; ⑥Ensure the quality and accessibility of health services.

The tasks of clinicians in environmental health are the following: helping patients interpret the dangers of environmental risks which they are concerned, exploring the possibility of environmental and occupational causes of acute and chronic disease in patients by performing historic and physical examinations that are environmentally sensitive, and reporting diseases that might have an environmental source to public health agencies. To accomplish these, the clinician needs to know what environmental hazards are likely for different patients, how they are likely to be exposed, and how the exposures threaten their health.

1.4   The achievements of Chinese public health

The development in the field of health services has brought concrete benefits to the Chinese people. The average life expectancy of the Chinese rose to 76.5 years in 2016 from 67.9 years in 1981; maternal mortality dropped from 88.9 per 100,000 persons in 1990 to 19.9 per 100,000 persons in 2016; and infant mortality declined from 34.7 per 1,000 in 1981 to 7.5 per 1,000 in 2016. The main health indicators of the Chinese are generally better than the average level of middle–and high–income countries, and China has achieved the UN's Millennium Goals in this regard ahead of schedule. Furthermore, China has established a complete medical and health system that is guided by the Constitution, based on civil laws and regulations, laws and administrative regulations on health, and local regulations, and directed by the outlines, programs, and plans of the health sector. The system has proved effective in maintaining sound doctor–patient relations, addressing medical disputes with impartiality, and ensuring citizens' right to health.

The reform of the medical sector has produced noticeable results. Within a short period of time, China was able to achieve the following: developing the world's largest basic medical insurance network that covers all citizens, providing insurance for patients of serious diseases, enabling patients to receive emergency medical services, and improving medical assistance. All of this has provided institutional guarantee that patients have access to medical services. The state has gained effective control over serious infectious diseases, has kept the spread of AIDS at a low level, has achieved the tuberculosis control target of the UN's Millennium Goals ahead of schedule, has reduced the number of schistosome infections to the lowest level in history, and became a polio–free country in 2000. China set up the world's largest online direct reporting system of notifiable epidemics and public health emergencies in 2015, and the average reporting time has been shortened to four hours from five days before the introduction of the system.

Significant progress has been made in developing a system of medical and healthcare services. A basic medical services network covering both urban and rural areas has been put in place, with 980,000 medical and health institutions at all levels, 11 million health workers, and seven million beds at medical institutions. The state has increased its efforts to foster more medical professionals. A standardization training system for resident doctors is being established, and outstanding figures such as Nobel Prize laureate in Physiology or Medicine Tu Youyou have made significant contributions to the society. As more social resources flow into the medical sector, private hospitals now account for over 57% of all hospitals, making medical services more diverse. China's medical and health emergency rescue capability is among the world's best. It stood the severe test of the Ebola epidemic, blocking all infectious sources from outside its territory and achieved zero infection while Chinese medical teams went on assistance missions in Africa.

After many years of hard work, a new stage has been reached in China's medical and health services. This has not only made the Chinese people healthier, but has also created a model suited to the country's prevailing conditions that is able to ensure people's right to health. This model has the following features.

(1) Prioritizing health and fitness. The government places people's health at the forefront of its development strategies, based on China's prevailing reality, incorporates the awareness of maintaining and improving people's health into the decision—making process of policies and the formulation and implementation of laws and regulations, and strives to achieve sound and coordinated development between healthy lifestyles, working conditions, the natural environment, and the economy and society.

(2) Focusing on prevention. The focus on healthcare has been shifted from treating illnesses to enhancing people's health. Equal emphasis has been put on disease prevention and treatment, and the well—being of both mind and body. Western medicine and TCM have been made complementary to each other. More efforts have been focused on the prevention and control of chronic, endemic and occupational diseases. In order to reduce the occurrences of illnesses, China's medical sector is striving to learn more about the patterns and development of health—related issues, emphasizing early diagnosis, treatment and recovery.

(3) Nonprofit services. The basic medical and healthcare services will continue to be basically nonprofit, and made available to all citizens as a public product. Public hospitals are the pillar of the medical service system, and steps will be taken to ensure universal access to public—health services.

(4) Equality and benefit for all. The state will continue to ensure full coverage of health and medical services. Focusing on rural areas and communities, the gaps in health conditions between urban and rural areas, between different localities and between different groups will be gradually narrowed, so that everyone has equal access to basic health services.

(5) Universal participation and sharing of benefits. The government will continue to assume the leading role, while private organizations and individuals are encouraged to participate. The goal is to involve all citizens in the building and development of the medical care system, with the benefits jointly shared by all. The government will appropriately handle its relationship with the market, so that the former can play its due role in the basic medical and healthcare sector and that the market can provide more choices in the nonbasic medical care sector.

1.5   Levels of prevention

1.5.1   Primary prevention and predisease

Most non infectious diseases can be seen as having an early stage, during which the causal factors start to produce physiologic abnormalities. During the predisease stage, atherosclerosis may begin with elevated blood levels of the "bad" low—densitylipoprotein cholesterol and may be accompanied by low levels of the "good" or "scavenger" high—density lipoprotein cholesterol. The goal of a health intervention at this time is to modify risk factors in a favorable direction. Lifestyle—modifying activities, such as changing to a diet low in saturated and trans fat, pursuing a consistent program of aerobic exercise, and ceasing to smoke cigarettes, are considered to be methods of primary prevention because they are aimed at keeping the pathologic process and disease from occurring.

1.5.1.1   Health promotion

Health—promoting activities usually contribute to the prevention of a variety of diseases and enhance a positive feeling of health and vigor. These activities consist of nonmedical efforts, such as changes in lifestyle, nutrition, and the environment. Such activities may require structural improvements in society to enable most people to participate in them. These improvements require societal changes that make healthy choices easier. Dietary modification may be difficult unless a variety of low−fat, low−salt, low−sugar, yet (tasty) and nutrient−rich foods are available in stores at a reasonable cost. Exercise would be more difficult if bicycling or jogging is a risky activity because of automobile traffic or social violence. Even more basic to health promotion is the assurance of the basic necessities of life, including freedom from poverty, environmental pollution, and violence.

1.5.1.2   Specific protection

If health−promoting changes in environment, nutrition, and behavior are not fully effective, it may be necessary to employ specific protection. This form of primary prevention is targeted at a specific disease or type of injury. Examples include immunization against poliomyelitis; pharmacologic treatment of hypertension to prevent subsequent end−organ damage; use of ear−protecting devices in loud working environments, such as around jet airplanes; and use of seat belts, air bags, and helmets to prevent bodily injuries in automobile and motorcycle crashes. Some measures provide specific protection, while contributing to the more general goal of health promotion. Fluoridation of water supplies not only helps to prevent dental caries, but it also is a nutritional intervention that promotes stronger bones.

Three major goals of primary prevention by specific protection are prevention of specific diseases (e. g., by using vaccines and antimicrobial prophylaxis), prevention of specific deficiency states (e. g., by using iodized salt to prevent iodine deficiency goiter and by using fluoride to prevent dental caries), and prevention of specific injuries and toxic exposures (e. g., by using helmets to prevent head injuries in construction workers, goggles to prevent eye injuries in machine tool operators, and filters and ventilation systems to control dusts). Vaccines are discussed as the prototype of a scientifically developed specific method of protection.

1.5.2   Secondary prevention and latent disease

Sooner or later, depending on the individual, a disease process such as coronary artery atherosclerosis progresses far less enough to become detectable by medical tests, such as cardiac catheterization, although the individual is still asymptomatic. This may be thought of as the latent (hidden) stage of disease. For many infectious and noninfectious diseases, the development of screening tests has made it possible to detect latent disease in individuals considered to be at high risk. Presymptomatic diagnosis through screening programs, along with subsequent treatment when needed, is referred to as secondary prevention because it is the secondary line of defense against disease. Although screening programs do not prevent the causes from initiating the disease process, they may allow diagnosis at an earlier stage of disease, when treatment is more effective.

Secondary prevention is concerned with early detection of disease, through either screening or case finding, followed by treatment. Screening is the process of identifying a subgroup of people in whom there is a high probability of finding asymptomatic disease or a risk factor for developing a disease or becoming injured. In contrast to case finding, which is defined subsequently, screening occurs in a community setting and is applied to a community population, such as students in a school or workers in an industry. Because a positive screening test result usually is not diagnosis of a disease, it must be followed by a diagnostic test (e. g., a positive finding on a screening mammogram examination must be followed by additional diagnostic imaging or a biopsy to rule out cancer). In this regard, initiating a screening program is similar to getting on a roller coaster, and those involved must continue until the end of the process is reached. Screening usually is distinguished from case finding, which is the process of searching for asymptomatic diseases and risk factors among people in a clinical setting (i. e. , among people who are under medical care).

The goal of secondary prevention is the detection of disease or risk factors in the presymptomatic stage, when medical, environmental, nutritional, and lifestyle interventions can be most effective. Screening is done in a community setting, whereas case finding is done in a clinical setting. For community screening programs to be beneficial and cost-effective, they must fulfill various requirements concerning the health problem to be detected, the screening test to be used, and the system available to provide health care for people with positive screening results. Biases such as lead-time bias and length bias can cause health care personnel and analysts to overestimate the benefit produced by a screening program, particularly when the program is aimed at detection of cancer. Although multiphasic screening seeks to make the process efficient by searching for many conditions at the same time, the high incidence of false-positive test results and other associated problems have made this technique less successful than was originally anticipated. Historically, the periodic health examination has been the most common method of case finding. Because it has provided disappointing benefits when examined carefully, it is now being replaced by lifetime health monitoring. This approach focuses on monitoring individuals for the specific set of conditions and diseases most likely to be found in persons of a certain age and gender, and its use has been advocated by experts on preventive medicine in Canada and the US. Many practitioners who emphasize preventive medicine prefer to see their patients for checkups more often than may be recommended, such as 1 or 2 years, to maintain a relationship of trust and to repeat health promotion messages that are important for efforts to change behavior.

1.5.3 Tertiary prevention and symptomatic disease

Tertiary prevention includes the control of existing disease (e. g. , heart disease, hypertension, and diabetes) and the control of (toxemia) during pregnancy.

When disease has become symptomatic and medical assistance is sought, the goal of the clinician is to provide tertiary prevention in the form of disability limitation for patients with early symptomatic disease or in the form of rehabilitation for patients with late symptomatic disease.

In practice, tertiary prevention and treatment of established disease are similar. The difference is in perspective. Treatment is expressly about fixing what is wrong, whereas tertiary prevention looks ahead to potential progression and complications of disease and aims to forestall those developments. Treatment and tertiary prevention often share methods, but they diverge in terms of motives and goals.

Methods of tertiary prevention are designed to limit the physical and social consequences of an injury or disease after it has occurred or become symptomatic. There are two basic categories of tertiary prevention. The first category, called disability limitation, has the goal of halting the progress of the disease or limiting the damage caused by an injury. This category of tertiary prevention is probably better thought of as "the prevention of further impairment. " The second category, called rehabilitation, focuses on reducing the social disability produced by a given level of impairment, by strengthening the patient's remaining functions and by helping the patient learn to function in alternative ways. Disability limitation and rehabilitation ordinarily should be initiated at the same time (i. e. , when the disease is detected or the injury occurs), but the emphasis on one or the other depends on factors such as the type and stage of disease, the type of injury, and available methods of treatment. This chapter discusses opportunities for tertiary prevention and provides specific clinical examples of disability limitation and rehabilitation.

The goal of tertiary prevention is to limit the physical and social consequences of an injury or disease after it has occurred or become symptomatic. The two major categories of tertiary prevention are disability limitation and rehabilitation. Methods of disability limitation include therapy, which seeks to undo the threat or damage from an existing disease, and symptomatic stage prevention, which attempts to halt or limit the future progression of disease. The strategies of symptomatic stage prevention are taken from primary prevention (e. g. , modification of diet, behavior, and environment) and from secondary prevention (e. g. , frequent screening for incipient complications, followed by treatment when complications are discovered). The effective management of chronic diseases such as coronary artery disease, hyperlipidemia, hypertension, and diabetes mellitus requires a combination of therapy and symptomatic stage prevention. This approach also can be used in the management of many other diseases, including stroke, chronic obstructive pulmonary disease, arthritis, and some cancers and infectious diseases. Rehabilitation should begin in the early stages of treatment. Depending on the needs of the patient, the rehabilitation team may include a rehabilitation counselor; physical therapist; speech therapist; occupational therapist; and psychiatric, emotional, or spiritual counselor. Under most state laws concerning workers' compensation, several categories of job related illnesses or injuries are recognized: permanent total disability, permanent partial disability, temporary total disability, temporary partial disability, and death. The goal of rehabilitation for workers, whether their impairment is temporary or permanent, is to minimize the social and occupational consequences of the impairment. Although it might seem that the opportunity for prevention is lost when a disease appears or an injury occurs, this is often not the case. The appearance of symptoms or the threat of severe complications may lead patients to take an active interest in their health status, seek the health care that they need, and make positive changes in their environment, diet, and lifestyle.

Lyu Quanjun

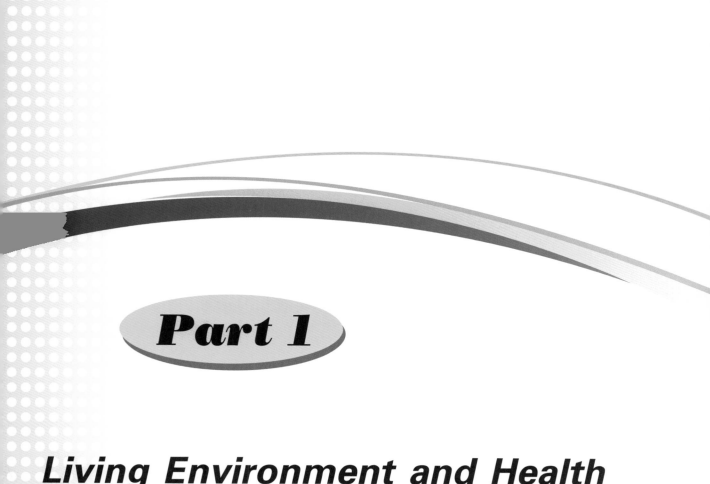

Part 1

Living Environment and Health

Chapter 2

Basic Concepts and Principles of Environmental Health

2.1   Classification of human environment

Environment refers to the human-centered external world. It is the unity of various natural and social elements that interact with the material and phenomena on the surface of the Earth and the material basis for the survival and development of mankind. It is also closely related to important condition of human health. The human environment refers to the human space around the earth and the various physical and social factors that directly and indirectly affect human life and development.

Environment is a complex system, generally classified according to the nature of the environment, the attributes and characteristics of the environmental elements, and the scope of the environmental space. According to the attributes and characteristics of environmental factors, human environment can be divided into natural environment, man-made environment, and social environment. Natural environment includes all kinds of things that exist in nature. They are naturally formed and existed before human beings, such as sunlight, atmosphere, land, sea, river, various animals and plants. Human environment is transformed through human processing and transformation, during which change its original appearance and structural characteristics of the material environment, such as cities, villages and towns, gardens, farmland, mines, airports, railway stations, railways and highways. The social environment is the environment formed by the material production system created by the long-term conscious social labor and the accumulated culture. The social environment consists of social politics, economy, culture, education, population, customs, and so on. These three types of environment can be further classified according to the attributes or characteristics of their constituent elements. For example, the natural environment can be divided into atmospheric environment and aquatic environment according to the components.

During the formation of the earth, gravity separates materials with different densities. Materials with lower density gradually float up and stay on the surface where as those with higher density gradually sink to the geocentric center. The air, liquid water, and rocks are arranged in concentric layers and formed three basic laps: atmosphere, hydrosphere, and soil lithosphere. Subsequently, organisms were created at the interface between the atmosphere and the oceans, and between the surface of the atmosphere and the solid land.

The long-term proliferation of living organisms formed the biological map. The atmosphere, hydrosphere, soil lithosphere and biosphere make up the human environment.

In addition, according to human influence on the environment, the environment can be classified into the primary environment and secondary environment.

2.1.1 Natural environment

2.1.1.1 Atmosphere

The atmosphere mainly refers to the atmosphere above the surface of the Earth and can be divided into troposphere, stratosphere, thermal stratification, and dissipation layer. The majority of the remaining hydrogen that forms the Earth's original substance, except for most of its emissions, is combined with oxygen to form water, so there is very little elemental hydrogen in the atmosphere. Nitrogen, as the main component of the atmosphere (about 78%), exists in the atmosphere in elemental form due to its inert. Negatively charged oxygen can form oxides with most elements, such as H_2O, CO_2, SiO_2, CaO and FeO. In the stratosphere, ozone (O_3) is generated by photochemical reactions with oxygen due to intense solar radiation. Ozone absorbs<340 nm of UV light and is decomposed into oxygen atoms, which in turn reacts with oxygen molecules to regenerate ozone. So in the stratosphere, a unique ozone layer is formed. The ozone layer absorbs the bio-devastating short-wave UV rays of solar radiation and thus protects the creatures on the surface of the Earth to survive and evolve.

2.1.1.2 Hydrosphere

Earth's water exists in the air, surface and underground in three forms: gaseous, liquid and solid. It is called atmospheric water, seawater, and terrestrial water (including rivers, lakes, groundwater, ice, and snow), and together they form the hydrosphere. The total amount of water in the hydrosphere is estimated at 1.38×10^9 km^3, of which 97.41% of the sea water covers 71% of the Earth's surface area. However, the fresh water, such as water in river, lake, and shallow ground accounts for only about 0.2% of the total. In the biosphere, the water in oceans, lakes, rivers, plant stems, and leaves evaporates and transforms into water vapor, rises to the atmosphere, and returns back as air currents transfer and rainfall, and penetrates from the surface to the ground. This cycle of movement is known as the water cycle. When a body of water is contaminated, the contaminants also enter the atmosphere, soil, food and the human body through the water cycle.

2.1.1.3 Lithosphere

The crust is mainly composed of three types of rocks: magma, sedimentary and metamorphic rocks. Crustal rocks are formed by long-term weathering of the parent material and soil is formed by the parent material through the role of microorganisms and plants. Soil lithosphere is the soil that covers the surface of the Earth, with loose layer containing minerals, organic matter, microorganisms, water, air, and other ingredients, for plant growth and biological activity to provide favorable space and material. Soil plays an important role in linking the organic and inorganic sectors. When soil is polluted, pollutants may be transferred to plants, air, and water through biological enrichment, water evaporation, and infiltration. Due to the differences of climate, geography and provenance in different periods of history, the quality of parent material, biological growth, and hydrosphere (especially groundwater) in different regions and the composition and the solubility of rock formed in different periods are quite different. For example, when groundwater in a certain area flows through high-fluorine deposits or fluorite-bearing rocks, the amount of groundwater fluoride will obviously increase and become the cause of endemic fluorosis. When soil is contaminated, it is possible to transfer contaminants to plants, atmosphere, and water through bio-concentration, evaporation of water, and submarines.

2.1.1.4 Biosphere

Biosphere refers to the whole body of living things and living environment on Earth. Its scope includes the lower atmosphere, upper lithosphere, hydrosphere, and pedosphere, usually from 12 kilometers below the horizontal to about 10 kilometers above the water level. In the biosphere, the material, energy, information recycling, and exchange are kept on. The birth, multiplication, and development of life make the biosphere full of vigor and vitality. In the process of interacting with environment, organism are affected by different environments and form different types of biological communities. On the contrary, biological activities can also influence the environment of different regions and change the quality of the natural environment.

2.1.2　Ecosystem

Ecological environment refers to the sum of the biological and various natural factors and conditions of living and breeding, and is the natural environment composed of ecosystems related to the existence and development of human being. There are not only many kinds of organisms in the biosphere, but also a large number of biological features. Moreover, creatures are the most biologically active organisms in the biosphere, with the most complex relationships and complexities that hide too much mystery. From the perspective of ecology and methods, it is necessary to study and understand this natural environment in depth.

2.1.2.1 Basic composition of the ecosystem

Ecosystem refers to the natural system composed of biological communities (including microorganisms, animals, plants, humans, etc.) and abiotic environment (air, water, inorganic salts, amino acids, etc.). Biotic factors can be divided into three parts: producers (green plants, synthetic bacteria, etc.), consumers (herbivorous, carnivorous, large carnivore), and decomposers (bacteria, fungi, and actinomycetes). These three components together with abiotic factor form were recognized as an ecosystem. Through their own functions, they maintain the exchange and circulation of material, energy and information in ecosystems, thus forming an indivisible unity. Due to the differences in geographical location and spatial distribution, there may exist independent large and small ecosystems, such as ponds, forests, supermarkets, lakes and other natural ecosystems as well as artificial ecosystems, such as cities, mining areas and factories. Numerous small ecosystems form the largest ecosystem on earth, namely the biosphere, also known as the human ecosystem. Humans are unusually special in the entire ecosystem. Humans are omnivorous, possess the characteristics of consumers at all levels, and at the same time, have the ability to influence the environment and are the most influential factors in the biosphere.

2.1.2.2 Ecosystem health

The various components of the ecosystem are constantly changing and moving. Due to the long-term evolutionary process, mutual compensation has gradually been established, so that the mutual compensation between outputs and inputs of producers, consumers and decomposers, biomes and abiotic environments, material and energy in the whole ecosystem always maintain a dynamic balance, which is called ecological balance. Ecological balance is the basis for the biological survival, activity, and reproduction to proceed normally. Affected and destroyed ecological balance will have different degrees of harm to creatures and even to human beings.

Ecosystems not only provide humans with all kinds of valuable products, but also provide a variety of important and irreplaceable services by manpower. However, the ecosystem must be in perfect and good condition to realize these functions.

In the 1990s, ecosystem management was referred to the important agenda of mankind. The concept of human "health" began to be borrowed to illustrate the state of complex structure and wide range of functions of ecosystem. Scientists began to borrow examples of human health to protect ecosystem health and to establish a good ecological goal based on the metaphor of human health. Ecosystems that are energetic, structurally stable, and self-regulating are often viewed as healthy ecosystems. Vitality refers to the function of the ecosystem, including the function of maintaining the complex nature of the system itself and the function of serving human beings. The structural stability refers to having a balanced and intact biological community and diverse biological populations. The self-regulation function of the ecosystem mainly depends on its feedback. Through the interaction of positive and negative feedbacks and transformation, the healthy system can maintain the normal structure and function under stress and has the ability to resist the "disease" to ensure that the system reaches a certain steady state. An unhealthy and morbid ecosystem is often in a recession and tends to collapse irreversibly.

Ecosystem health is an important prerequisite for achieving sustainable development. A healthy ecosystem is the material basis for human survival and development, as well as the basis for human health. Emphasis should be placed on the inter-linkage between ecosystem health and human health. The impact of the environment on human health is more indirect but more macroscopic, more complex, and far-reaching. Maintaining and preserving the structure of the ecosystem, the sustainability of the function, restoring the creation of the ecosystem, rebuilding the destroyed life support system of the Earth, and realizing the health of the ecosystem are the future important missions for professionals of environment and environmental management.

2.2   Environment and human health

All kinds of material in human living environment are made up of chemical elements. The body continue to carry out the exchange of material and energy flow through the metabolism with the external environment, making the structural components of the body and the environment in a dynamic balance. Furthermore, a complex unity between human and environment is formed. In order to survive and better develop, human beings must adapt themselves to the changes of environmental conditions as soon as possible, and absorb certain elements from the environment continuously to meet the needs of the body to complete the process of its own activities. In the process of evolution, from low to high, creatures choose certain crucial elements in their living environment to ensure that they can evolve smoothly to a higher level. As a result, these elements become the essential material components for maintaining biological survival, reproduction, and other life process.

2.2.1   Human adaptability to the environment

In the process of long-term evolutionary development of mankind, various environmental conditions are constantly changing, and the human body forms a certain regulatory function to adapt the changes in environmental conditions. The body's climate adaptation, thermal adaptation, light adaptation are the best examples of the body to adapt to the external environment changes. For example, repeated heat exposure allows the body to generate thermal adaptations to the thermal environment, after which the body's temperature regulation, sweat gland secretion, water and salt metabolism, cardiovascular system, nervous system, endocrine function have been improved.

Long-term living in different regions, people have different adaptability in abnormal external environment. In the plateau environment, due to the sparse oxygen content in the atmosphere, the human body can maintain the normal physiological activities by increasing the quality of breathing air, accelerating blood circulation, increasing the number of red blood cells or hemoglobin to improve the oxygen carrying capacity. After affected by exogenous substances, the body will display some adaptive changes, such as detoxification and excretion function to remove toxic substances from the body, immune function to prevent the entry of harmful substances into the body. In addition, when environmental factors cause the loss of genetic material, the body can initiate a series of DNA repair mechanisms to maintain the stability of genetic characteristics. Of course, human body has limited adaptive capacity to environmental changes. If the abnormal changes (such as drastic weather changes, natural or man-made pollution) exceed the normal scope of human physiological adjustment, it will cause the body's abnormal reactions, and eventually lead to disease or even death.

2.2.2　The impact of environmental factors on health

In natural environment and living environment, there are many protective factors for human survival and health, such as clean and normal composition of the air, water and soil, adequate sunlight and the right climate, beautiful scenery and vegetation, comfort and elegant living conditions. These are the essential elements of the survival of humans and other creatures on Earth. At the same time, there are also some factors that adversely affect human health and survival in our living environment, such as extreme cold or hot climate, abnormal levels of some chemical elements in soil and drinking water, excessive UV radiation and various natural disasters. In addition, environmental destruction and pollution caused by mankind have increased the degree of harm to human health.

A large number of studies have found that environmental factors have both favorable and harmful effects on the health of the body. For example, UV light has the roles of bactericidal, anti-rickets disease and enhancing the body immunity and so on, but excessive ultraviolet radiation can cause erythema, skin pigmentation and even carcinogenic, and increase the incidence of eye cataracts. Appropriate temperature is essential for human survival, extreme weather conditions, such as heat waves during the heat summer season can significantly increase mortality, and cold weather can cause cardiovascular diseases. Moderate light is necessary for human beings' production and activities, but excessive light stimulation can lead to flash blind symptoms. And strong solar radiation can cause skin erythema, phototoxic reaction, or light allergic reaction.

In addition, studies have shown that even in the traditional sense of toxic, substances at very low doses may show beneficial effects on the body, also known as the "hormesis" effect. Because some substances at low doses has a stimulating effect on the biological system, while at high doses has an inhibitory effect. For example, long term consumption of a larger amount of alcohol can increase the risk of esophageal cancer, liver cancer, and mortality, but moderate consumption of alcohol can reduce the incidence of coronary heart disease, stroke, and overall mortality. Low dose X-rays prolong the lifespan of mice and guinea pigs. Low doses of ethanol and acetaldehyde prolong the lifespan of fruit flies. In addition, low doses of arsenic trioxide can treat leukemia, while higher doses can lead to health hazards and even death. There are many more environmental chemicals that have such biological effects, such as cadmium, lead, mercury, and saccharin.

2.2.3　The coordinated development between humans and environment

Nature, human society, and science and technology are the three relatively independent fields that are mutually distinguishable, interrelated, and indivisible. The history of human evolution and development depends on the environment, adapt to the environment, and change the environment. It is a dynamic process of an interaction between people and the environment. People can make use of and change the environment and the environment can provide favorable conditions for the development of mankind to achieve a coordinated development of man and the environment.

2.3 Environmental changes and body response

The body is actively responding to environmental changes. The quality and quantity of the reaction depends both on the changing environmental factors and the state of the body.

2.3.1 Exposure of environmental media and environmental factors

Exposure to environmental chemicals generally occurs to environmental media containing these substances. However, it is anthropogenic emissions or natural environmental chemicals, a series of complex changes in morphological characteristics or chemical properties will take place after the chemicals enter the environment. These changes can lead to two outcomes: one is to through the environment self-purification gradually return to the state before the pollution and the other one is to pollute the environment and harm the human body.

Migration of environmental material in environmental media: the transfer of environmental material refers to the process of spatial displacement of environmental material in the environment. Once material enters into environment, the substance first migrates within a single medium (air, water or soil) that receives the substance (such as chemical pollutants) and then enters other environmental media, including organisms.

2.3.1.1 Migration within a single media

In the air, material movement is mainly by diffusion and convection. Because air has a low viscosity, it diffuses rapidly in the air, about 100 times faster for the same substance than in water. Air convection has the strongest migrating effect. In the troposphere, there are regular convection and irregular turbulence, and migration of direct viewable substance. The movement of compounds in water is achieved by diffusion, dispersion and water flow, mainly by the turbulence and advection of water. The movement of chemicals in the soil is achieved by diffusion within the liquid or by water movement through the interstices between the soil particles. The direction of diffusion is always from a high concentration area to a low concentration area.

2.3.1.2 Migration between different media

Once discharged, the chemical enters any of the four environmental media and can then be vaporized into the air, adsorbed into the soil, dissolved into the water, and absorbed into the body by absorption, inhalation, and ingestion. The movement of chemicals from one media to another is affected by many factors.

2.3.1.3 Biological mobility

Environmental chemicals enter into the body through the food chain and food web in the biological migration. During the migration process, chemicals may be stored and accumulated in the organism, increasing the content in the body, especially at upper trophic levels. In this process, the phenomenon that the concentration of chemical substances in the living body gradually increases with the trophic level is called biomagnification.

2.3.2 Transformation of environmental chemicals in environmental media

The process by which a contaminant is transformed into another substance by chemical or biological means in the environment is called chemical transformation. Secondary pollutants are new pollutants that are usually transformed by various reactions in the environment and usually have different physico−chemical properties as the original pollution. Pollutants discharged directly from sources are called primary pollutants.

2.3.2.1 Chemical conversion

Chemical conversion refers to the transformation of pollutants through various chemical reaction processes. In the atmosphere, pollutant conversion is mainly done by optical and catalytic oxidation. Atmospheric volatile organic compounds, such as nitrogen oxides and other pollutants generated by photochemical oxidation of ozone, peroxyacetyl nitrate, and its similar oxidizing substances, are collectively referred to as photochemical oxidants. The Los Angeles Photochemical Smog Incident, which took place in the United States in 1946, is a typical example of atmospheric pollution caused by photochemical reactions.

2.3.2.2 Biotransformation

Biotransformation refers to the process by which the environmental chemical changes through the catalytic action of the corresponding enzyme system in the organism. Under the catalytic action of the enzyme system, the chemical changes its chemical properties through various biochemical reactions. On the one hand, the results of biotransformation can reduce the toxicity of most substances. On the other hand, the biotransformation can increase toxicity of some substances, which becomes more easily absorbed and accumulated by the organism. For example, inorganic mercury in the river bottom can convert virulent methylmercury with the involvement of microorganisms.

Exposure characteristics and reactions environmental exposure is a determinant of harmful effects of environmental factors. Without environmental exposure, there is no corresponding effect. The routes, intensity, and timing of exposure are closely related to their effects.

The same kind of harmful compounds can come from different sources of pollution. Even if pollutants come from the same source of pollution, many environmental substances and harmful compounds will exist in different kinds of media because the material migration can be conducted between various media. These harmful compounds are often exposed in multiway, rarely single. Through these media, environmentally harmful compounds may enter into the body through the respiratory tract, mouth, and skin.

Dose−response relationships dosages usually refer to the amount of harmful substances that enter the body. The harmful effect is closely related to the amount of harmful substances to the body's target organs or tissues. However, there are many difficulties in the determination of the dose of target organs and tissues. Therefore, in the practice of environmental sanitation, the exposure amount of harmful substances in the environment is commonly used to reflect the human exposure dose. A dose−response relationship refers to a relationship when the dose of harmful agent increases, the number of individuals suffering a particular biological effect increases. The dose−response relationship is usually expressed as the percentage of individuals with the presence of biological effects. The dose−response relationship is a count of data, also known as quantitative response with a quantitative description, such as "negative or positive" "with or without" "death or survival" and so on. This is the general representation of the body's response to environmental stressors in the population.

2.3.2.3 Accumulation effects and tolerance

Under the action of a dose or intensity of environmental harmful factors, the duration of the action has an important influence on the severity of the organism's harmful biological effect. In particular, the presence of low doses of environmental pollutants takes a considerable amount of time to exert a detrimental effect on health. Prolonged exposure to environmental harmful factors, especially chemical pollutants, may accumulate in the body, and gradually reach the doses or concentrations for pathological damage in the target organ and tissue, thereby manifesting harmful biological effects. Accumulation of substances in the body is often affected by three factors: intake dose, biological half-life and intake time. In theory, the maximum possible amount in the body tends to stabilize after six half-life reduction of chemical pollutants. Since then, intake and discharge tend to balance. Therefore, the lengths of intake time not only significantly affect the amount of accumulation of the harmful substances in the body, but also affect the biological effects. In the meantime, the intake also plays a decisive role in the change of the accumulation amount of the substance in the body, the greater the intake, the greater the maximum volume. If daily intake is reduced, the maximum volume in the body is also bound to decrease. The low intake may be considered acceptable if the intake is reduced to a level below the level at which the maximum amount of accumulation in the body occurs i. e. the long-term effect will not have a detrimental effect on the body. This dose or concentration of ingestion is then referred to as a dose/concentration or subliminal dose/concentration in which no detrimental effect is observed. It is an important basis for setting the maximum allowable concentration of harmful substances in the environment.

Some environmental harmful factors in the body can be quickly broken down and excreted in different forms, thus will not be accumulated in the body, but can gradually accumulate effect on functional changes in the target tissue or target organ. These changes can lead to the increase of body's reactivity to the substance and aggravation of the functional or biochemical metabolic changes, eventually resulting in organ or tissue damages. This is called functional accumulation. Due to the accumulation of functional changes, the degree of damage to the body is also significantly related to aging, the amount of intake, and the extent and timing of the functional changes. If each intake is small, it will not cause function changes in target tissue and organ or obvious accumulation or reactivity. This intake can still be used as the basis for the development of environmental hygiene standards.

2. 4 Environmental multi-factor exposure and joint effects

2.4.1 The diversity of environmental factors

Environmental hazards are diverse and include physical, chemical, and biological factors. Each major category contains many sub-categories and specific factors. Taking chemical substances as an example, there are millions of known compounds, thousands of carcinogens and teratogens. These substances probably enter into the environment and exist in a variety of environmental media. At the same time, pollutants that are continuously released from human activities and living activities, such as atmospheric exhaust, automobile exhaust and various industrial wastewaters, have complex mixtures. More than 200 types of chlorinated disinfection by-products are produced by drinking water chlorination disinfection; there are more than 200 ingredients for cooking fumes; and more than 3,800 substances are produced from tobacco combustion, of which,44 are carcinogenic. These substances continue to enter the environment and human may be exposed to various media. Therefore, the pollutants of body intake from air, drinking water, and food are not single, but a co-existence of variety of substances.

The effects of multiple environmental substances on the human body are different from those of any one of them alone. They often play a very complex role in the body and affect each other in the process of biological transport, transformation, protein binding or excretion, and have toxic effects on human body. When two or more chemicals simultaneously acting on the organism, they may have acomprehensive toxic effect, known as the joint-or combined toxic effect. With the increase in environmental pollutants, the joint toxicity has drawn more and more attention.

2.4.2　The type of joint effect

Depending on the nature of the toxic effects of multiple chemicals acting simultaneously on the body, the combined effects of chemicals can be divided into the following categories.

2.4.2.1　Additive effect

If the interacting compounds are homologs in their chemical structure or their toxic effects act on same target organs, their total effect on the body is equal to the sum of the individual effects of the each compound. This is the compound additive effect. It is known that the interaction of some compounds, such as stimulation of most irritating gases, often has additive effect. Compounds that have an anesthetic effect also usually have additive interaction.

2.4.2.2　Independent effect

When two or more compounds acting on the body simultaneously, the biological effects of the chemicals do not interfere with each other, so that there is not interaction of the respective compounds, but each has their individual toxicity effect, is called an independent effect. For example, after rats exposed to both alcohol and vinyl chloride for a certain period of time, liver homogenate occurs lipid peroxidation, while vinyl chloride causes microsomal lipid peroxidation. The two compounds in a certain dose have no significant interactive effect, but independent effect.

2.4.2.3　Synergistic effect

Interactions between the compounds result in increased toxicity, i. e. , the combined effects of the compounds is greater than the sum of the individual effects of the individual compounds, is called synergistic effect of the compounds. The mechanism by which multiple compounds interact synergistically is complex and diverse. It may be related to the rate of absorption among compounds, the accelerated absorption, the delayed release, the *in vivo* degradation process and the in vivo metabolic kinetics.

2.4.2.4　Enhancement effect

A chemical is nontoxic to an organ or system but increases its toxic effect when exposed simultaneously or sequentially to another chemical is called potentiation. For example, isopropanol is non-toxic to the liver, but when it enters the body simultaneously as carbon tetrachloride, the toxicity of carbon tetrachloride can be significantly higher than its sole effect.

2.4.2.5　Antagonism effect

The phenomenon that the total effect of interaction of each compound in the body is lower than the sum of their individual effects is called antagonism. There are several possible forms of antagonism of compounds *in vivo*. One is the competition between compounds. For example, the competition combination between oxime compounds and organophosphorus compounds with cholinesterase results in weakened toxicity effect of organophosphorus compounds. One is caused by changes in the metabolic process between compounds, such as 1,2,4-tribromobenzene, 1,2,4-trichlorobenzene, and some other halogenated benzene compounds, and cause some metabolism inducements of the organophosphorus compounds to reduce its toxicity. Another one is functional or effector antagonism, a good example is poisoning therapy, atropine against muscarinic–like symptoms caused by organophosphorus compounds.

2.5 Environment pollution and human health

With the development of industry, urban construction and expansion, the natural environment of human existence has undergone tremendous changes. While developing and utilizing natural environment resources and creating new living environment, human beings also release wastes into the environment and pollute the environment. The amount of pollutants entering the environment exceeds the self–purification capacity of the environment, causing the environmental quality to deteriorate, directly or indirectly affecting human health, is called environmental pollution. A wide range of environmental pollutants, according to their properties, are generally divided into chemical, physical, and biological three categories. These pollutants can cause a variety of hazards on the body, including acute, chronic and carcinogenic, and teratogenic long–term hazards.

2.5.1　Acute and chronic health effect

2.5.1.1　Acute health effect

A large number of environmental pollutants are discharged into the environment in a short period of time, and exposures of population in a relatively short period of time exhibit adverse reactions, acute poisoning, and even death. In the process of industrialization, people in the developed countries are repeatedly exposed to acute poisonings caused by industrial pollution due to their lack of environmental protection. In the mid–to–late 20th century, due to the rapid development of industrial production, the occurrence of air pollution and smoke incidents occurred more frequently. The London Smoke Incident in the United Kingdom, Los Angeles Photochemical Smog Event in the United States, and the Yokkaichi Asthma in Japan happened in that period. In London Smoke Incident, patients with pulmonary and cardiovascular disease became exasperated and died. Photochemical smog can cause eye and upper respiratory tract irritation and dysfunytion. The occurrence of Atmospheric Pollution Event is close related to serious air pollution, and is meteorological conditions or special topographical conditions that are not conducive to the diffusion of pollutants in the environment.

Acute poisoning incidents occurred in the residents living near the factory because of unreasonable industrial design, overloaded, or accidental exhaust gas and wastewater discharge. It is not uncommon for acute poisoning of people and animals when the factories discharge excessive quantities of pesticides, fluorides, chromates, and arsenides, such as Cl_2, NH_3, H_2S, HCN and other toxic substances into the atmosphere or surface water or groundwater. In addition, toxic and harmful raw chemical materials, products, etc., enter the environment due to accidents and cause pollution events during production, storage and transportation. Incidents such as the leakage of methyl isocyanate (CH_2CNCO) at the Bhopal Pesticide Factory in India in 1984 led to the death of more than 2,500 people due to the exposure to this gas.

Due to the rapid development of nuclear industry, the application of atomic energy in industry has increased dramatically. On March 11, 2011, a nuclear leak in Fukushima occurred in Japan, where the scope of the damage was extremely rare. Together with the 1986 Chernobyl accident in Soviet Union and the 1979 Three Mile Island nuclear accident in the United States, they are the three most serious nuclear accidents in human history. Nuclear accidents have caused heavy casualties for the residents around. Their long half–life of radionuclides, which contain radioactive particles floating in the sky, can spread to far off places. Radioactive materials can enter the body through respiratory inhalation, skin contact and digestive tract absorption, causing external and internal radiation damage and radiological disease. They can also increase the incidence of cancer, aberrations, and hereditary lesions, which can also affect the health of later generations.

In addition, when drinking water is contaminated with pathogenic microorganisms, acute infectious diseases may occur. After the centralized water supply system is polluted by the pathogen, it may cause some outbreak of waterborne infectious diseases in the water supply area. For example, the outbreak of waterborne disease caused by Cryptosporidium in Wisconsin in 1993 led to 403,000 sick people, over 4,000 hospitalizations and 112 deaths. In crowded, poorly ventilated, dark and humid air, pathogenic microorganisms can be spread through the air to susceptible populations. For example, in the Worldwide SARS epidemic in the spring of 2003, respiratory droplets of patients with respiratory is an important route of transmission.

2.5.1.2　Chronic hazards

Long-term repeated effects of low concentrations of harmful substances in the environment on the body is called chronic hazards. Chronic hazards can result from long-term exposure to environmental chemical contaminants or harmful physical factors. The occurrence of chronic hazards is related to the exposure dose, exposure time, biological half-life, and chemical characteristics of chemical pollutants, as well as the body's responses. The gradual accumulation of low levels of environmental pollutants, including the substance or function of the substance, in the body is the root cause of chronic harm. Chronic harm caused by environmental pollutants have the following characteristics.

(1) Non-specific effects

Chronic hazards caused by environmental pollutants often do not have typical clinical manifestations. Under the action of environmental pollutants for a long time, the body's physiological function, immune function, and resistance to environmental harmful factors may be significantly weakened, the sensitivity to biological infection is increased, consequently, morbidity and mortality are increased, and children's growth and development are affected.

(2) Chronic diseases

The long-term effect of low-dose environmental pollutants can directly cause some chronic diseases, such as chronic obstructive pulmonary disease (COPD), a group of lung diseases associated with the long-term effects of air pollutants and changes in meteorological factors. It includes chronic bronchitis, bronchial asthma, asthmatic bronchitis, and emphysema and their recurrence. And the long-term exposure of inorganic fluoride can cause skeletal system and enamel damages of tooth.

(3) Persistent accumulative hazards

In the environmental pollution, some pollutants, such as lead, mercury, cadmium, arsenic, fluorine and its compounds, as well as some fat soluble and uneasily degradable organic compounds, such as organic chlorine (DDT, TCDD, PCBs, etc.), can be stored in the tissues and organs of human body for a long time. Despite their low concentrations in the environment, their concentration in the contaminated population is significantly increased due to their persistent accumulation in the human body. After the use of organochlorine pesticides in various countries, the residual organic chlorine in the environment enters the human body through the respiratory tract, digestive tract, and skin, and gradually increases in the body fat. It may even pass through the placental barrier to embryos or through breastfeeding to infants, damaging the health of the next generation.

(4) Chronic joint effects

Under long-term effects, when there are many kinds of harmful pollutants in the environment at the same time, chronic joint effects of pollutants may appear, such as the combined effect of fluorine and arsenic. The role of the food chain and biomagnification is of great significance in environmental health hazards to people's health. For example, nuisance disease "Minamata disease" and "itai–itai disease" are closely related to the role of the food chain and biomagnification. Adverse reactions of the body caused by chronic hazards from environmental pollution do not have specific damage characteristics. Due to a long duration of exposure, the factors that affect the body's reaction are complex, so it is not easy to determine the causal relationship between the pollutants and chronic damage in the body. Once more obvious symptoms occurred, the damage often has become irreversible, may have serious health consequences.

2.5.2   Environmental pollution and carcinogenic harm

In 1775, Pott, a British surgeon, found that the occurrence of scrotal cancer in chimney sweeper in London, England, was related to the deposition of soot on the scrotum. After nearly a century of medical research, scientists confirmed the carcinogenicity of coal tar in soot. The existence of chemical carcinogens in the environment, as well as the relationship between environmental pollution and the occurrence of cancer has drawn more and more attention. Over half a century, the rankings of the spectrum of disease and causes of death in all countries in the world have been significantly changed. The top two leading causes of deaths from developed countries have changed from acute infections and infectious diseases to cardiovascular disease and tumor. Tumor has gradually become a common disease that threatens the health of the population. In the 1970s, the World Health Organization (WHO) published data on the causes of death in 45 countries or regions and showed that tumor death rates in 32 countries accounted for the first and second places in the cause of death.

Classification of carcinogens: the International Agency for Research on Cancer (IARC, 2002) states that chemical carcinogens are chemicals that can cause an increase in the incidence of malignancies. In some cases, chemicals that can induce benign tumors can also be considered as chemical carcinogens. There are currently about 7,000 kinds of chemicals, of which more than 1,700 kinds of them have positive results in animal carcinogenesis test. Based on their carcinogenic risk to human beings, carcinogens are classified into four categories in the 985 chemicals reported by IARC (2011).

Category 1: carcinogenic to humans, 118 substances. Such substances have full and clear proof of carcinogenicity to humans and animals.

Category 2A: probably carcinogenic to humans, 75 substances. Such substances have limited evidence of carcinogenicity to humans and sufficient evidence of carcinogenicity in experimental animals.

Category 2B: possibly carcinogenic to humans, 288 substances. Such substances have limited evidence of carcinogenicity to humans, insufficient evidence of carcinogenicity in laboratory animals, or insufficient evidence of carcinogenicity in humans and sufficient evidence of carcinogenicity in experimental animals.

Category 3: unclassifiable as to carcinogenicity to humans. A total of 503 substances that are suspicious of human carcinogen.

Category 4: probably no carcinogenic to humans, Such substances are based on information available to confirm that the substance is not a carcinogen.

The occurrence of cancer is a complex and dynamic process of interaction between the host and the environment. Important host factors include genetic makeup and health status, while major environmental factors include air pollution, water pollution and food contamination. Therefore, the study of the role of different environmental factors and the occurrence of cancer is of great significance.

Wang Baiqi

2.6   Susceptibility of population

2.6.1   Susceptible population

There are differences in response to environmental hazards, and people who are more sensitive are often referred to as susceptible populations.

2.6.1.1   Age and gender

Pregnant women, infants, young children, and older adults have long been recognized as susceptible populations by the scientific community. Because the fetus will absorb the maternal nutrition during pregnancy, the general resistance of pregnant women will be lower. Therefore, all kinds of nutrition should be supplemented to improve the immunity of pregnant women during pregnancy. Infants born more than 6 months old are susceptible to many diseases because of the gradual disappearance of their antibodies from the mother, plus whose acquired antibodies have not been formed. Further, the detoxification enzyme system in infants is not yet mature, and immunoglobulin levels in serum are low. In contrast, older adults' immune function and DNA damage repair ability decrease. Therefore, in many environmental pollution events, the number of older people and infants with pathological changes and even deaths is more than the general population.

2.6.1.2   Nutrition and health condition

Nutrition is very important in determining various states of health. Human immunity is influenced by many factors, in which nutrition plays a very important role. It is the material basis for maintaining normal immune function and health of the human body. Nutrient deficiency increases the risk of many diseases. People with anemia, diarrhea, diabetes, cancer, and tuberculosis may have weakened immune system and thus may be more vulnerable. According to the existing nutrition research results, adequate nutrient supplement may greatly improve the human body's immunity and decrease the susceptibility to certain diseases.

2.6.1.3   Income

People with low income refer to those with low level of education, mainly engaged in low skilled work, and with poor working environment. They are more likely to be exposed to toxic and harmful substances due to the nature of their work. Because of poor medical conditions and economic status, diseases are often not timely discovered in these people, and they do not have regular health monitoring. Therefore, they are considered as vulnerable groups in society.

The factors that affect susceptibility are not always permanent for individuals, especially for those caused by bad habits; susceptibility will be reduced, and even returned to normal level after correction.

2.6.2   Susceptible gene

Abnormal genetic material is the internal cause and basis of disease. These abnormalities may arise from parental genetic predisposition, and may also be induced by harmful environmental factors in the acquired life. The results of modern medical research showed that most diseases are the results of many environmental factors and genetic constitutions. The genetic predisposition to health is associated with a number of genotypes that are associated with disease, which we call disease susceptibility genes. It should be emphasized that susceptible gene is a relative concept, that individuals with this genotype are more susceptible to disease than the general population.

SNPs may have no effect on gene expression, or they can change the function of a gene completely. Many gene variants have been identified to be associated with environmental pollution related diseases, including DNA repair related genes, receptor related genes, cell cycle related genes, and genes involved in the oxidation process in a large number of genome-wide association studies and candidate gene studies performed in diverse populations around the world. These polymorphisms lead to changes in the activity of the corresponding protein or enzyme. The mounting evidence suggests that these gene variants interact with multiple environmental factors and increase susceptibility to some diseases.

Public health genomics is the use of genomics information to benefit public health, and this field is less than a decade old. It is an emerging field that assesses the impact of genes and their interaction with behavior, diet, and the environment on the population's health. Advances in genomic sciences are increasingly being used to improve health and prevent disease, which provides more effective personalized preventive care and disease treatments with better specificity.

The interface between public health and genetics consists of working toward an understanding of how genes and the environment acting together to cause these diseases. Many disorders and diseases that affect humans reflect the interplay between the environment and their genes, however we are still in the initial stage of understanding the specific role of genes which play in common disorders and diseases.

2.6.3   Population-related diseases

Pollution, not disease, is the biggest killer in the developing world. Diseases caused by pollution lead to millions of people deaths each year. Pollution can come from traffic, factories, power generation, wild fires, or even cooking with a wood stove. But these chemicals don't stay put, rain washes them into soils and waterways, and wind blows toxic particles to long distances, sometimes coating crops and food.

Pollution-related diseases are caused by environmental pollution-related pathogenic factors. There are many different types of pollution-related diseases, which are attributed to exposure to toxins in the air, water, and soil. Several representative environmental pollution diseases in the field of environment and health are expounded here.

2.6.4   Air pollution and diseases

Air pollution is the introduction of harmful substances into the atmosphere and cause adverse effects on human health. Classification from morphology, these substances include solid particles, liquid droplets, or gasses suspended in the air.

2.6.4.1   Sources

They can have a natural origin (windblown dust, wildfires, volcanoes and dust storms) or be man-made (power plants, industrial processes, agricultural operations, vehicular traffic, domestic coal burning, as well as industrial and municipal waste incinerators).

2.6.4.2   Industrial and agricultural production

The emission of pollutants from industrial enterprises mainly comes from the combustion of fuels and the process of industrial production. Industrial fuel in China is mainly coal, followed by oil. In agricultural production, the use of chemical fertilizer, pesticide spraying, and burning of straw can also cause air pollution.

2.6.4.3   Life stove and heating boiler

Coal or oil is fuel for heating boiler, and the fuel of cook stove is mainly natural gas, gas, liquefied petroleum gas, and coal, all of which are the sources of air pollution.

2.6.4.4 Vehicular traffic

At present, the main fuel for transportation is gasoline and diesel. A large amount of particulate matter can be produced after combustion, such as nitrogen oxides, polycyclic aromatic hydrocarbons, and aldehydes, which has become an important source of air pollution in China.

2.6.4.5 Adverse health effect

The composition of air pollutants varies in time and space, and can lead to different toxicity. Small particles can adsorb and retain toxic substances.

Air pollution is known to cause a variety of health problems, including effects on respiratory tract, COPD, nervous, and vascular system when the content of pollutants in air exceeds its self-purification capacity. Research has demonstrated increased risk of developing asthma and COPD from increased exposure to air pollution. Data are accumulating that air pollution affects the central nervous system, short-term memory, learning ability, and impulsivity.

Pollution is believed to have adverse effects on the heart, chronic cardiovascular problems, a risk factor for stroke. People with atherosclerosis or building up of fatty deposits on the inner lining of the arteries, may experience immediate trouble when air pollutants play a role in causing plaque in a blood vessel to rupture, triggering a heart attack.

Air pollution is found to be associated with a high incidence of cancer. There is no doubt that there is a close relationship between air pollution and lung cancer. In addition, the incidence of bladder cancer was found increased by air pollution. The function of several other organs can be also influenced; kidney disease was already added to the list of health problems associated with air pollution.

The WHO estimated in 2014 that air pollution causes the premature death of some 7 million people worldwide each year.

2.6.4.6 Mechanism

The mechanisms of air pollution-induced health effects involve oxidative stress and inflammation. The molecular pathways through which airway inflammation induces lung injury have not been fully elucidated, but IgE-mediated sensitization to airborne allergens and toll-like receptor (TLR)-mediated innate immune responses are conformed to be involved.

Due to oxidative stress, pollutants can cause lung damage by acting directly on the production of free ROS, or indirectly by inducing inflammation. Glutathione is antioxidant that help to reduce the epithelial cell inflammation and tissue injury generated by ROS, and research found that people with GSTM1 null genotypes show reduced glutathione-S-transferase (GST) activity and consequently have higher sputum neutrophil and macrophage counts following ozone exposure. Besides glutathione, catalase and myeloperoxidase are the other two antioxidant enzymes that may be relevant to the impact of pollution on airway disease.

2.6.4.7 Prevention

Since a large share of air pollution is caused by combustion of fossil fuels, the reduction of these fuels can reduce air pollution drastically. Transition to renewable energy is very effective and some clean power sources have been used, such as wind power, solar power, and hydro power. According to a study published in 2015, the switch to 100% renewable energy in the United States would eliminate about 62,000 premature deaths per year and about 42,000 in 2050.

Additional strategies to improve air condition include improving production process to reduce exhaust emissions, choosing coal with low sulfur and low ash, and energetically develop and popularize gaseous energy, etc.

Although there are various technologies and strategies available to control air pollution, it is very necessary for the government to provide legal support and strengthen supervision at the same time.

2.6.5 Chronic methyl-mercury poisoning

In the early 1950s, massive methyl mercury (MeHg) poisoning of residents living around Minamata Bay, first raised awareness of the resulting severe neurological disease. This neurological disorder was named Minamata disease (MD) because the victims lived near the Bay. It was caused by the release of methylmercury in the industrial wastewater from the Chisso Corporation's chemical factory, which continued from 1932 to 1968. While cat, dog, pig, and human deaths continued for 36 years, the effect was severe enough in cats that it came to be named as "dancing cat fever".

2.6.5.1　Sources

Mercury poisoning is a type of metal poisoning due to mercury exposure. It is mainly caused by mercury in water and food contamination caused by fish, shellfish, and so on. The consumption of fish is by far the most significant source of ingestion-related mercury exposure in humans, although plants and livestock also contain mercury due to bio-concentration and bio-magnification by ingesting other mercury-containing organisms. Consumption of whale and dolphin meat is the practice in Japan, the meat is a source of high levels of mercury poisoning, it's mercury level was found to be more than 20 times of the acceptable Japanese standard.

2.6.5.2　Symptoms and diagnosis

Methylmercury accumulates and exceeds a threshold value, leading to system damage in ingested people. Symptoms related to toxicity are typically neurologic, such as ataxia, visual disturbance, hearing loss, paresthesia (early signs), dysarthria, mental deterioration, muscle tremor, movement disorders, paralysis, and even death. It depends upon the type, dose, method, and duration of exposure. Mercury poisoning may also cause cardiovascular diseases, symptoms are as follows: abnormal heart rhythm, abnormal blood pressure, abnormal changes in the ST segment, lower broadened P wave, unexplained elevated serum triglyceride, and unexplained elevated cholesterol.

Other symptoms may include kidney dysfunction or decreased intelligence. Affected children may show red cheeks, lips and nose, loss of hair, nails and teeth, transient rashes, muscle weakness, and increased sensitivity to light. The effects of long-term and low-dose exposure to methylmercury are unclear.

Diagnosis of elemental or inorganic mercury poisoning involves determining the history of exposure, physical findings, and an elevated body burden of mercury. If methylmercury intoxication is suspected, information regarding the patient's diet, including the amount of fish consumed, frequency, types, source of fish, and source of water supply should be inquired. Further information about classic symptoms, including: perioral and facial paresthesia, extremity numbness, dysarthria, headache, constriction of the visual fields, difficulty in hearing, memory loss, problems with walking, and so on are also needed.

There are three ways to diagnose organic mercury poisoning. Whole-blood mercury concentrations are typically less than 6 μg/L, but because of its short half-life in the blood, this measure is not useful for suspected cases. To obtain chronic exposure value, urine 24-hour levels are more reliable than spot collections. Mercury concentration in hair is more reliable and it is normally 5 μg/g. Thus, hair analysis is more reliable than urinary mercury levels, whole-blood test is also better than urinary examination.

2.6.5.3　Mechanism

Mercury is the most poisonous, non-radioactive, and naturally occurring substance on our planet. Compounds of mercury tend to be much more toxic than either the elemental form or the salts. These compounds have been implicated in causing brain and liver damage. Dimethyl–mercury is the most dangerous mercury compound.

Mercury irreversibly inhibits selenium – dependent enzymes. High mercury exposures deplete the amount of cellular selenium for the biosynthesis of thioredoxin reductase and other selenoenzymes that prevent and reverse oxidative damage. If the depletion is long lasting, it can result in brain cell dysfunctions which can ultimately cause death. Cell culture and animal experiments have shown that methylmercury can induce excessive expression of apoptosis related genes in nerve cells, thereby mediating apoptosis. Mercury may also inactivate S–adenosyl–methionine, which is necessary for catecholamine catabolism by catechol–O–methyl transferase.

Methyl–mercury can also inhibit β–tubulin and interfere with the internal structure of neurons and the dynamic balance of biochemical reactions. The structure and function of mitochondria can be destroyed obviously, thus disturbing the release of neurotransmitters.

Improving the production process and eliminating the waste water containing mercury to the environment are the most fundamental measure to prevent chronic mercury poisoning. To this end, many governments and private agencies have made efforts to regulate heavily the use of mercury. The United States Environmental Protection Agency (EPA) issued recommendations in 2004 regarding exposure to mercury in fish and shellfish. Considering the great impact on children, EPA also developed the "Fish Kids" awareness campaign for children and young adults.

2.6.6   Chronic cadmium poisoning

Itai–itai disease is a serious environmental pollution disease found in cadmium polluted areas. The main symptom of a typical case of chronic cadmium poisoning is severe pain in the whole body. The cadmium was released into rivers by mining companies in the mountains, and the water in the river was mainly used for irrigation of rice fields, but also for drinking water, washing, fishing, and other uses by downstream populations.

2.6.6.1   Sources

Cadmium is widely used in industry. It is mainly used in electroplating, colourant, plastic stabilizer, alloy, battery, and ceramic manufacture, etc. Generally speaking, the cadmium in the atmosphere mainly comes from the smelting of non–ferrous metals, calcination, and sintering of ores. Cadmium in water mainly comes from industrial wastewater, and cadmium in soil is mainly caused by irrigation of cadmium containing wastewater. Therefore, food is another source of cadmium. Cadmium content in rice, fish, and shellfish are increased, resulting in the cadmium accumulation of the intake.

Smoking is another significant source of cadmium exposure. A pack of cigarettes contains 15 μg of cadmium and the intake of passive smoking was higher than that of active smoking. Aside from smokers, people who live near hazardous waste sites or factories that release cadmium into the air have the potential for exposure to cadmium in air.

2.6.6.2   Symptoms and diagnosis

One of the main effects of cadmium poisoning is weak and brittle bones, with progressive aggravation. Lumbago and knee pain in the early stage of onset, then spread throughout the body. The victims experience sharp tingling during activity and relief during rest. The skeleton is severely deformed and brittle. Most of the patients are women over 40 years of age. Pregnancy, lactation, malnutrition, and so on are vulnerable groups to be affected.

Increased concentrations of urinary beta-2 micro-globulin (>9.6 μmol/mol creatinine) can be an early indicator of renal dysfunction in persons chronically exposed to low levels of environmental cadmium. Chronic severe poisoning is associated with chronic renal insufficiency, accompanied by osteoporosis and osteomalacia. Domestic and international studies have found that urine enzyme content changed in patients with chronic cadmium poisoning.

2.6.6.3 Mechanism

Acute exposure to cadmium fumes may cause flu-like symptoms, including fever, shivering, and muscle ache. Inhaling cadmium-laden dust quickly leads to problems in respiratory tract and kidney. Ingestion of any significant amount of cadmium can cause immediate poisoning and damage to the liver and the kidneys.

Chronic cadmium poisoning occurs after prolonged exposure to the dust or fumes of cadmium-containing compounds. Cadmium mainly passes through the respiratory tract, the digestive tract and the blood circulation into the whole body, and selectively accumulated in the liver and kidney. Renal function impairment in patients of chronic cadmium poisoning was obvious, inspection was found with increased sugar and calcium in urine, and changed urinary enzyme. Compounds containing cadmium are also carcinogenic. Animal experiments and epidemiological survey of population found that cadmium can cause chromosome aberrations.

2.6.6.4 Prevention

Once cadmium is discharged into the environment, it is extremely difficult to eliminate. Therefore, the most fundamental way to prevent cadmium poisoning is to control cadmium emission. We should also strengthen the detection of cadmium content and control the intake, and keep regular health examination for residents in cadmium polluted areas and health monitoring for high-risk and susceptible population. Vitamin D supplementation and high protein diet can alleviate the disease in patients with chronic cadmium poisoning. At present, there is no safe method for cadmium removal, and the effect of metal chelating agent on cadmium removal is not significant, and it may also lead to redistribution of cadmium in vivo.

2.6.7 Legionnaires' disease

Legionnaires' disease is a severe form of pneumonia infection caused by the bacterium legionella, which gets its name from an outbreak that killed 29 people attending an American Legion at a Philadelphia hotel in 1976. The bacteria can also cause a less serious infection called Pontiac fever that has symptoms similar to a mild case of flu.

2.6.7.1 Sources

Legionella infection is more related to artificial water environment. The bacteria grow best at warm temperatures between 25 ℃ and 45 ℃. Therefore, it is found naturally in cold and hot water piping system, air conditioning cooling tower circulating water, and air humidifier, which provide a good living environment for it. Water sources in buildings, offices, hotels, and hospitals are main sources of contaminated water.

Most people get legionnaires' disease from inhaling instead of person-to-person contact. Many people exposed to legionella do not become sick, older people and those with weakened immune systems are more susceptible than others.

2.6.7.2 Symptoms and diagnosis

The illness takes two distinct forms: Legionnaires' disease and Pontiac fever. The main symptom of Legionnaires' disease is systemic multiple organ damages caused by lung infection. It frequently begins with the following signs and symptoms: chills, myalgia, dizziness, headache, and dysphoria. Soon later, it will develop other signs and symptoms that may include: cough, shortness of breath, chest pain, gastrointestinal symptoms, confusion, or other mental changes. Pontiac fever symptoms are primarily fever and muscle aches; it is a milder infection than Legionnaires' disease. No pneumonia has been found, but pleurisy and exudative inflammation present. The over all prognosis is good and few death will occur.

It is difficult to distinguish pneumonia only based on nonspecific laboratory diagnosis and chest X-ray examination due to early Legionnaires' disease and other causes. Additional specific tests are required for diagnosis. One of the useful tests is to detect identifiable proteins of the Legionnaires' bacterium in urine. Besides, a culture of the sputum may be helpful to detect the bacteria. Of all the available tests, the most specific one is isolation and culture of the bacterium secreted by the respiratory tract.

2.6.7.3 Mechanism

The pathogenesis of Legionella remains unclear. It was found that legionella blooms and releases in epithelial cells, macrophages, and neutrophils, leading to cell death.

The incidence of inhalation is closely related to the virulence of pathogenic bacteria and the immunity level of human body. People with decreased immunity are particularly susceptible to this disease. Alveolar macrophages are lysed and release a large number of bacteria, leading to acute damage to the alveolar epithelium and endothelium.

The pathogenicity of Legionella is also related to the surface structure of bacteria and the production of various toxins. The outer membrane proteins of Legionella can promote the uptake of bacteria by phagocytes and destroy their bactericidal function. The enzymes produced by Legionella generally have three kinds of activities, protein decomposition, hemolysis, and cytotoxicity. In addition, it can induce the production of pre-clotting factor active substances in human peripheral blood monocytes, which may contribute to disseminated intravascular coagulation in the course of infection.

Prevention to date, there is no vaccine for this bacterium. Prevention mostly depends on good maintenance of water systems to limit the growth of bacteria and the formation of biological aerosols. The sanitary management of cooling water in public places and circulating water system of large buildings should be strengthened and disinfected regularly. Exercise may improve the body's ability to resist disease, and closely monitoring vulnerable groups to protect them against the disease are warranted.

Jiang Bijie

2.7 Prevention and control

2.7.1 Environmental protection standard system

2.7.1.1 Environmental protection law

In order to protect the environment, all countries have formulated environmental protection law. *Law of Environmental Protection of the People's Republic of China* has been adopted in 1989, and revised in 2014. The highly anticipated law revision aimed at improving the current law by providing more specific details and mechanisms for enforcement to protect and improve the environment, prevent pollution and other public hazards and ensure public health.

The key principles outlined in the law include the following.

(1) Clearly identify environmental protection responsibilities of the governments, and all units and individuals have the obligation to protect the environment.

(2) Source – control and co – control of multiple pollutants through planning, clear standards, and strengthened environmental protection requirements for construction projects and emitters.

(3) Citizens should enhance the awareness of environmental protection, adopt a low carbon and frugal lifestyle, and conscientiously fulfill their environmental protection obligations.

(4) To improve total emission control system and emission permit system.

(5) To improve legal responsibility and increase the strength of penalties.

(6) To support the development and application of environmental protection technology, encourage the development of related industries, and improve the level of science and technology in environmental protection.

The governments at all levels should strengthen the publicity and popularization of environmental protection.

2.7.1.2　The ministry of environment

The ministry of environment explored measures against the heavy pollution and the local governments implemented plans according to warnings and instructions from the ministry.

2.7.2　Pollution source control and monitoring

2.7.2.1　Reasonable urban planning

The relevant urban planning laws and regulations should be promulgated to regulate urban construction and economic development. In the prevention and control of urban or regional pollution, it is very important to take reasonable both planning and technological measures. At its most basic level, land–use planning is likely to involve zoning and transport infrastructure planning. It is an important part of social policy in most developed countries, ensuring that land is used efficiently for the benefit of the wider economy and population, as well as to reduce the environment pollution. In addition, great importance should be attached to the green spaces in the city, together with surrounding areas of the city. Grassland not only beautifies the environment, but also plays an important role in improving the environmental quality of the city.

2.7.2.2　Production process reform

To improve energy structure, enterprises with high pollution and high energy consumption should be closed. Besides, transition to renewable energy is effective in reducing energy consumption. For the soil and water protection, pollutants emission from the source control is critical. Wastes containing heavy metal pollutants are prohibited into water or soil before treatment.

2.7.2.3　Monitoring of pollution status

The purpose of pollution monitoring is to understand the status of pollution control, get to know the temporal and spatial distribution of pollutants, predict the development trend of pollution, so as to achieve more effective environmental protection purposes.

It is worth noting that, although the current environmental pollution is mainly divided into three parts, air pollution, water pollution and soil pollution, they are not separate and always interact with each other. Therefore, comprehensive prevention and management are necessary.

2.7.2.4　Protection of susceptible population

In epidemiology, a susceptible individual is a member of a population who is at risk of becoming infected by a disease. Therefore, susceptible populations always require special consideration.

Improve Immunity: It is very important to enhance the resistance to disease through good nutrition to improve the immune status of the human body. Protein, vitamin A, vitamin C, vitamin E, iron, zinc and selenium are nutrients closely related to the immune function of the body. Taking part in physical exercise is another way to improve the physical immunity. The most effective way is aerobic exercise, such as jogging, yoga, cycling, and swimming are all very good aerobic exercises.

Vaccination is the administration of antigenic material (a vaccine) to stimulate an individual's immune system to develop adaptive immunity to a pathogen. It is used to help you adjust the environmental factors that induce disease, so as to delay or avoid the occurrence of disease.

2.7.2.5 Susceptibility gene detection

Detection of disease susceptibility genes is the detection of hidden "gene mines" in health, predicting the risk of future possible diseases. Variations within the Genome are being studied to determine susceptibility to diseases. Genetic testing is the process of detecting genetic abnormalities using genetic and molecular biological techniques. Accurate and sensitive prediction of disease, or detection of early stages of disease, could allow the prevention or arrest of disease development as immunotherapy treatment is available. Through genetic testing, we know whether we are susceptible to some common diseases (susceptibility risk), such as cardiovascular and cerebrovascular diseases, autoimmune diseases, and tumors. It can help to avoid harmful substance exposures associated with specific diseases, delay the occurrence and development of diseases, and improve the diagnosis and regular monitoring of the disease. Early diagnosis and early treatment may minimize the damage caused by the disease.

Genetic testing is not the same as disease diagnosis. Positive results suggest a person at a high risk of illness, but it does not mean that the individual will suffer from this disease in the future. Indeed, there are many diseases which will only develop when the existing predisposing genetic factors, interact with external environmental factors or with other genetic factors.

2.7.2.6 Risk assessment

Environmental risk assessment is the process of evaluating the likelihood that adverse human health and ecological effects may occur as a result of exposure to one or more agents. The purpose of the assessment is to provide relevant and useful information to inform the remedial decision. Risk assessments conducted and used by regulators are the most objective and scientific ways to understand the potential adverse health outcomes of environmental hazards, through which we can better understand the risks faced by susceptible populations. Risk assessments can help regulators apply science in policy and decision-making.

2.8 Research methods

The relationship between environment and health is the core content of environmental hygiene research. The common research means are environmental epidemiology and environmental toxicology. With the development of life science and environmental science, some new research methods have emerged in the field of environmental hygiene. Omics is a new technology in molecular biology, characterized by high resolution, high sensitivity, and high throughput. Therefore, it has broad application prospects in the field of environment and health.

2.8.1 Environmental epidemiology

Environmental epidemiology is a branch of epidemiology concerning the discovery of the environmental exposures that affect human health and the identification of public health and health care actions to manage the risks associated with harmful exposures. It studies the relationship between external environmental factors and the population health from the macro level.

Similar to those used in traditional epidemiology, descriptive studies (ecological research and current situation research), analytical studies (case-control studies, cohort studies), and experimental epidemiological studies are adopted in environmental epidemiology. The selection of different epidemiological methods is based on the content of environmental epidemiological studies.

For environmental epidemiological investigation, it is necessary to avoid separating the environment from the body and studying isolated and unilateral effect. In general, the following principles should be followed:

Sample should be representative. The larger the sample, the more it can reflect the actual situation. But it takes a lot of manpower and material, and needs a long time. In general, survey sampling method is adopted, and representative samples are extracted randomly.

Survey design should be contrastive. There is a significant difference in health reaction between exposed and unexposed people.

Paying attention to the availability of information. Interference factors should be excluded, and the combination of multiple factors in the environment should be considered carefully.

2.8.2   Environmental toxicology

Environmental toxicology is a multidisciplinary field of science, it studies the biological effects, mechanisms, and early damage indicators of environmental pollutants on the body, so as to provide scientific basis for developing environmental hygiene standards and environmental protection work. The study of the toxic effects of environmental pollutants is mainly through animal experiments.

The main tasks of environmental toxicology research include the following.

Study of the damage and mechanism of the pollutants to the body, including their degradation and transformation products.

Exploring the early indicators of environmental pollution on human health.

Detecting the biological changes that occur initially after the action of environmental pollutants with the most sensitive detection means.

Quantitative assessment of the impact of toxic environmental pollutants on the body, determining the effect of dose and dose-response relationship.

Confirming the cause of the suspected pathogenic factors by established animal model.

The study of environmental toxicology is mainly based on animal experiments, observing the various biological changes of experimental animals exposed to different doses of environmental pollutants through various ways. Experimental animals are generally mammals and other vertebrates, but insects, and microbes and animal cell lines can also be used. According to the purpose of the study, it can be divided into the following five categories (Figure 2-1).

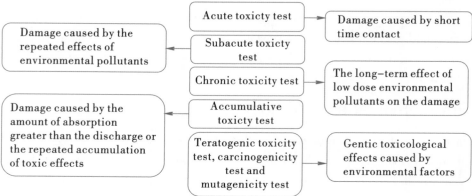

Figure 2-1   Common test methods for environmental toxicology

2.8.3　Environmental Omics

Omics refers to a field of study in biology ending in－omics, such as genomics, proteomics, metabolomics, transcriptomics, immunomics, glycomics, and RNAomics.

In recent years, omics has also been applied in the field of environmental hygiene.

2.8.3.1　Environmental genomics

Environmental microbiology has developed rapidly in recent years as a result of the study on environmental changes and the needs of microbial communities. Metagenomics, may also be referred to as environmental genomics, is the study of genetic material recovered directly from environmental samples.

With this technology, scientists can also study the cellular structure of human tissue, the interaction of genes, proteins, and molecules as a whole, and thus explore the relationship with the health of the body. The environmental genome project (EGP) was first proposed by the National Institute of Environmental Health Sciences in 1997. EGP scientists want to determine how these genes change among individuals and whether these changes are associated with disease susceptibility.

2.8.3.2　Environmental proteomics

Environmental proteomics mainly studies the toxicity and production process of biological molecules caused by environmental pollution factors, and finds the target protein of pollutants. The content mainly includes two kinds of studies; one is the study of protein expression in contaminated environment, including protein identification and quantification, as well as cell location and modification. Second is the study of protein function in contaminated environment, including protein interaction and network relationship.

Proteomics will be one of the most effective ways to find molecular markers and drug targets for disease. Proteomics technology also has a very attractive prospect in clinical diagnosis and treatment of cancer, Alzheimer's disease, and other important human diseases. Now many large drug companies are investing numerous manpower and material resources in proteomics research.

Wang Baiqi

Chapter 3

Air and Health

3.1   Composition of the atmosphere

Air lets our living planet breathe—it is the mixture of gases that fills the atmosphere. The air contains a variety of substances that not only affect the health, longevity, and quality of life for people and plants, but also have positive and negative effects on nonliving aspects of the environment.

3.1.1   Atmospheric structure and chemical composition

By volume, dry air contains 78.09% of nitrogen, 20.95% of oxygen, 0.93% of argon, 0.04% of carbon dioxide, and small amounts of other gases including neon, helium, krypton, and xenon. Air also contains a variable amount of water vapor on average around 1% at sea level, and 0.4% over the entire atmosphere. The atmosphere is divided into layers according to major changes in temperature. Gravity pushes the layers of air down on the earth's surface and 99% of the total mass of the atmosphere is within 32 km of the distance above the earth surface.

The layer of air closely adjacent to earth's surface is called the troposphere. Ranging in depth from 16 km over the equator to about 8 km over the poles, this zone contains 75% of the total mass of the atmosphere and where most weather events occur. Air temperature drops rapidly with increasing altitude above the Earth's surface, reaching about −60 ℃ at the top of the troposphere. A sudden reversal of this temperature gradient creates a sharp boundary, the tropopause, which the temperature remains fairly constant here. Human is most directly concerned with this layer.

The stratosphere extends from the tropopause up above 50 km. Air temperature in this layer remains fairly constant. Although more dilute than the troposphere, the stratosphere has a with troposphere except for two important components, water and ozone. The fractional volume of water vapor is about one thousand times lower, and ozone is nearly one thousand times higher than in the troposphere. Ozone is formed from dioxygen by the action of ultraviolet light and also atmospheric electrical discharges. The ozone within stratosphere is beneficial, shielding plants and animals from the damaging of ultraviolet rays.

Above the stratosphere, the temperature drops again as the altitude increases, creating the mesophere. This layer is the coldest region of the atmosphere due to decreasing of solar heating and increasing cooling by carbon dioxide radioactive emission. Temperatures in the upper mesosphere fall as low as -101 ℃, varying according to latitude and season.

At the altitude of 80 km, another abrupt temperature change occurs. This is the beginning of the thermosphere, a region contains highly ionized gases, extending to about 1,600 km. The temperature increases dramatically in the thermosphere because molecules are constantly bombarded by high-energy solar and cosmic radiation. Ionosphere is the lower part of the thermosphere. The particles of gas there become electrically charged due to absorbing ultraviolet and X-ray radiation from the sun. There is no sharp boundary marking the end of the atmosphere.

3.1.2　Physical composition of the atmosphere

The atmosphere functions as a highly effective regulator of heat and radiation, and is the principal sources of energy for life. Sunlight that travels through space and shines on the Earth is termed solar radiation. On Earth, sunlight is filtered through Earth's atmosphere, and is obvious as daylight when the sun is above the horizon. When the direct solar radiation is not blocked by clouds, it is experienced as sunshine, a combination of bright light and radiant heat. When it is blocked by clouds or reflects off other objects, it is experienced as diffused light. Solar radiation includes an infinite array of radio, microwave, infrared, visible-light, ultraviolet (UV), X-ray, and gamma-ray emissions (Figure 3-1).

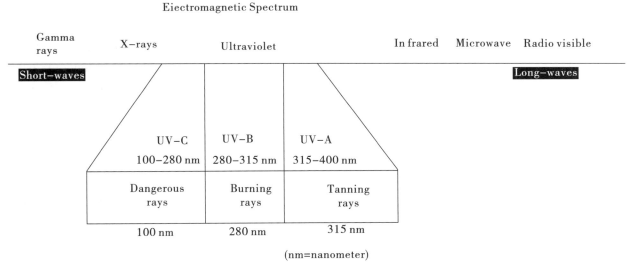

Figure 3-1　**Four layers of the earth's atmosphere**

The atmosphere protects the biosphere from harmful incoming solar radiation. Incoming solar radiation fluctuates from time to time and on average, about half of this radiation is reflected or absorbed by atmosphere. The absorption of solar radiation by the atmosphere is selective. Visible light passes through almost undiminished, whereas ultraviolet light is absorbed mostly by stratospheric ozone.

Although the solar corona is a source of extreme ultraviolet and X-ray radiation, these rays make up only a very small amount of the power output of the Sun (see spectrum at right). The spectrum of nearly all solar electromagnetic radiation striking the Earth's atmosphere spans a range of 100 nm to about 1 mm (1,000,000 nm). This band of significant radiation power can be divided into 3 regions in increasing order of wavelengths: UV range, visible range, and infrared range.

UV rays are an electromagnetic radiation with a wavelength from 10 nm to 400 nm, shorter than that of visible light but longer than X-rays. There are mainly three categories of UV radiation: UV-A (315-

400 nm) , UV-B (280-315 nm) , and UV-C (100-280 nm). UV-A is the least damaging (longest wavelength) form of UV radiation and reaches the Earth in greatest quantity. Most UV-A rays pass right through the ozone layer in the stratosphere. UV-B radiation can be very harmful. Fortunately for life on Earth, most of the sun's UV-B radiation is absorbed by stratospheric ozone. UV-C radiation is potentially the most damaging because it is very energetic. When UV-C light reaches the stratosphere, it is completely absorbed by oxyen molecules and unable to reach the Earth's surface.

The ultraviolet radiation in sunlight has both positive and negative health effects, as it is both a principal source of vitamin D_3 and a mutagen. UV light causes the body to produce vitamin D, which is essential for life. The human body needs some UV radiation to maintain adequate vitamin D levels. An appropriate amount of UV-B (which varies according to skin color) leads to a limited amount of direct DNA damage. This is recognized and repaired by the body, and then melanin production is increased, which leads to a long-lasting tan. This tan occurs with a 2-day lag phase after irradiation. Ultraviolet radiation has medical applications in the treatment of skin conditions, such as psoriasis and vitiligo, UV light with wavelength of 311 nm is most effective for these conditions.

The International Agency for Research on Cancer(IARC) of the World Health Organization (WHO) classified all categories and wavelengths of Ultraviolet Radiation as a Group 1 carcinogen in 2011. This is the highest level designation for carcinogens and means that "there is enough evidence to conclude that it can cause cancer in humans". Excessive UV exposure results in a number of chronic skin changes. These include various skin cancers of which melanoma is the most life-threatening. United Nations Environment Programme (UNEP) has estimated that more than 2 million nonmelanoma skin cancers and 200,000 malignant melanomas occur globally each year. The worldwide incidence of malignant melanoma continues to increase, and is strongly related to frequency of recreational exposure to the sun and to the history of sunburn. There is evidence that risk of melanoma is also related to intermittent exposure to UV, especially in childhood. In the event of a 10% decrease in stratospheric ozone, an additional 300,000 non-melanoma and 4,500 melanoma skin cancers could be expected worldwide. Caucasians have a higher risk of skin cancer because of the relative lack of skin pigmentation. Other UV-related skin disorders include actinic keratoses and premature aging of the skin.

UV exposure of the eye depends on many factors : ground reflection, the degree of brightness in the sky leading to activation of the squint reflex, the amount of atmospheric refection, and the use of eyewear. The acute effects of UV on the eye include the development of photokeratitis and photoconjunctivitis, which are like sunburn of the delicate skin-like tissue on the surface of the eyeball and eyelids. While painful, they are reversible, can be easily prevented by protective eyewear, and have not been associated with any long-term damage.

Chronic effects include the possible development of pterygium (a white or cream colored opaque growth attached to the cornea) , squamous cell cancer of the conjunctiva (scaly or plate-like malignancy) , and cataracts. Some 20 million people worldwide are currently blind as a result of cataracts. WHO estimates that as many as 20% of them may be due to UV exposure.

UV intensity can be higher or lower for surfaces at different angles to the horizontal. Likewise, UV intensity can nearly double with reflection from snow or other bright surfaces like water, sand, or concrete. The UV Index provides a daily forecast of the expected intensity of UV radiation from the sun. The UV Index scale explains the UV Index and steps ; which one can take to minimize the risks from harmful exposure to the sun's rays. It predicts the ultraviolet radiation levels on a 1-11+ scale, helping people determine to applying proper sun protection.

3.2   Sources and types of ambient air pollution

Air pollution worldwide is a growing threat to human health and the natural environment. Air pollution may be described as contamination of the atmosphere by gaseous, liquid, or solid wastes, or by-products that can endanger human health and welfare of plants and animals. The air pollution problem is encountered outdoor as well as indoor.

3.2.1   Sources of air pollution

In order to understand the causes of air pollution, several divisions can be made. The source of air pollution can be dichotomized into natural and anthropogenic sources. Natural sources include dust blown by wind, pollutants from wildfires and volcanic eruptions. Anthropogenic air pollution, contamination produced by humans, may also adversely affect human health. Sources of air pollution may also be classified by the ways they generate emissions: transportation, stationary combustion sources, industrial processed, solid waste disposal facilities, and miscellaneous.

3.2.2   Types of ambient air pollutant

Any undesirable substance mixed with open air could be termed as an air pollutant, whether it is man-made or natural, which exceeds international environmental health standard in concentration and self-purification capacity in total air amount. The major pollutants which contribute to ambient air pollution are sulphur dioxide, carbon dioxide, nitrogen oxides, ozone, suspended particulate matter, lead, carbon dioxide, and toxic pollutants. There are two basic physical forms of air pollutants. The first is gaseous form, such as sulfur dioxide, ozone, and hydrocarbon vapors in the form of gas. The gasses lack definite volume and shape and the molecules are widely separated. The second form of air pollution is particulate matter, such as smoke, dust, fly ash, and mists.

Most human inputs of ambient air pollutants come from the burning of fossil fuels in power plants, industrial facilities, and motor vehicles. The outdoor air pollutants are also classified as primary pollutants and secondary pollutants. The primary pollutants are harmful chemicals emitted directly into the atmosphere from natural processes and human activities. They remain in the same chemical form as they are released, such as sulfur dioxide and hydrocarbons emitted from factories. Secondary pollutants are not emitted directly, rather, they react with one another and with other normal components of air to form new harmful chemicals. Ground level ozone is a prominent example of a secondary pollutant.

3.2.3   Influences of climate, topography, and atmosphere processes

Topography, climate, and physical processes in the atmosphere play an important role in transport, concentration, dispersal, and removal of air pollutants. Wind speed, mixing between atmospheric layers, precipitation, and atmospheric chemistry all determine whether pollutants will remain in the locality where they are produced or go elsewhere. The following part will mainly introduce how the temperature inversion affects air pollution levels.

The accumulation of chemically active compounds in the atmosphere is greatly affected by land features and atmospheric movements. Valleys nearby mountain areas, and the lack of open space (parks, forests, wild environment areas, and bodies of water) strongly increase the severity of air pollution in a locale. These features hold the air mass like a container and prevent dilution and mixing. Stagnant air masses may receive emissions for days on end. When conditions are right, usually in the morning or when there is descent of air from higher altitudes, a special atmospheric condition is created, which is called temperature inversion. In an inversion, the temperature rises with increasing altitude rather than falling, which is normally the case. An inversion layer is a mass of air with an inverted temperature gradient (warmer above, cooler below). The motion of air in an inversion layer is suppressed and it limits the mixing and dilution of air pollution. Inversions are very common, especially in valleys and coastlines. There are two types of temperature inversions: surface inversions that occur near the Earth's surface, and aloft inversions that occur above the ground. Surface temperature inversions play a major role in air quality. The worst episodes of air pollution usually occur when inversions stay in place for days on end and the atmosphere underneath receives air pollution day after day with no mixing or wind to dilute it.

3.3　Harmful effect of air pollution

Air pollution can harm the health of people and animals, damage crops or stop their growing properly. We can distinguish between direct damage and indirect damage of air pollution.

3.3.1　Direct damage of air pollution

Generally if one is young and in a good state of health, moderate air pollution levels are unlikely to have any serious short term effects. However, elevated levels and/or long term exposure to air pollution can lead to more serious symptoms and conditions affecting human health. Different people will be affected by air pollution in different ways depending on: their age and general health; the type of pollutant; the duration of exposure to the pollutant; what they are doing at the time they are exposed and etc. Polluted air can cause damage to health and affect health in both acute and long—term way. Acute effects may be brought on, for instance, by pollution episodes, while chronic and long—term effects may generally affect a greater proportion of the population.

3.3.1.1　Acute poisoning

If the concentration of pollutants rapidly increases in short—term and a lot of pollutants (fume, exhaust gas) are absorbed by population, It will induce acute poisoning. Respiratory symptoms are the most common acute health effects from air pollution. Common symptoms include cough, irritation of nose and throat, and mild shortness of breath. These respiratory symptoms are often associated with eye irritation and a sense of fatigue. Other symptoms include headach, nausea, and allergic reactions. Short—term air pollution can aggravate the medical condition of individuals with asthma and emphysema.

Smog episode is the main sort of air pollution that causes acute poisoning, this sort of accident is usually caused by smoke from burning fuel and pollutants produced during production. According to formation reason, there are two major sorts of smog: soot smog and photochemical smog. Soot smog, namely London smog type or reduction type, mainly contains sulfur dioxide (SO_2), particle, and carbon monoxide (CO). Soot and waste industrial gases get into atmosphere and cannot be diffused fully, thus causing soot smog. Since industrial revolution, using of coal increased rapidly, lots of smoke of burning coal polluted the air seriously. When the weather was foggy and wind was light, the pollution became trapped over the cities. The smoke and fog mix to produce smog. From the end of 19th century, soot smog issues were recognized and several episodes have been well—documented, including one in Belgium in 1930 (Meuse Valley), one in the United States in 1948 (Donora, Pennsylvania), one in Mexico in 1950 (Poza Rica), and one in England in

1952 (Landon).

　　Air pollution regulations in developed countries have resulted in reduced industrial smog events, but photochemical smog remains a persistent problem, largely driven by vehicle emissions. Photochemical smog is produced when sunlight reacts with nitrogen oxides and at least one volatile organic compound (VOC) in the atmosphere. Nitrogen oxides come from car exhaust, coal power plants, and factory emissions. VOCs are released from gasoline, paints, and many cleaning solvents. Photochemical smog, also namely oxidation type, mainly contains nitrogen oxides (NOx), hydrocarbon (CH), ozone, Peroxyacyl Nitrates (PANs), VOCs, and aldehyde. PANs cause watery eyes and can damage plants, ozone irritates eyes and deteriorates rubber and plants. Los Angeles in America is a good example of a city that has a big problem with photochemical smog. In 1943, 1946, 1954, and 1955, serious acute poisoning episodes occurred in Los Angeles America. During the accident in 1955, the air temperature reached up to 37.8 ℃ and continued for more than a week, asthma and bronchitis spreaded, mortality of population older than 65 increased, about 70-317 people died every day.

　　Industrial accidents may release a relatively large quantity of a specific type of air pollutant that becomes a local problem. Production accidents that cause acute poisoning don't occur often, but once it occurs, the harm is very serious. Event like the 1984 Baphol disaster in India often refers to as industrial accident because the release of a gas of methylhetrocyanic acid from local plant killed over 3,800 people.

3.3.1.2　Chronic and long-term effects

　　Mucosal irritation in the form of acute or chronic bronchitis, nasal tickle, or conjunctivitis is characteristic of high levels of air pollution, although individuals vary considerably in their susceptibility to such effects. Continual exposure to air pollution may affect the growing lungs of children and aggravate or complicate medical conditions in the elderly. Air pollution was the direct or indirect cause of inhabitant's respiratory tract diseases, such as chronic obstructive pulmonary diseases and other diseases.

　　Respiratory effects of air pollution, particularly in people who suffer from chronic bronchitis, may place an additional strain on the heart as well. Air pollution is associated with increased risk of death from heart and lung diseases, even at levels below those known to be acutely toxic to the lungs or heart. The stimulation of nerve reflexes connecting the heart and the lung may cause additional problems in patients with heart diseases.

　　In some regions, air is very seriously polluted by Cd, Se, Pb, F and other chemical materials, residents will suffer chronic chemical poisoning. Central nervous system dysfunction, and possibly learning disabilities in children, may result from accumulated body burdens of lead. Air pollution contributes a large fraction of lead exposure in many countries because of lead additives in gasoline. Even in countries where lead has been removed from gasoline, the lead remains in the environment as one source of exposure.

　　The link between cancers and ambient air pollution has always been a concern. Examples of cancer associated with community air pollution include point-source emissions from some poorly controlled smelters that release arsenic, which can cause lung cancer. In 2012, IARC has reclassified diesel engine exhaust from "probably carcinogenic to humans (Group 2A)" to "carcinogenic to humans (Group 1)". Outdoor air pollution was also classified as "carcinogenic to humans (Group 1)" in 2013.

　　There are also important examples of indoor air pollution in homes (radon) that are linked to lung cancer. Tobacco smoking is more carcinogenic than arsenic or radon in the air, multiplying the lung cancer risk from these toxins.

3.3.2　Indirect damage of air pollution

　　The major indirect damages of ambient air pollution are acid deposition, greenhouse effects, and ozone depletion.

3.3.2.1   Acid deposition

"Acid rain" is a broad term referring to a mixture of wet and dry depositions (deposited materials) from the atmosphere containing higher than normal amounts of nitric and sulfuric acids. The precursors, or chemical forerunners, of acid rain formation result from both natural sources (such as volcanoes and decaying vegetation) and man–made sources (primarily emissions of SO_2 and NO_x resulting from fossil fuel combustion). Acid rain occurs when these gases react in the atmosphere with water, oxygen, and other chemicals to form various acidic compounds, resulting in a mild solution of sulfuric acid and nitric acid. When sulfur dioxide and nitrogen oxides are released from power plants and other sources, prevailing winds blow these compounds across state and national borders, sometimes over hundreds of miles.

Wet deposition refers to acidic rain, fog, and snow. If the acid chemical in the air are blown into areas where the weather is wet, the acid can fall to the ground in the form of rain, snow, fog, or mist. As this acidic water flows over and through the ground, it affects a variety of plants and animals. Dry deposited gases and particles can be washed from these surfaces by rainstorms, leading to increased run off water. This run off water makes the resulting mixture more acidic. About half of the acidity in the atmosphere falls back to earth through dry deposition.

Acid rain causes acidification of lakes and streams, and contributes to damage of trees at high elevations and many sensitive forest soils. In addition, acid rain accelerates the decay of building materials and paints, including irreplaceable buildings, statues, and sculptures that are part of our cultural heritage. Prior to falling to the earth, SO_2 and NO_x gases and their particulate matter derivatives: sulfates and nitrates, contribute to visibility degradation and harm public health. Direct effects of acid deposition on humans have been difficult to study. However, the pollutants that cause acid rain: SO_2 and NO_x, do damage human health. Transregional transportation of pollution, as with acid deposition and the long range transport of air toxins, may result in increased airway reactivity and asthma.

3.3.2.2   Greenhouse effects

The greenhouse effect happens when certain gases, known as greenhouse gases, collec in earth's atmosphere. These gases include carbon dioxide (CO_2), methane, nitrous oxide (N_2O), fluorinated gases, and ozone. Greenhouse gases let the sun's light shine onto the earth's surface, but they trap the heat that reflects back into the atmosphere. In this way, they act like the glass walls of a greenhouse. This greenhouse effect keeps the earth warm enough to sustain life.

Most of the CO_2 in the atmosphere comes from burning fossil fuels. Cars, trucks and trains, and planes, as well as many electric power plants, all burn fossil fuels. Another way which humans release CO_2 into the atmosphere is by cutting down forests, because trees contain large amounts of carbon. People add methane to the atmosphere through livestock farming, landfills, and fossil fuel production, such as coal mining and natural gas processing. Nitrous oxide comes from agriculture and fossil fuel burning. Fluorinated gases include chlorofluorocarbons (CFCs), hydrochlorofluorocarbons (HCFCs), and hydrofluorocarbons (HFCs). These gases are used in aerosol cans and refrigeration. All of these human activities produce greenhouse gases to the atmosphere. The rise in earth's average temperature contributed by human activity is known as global warming.

Most scientists agree that we must reduce the amount of greenhouse gases released into the atmosphere. There are lots of ways of doing this, including: drive less, use public transportation and carpool, walk, fly less, reuse, recycle, use less electricity, eat less meat, or plant trees. Trees can absorb carbon dioxide, keeping it out of the atmosphere.

3.3.2.3   Ozone depletion

Ozone occurs naturally in the earth's upper atmosphere, 10–30 miles above the earth's surface, where it forms a protective layer that shields us from the sun's harmful ultraviolet rays. This "good" ozone is gradually being destroyed by manmade chemicals. An area where ozone has been most significantly depleted, for example, over the North or South Pole, is sometimes called "hole in the ozone." The production and emissions of CFCs are the leading causes of ozone layer depletion. Emission of CFCs accounts for roughly 80% of total depletion of ozone. Other ozone–depleting substances include HCFCs and VOCs. These are often found in vehicle emissions, byproducts of industrial processes, refrigerants, and aerosols. Every time 1% of the ozone layer is depleted, 2% more UVB is able to reach the surface of the planet. Ultraviolet rays of the sun are associated with a number of health and environmental issues. Exposure to ultraviolet rays poses an increased risk of developing several types of skin cancers, including malignant melanoma, basal and squamous cell carcinoma. Direct exposure to UV radiations can result in photo keratitis (snow blindness) and cataracts. Effects of UV rays include impairment of the immune system. Increased exposure to UV rays weakens the response of the immune system. Constant exposure to UV radiation can cause photoallergy, which results in the outbreak of rash in people with light skin. Ozone chemicals can cause difficulty in breathing, chest pain, throat irritation, and hamper lung functioning.

Wu Mei

3.4   Health effects of several major air pollutants

Some of the common ambient air pollutants, their sources, and their health effect are described further below. It is important to understand that these pollutants are seasonal in their patterns.

3.4.1   Sulfur dioxide (SO_2)

Sulfur dioxide, or SO_2, belongs to the family of sulfur oxide gases (SOx). SO_2 is a colorless gas with a sharp odor, and mainly comes from natural (such as volcanoes) and man–made sources (such as power plants and industrial sources). It is produced from the burning of fossil fuels (coal and oil) and the smelting of mineral ores that contain sulfur. The main anthropogenic source of SO_2 is the burning of sulfur–containing fossil fuels for domestic heating, power generation, and motor vehicles. SO_2 has been the major problem in inducing or acidifying air pollution during the period of rapid economic growth in many countries.

SO_2 in the air can affect the respiratory system and the function of lung, and cause irritation of eyes. SO_2 is associated with an elevated risk of mortality and morbidity (including cough and bronchitis), especially among vulnerable populations, such as asthmatics and elderly people. Sulfate, a major sulfur–containing ion in water, is a major constituent of air pollution capable of forming acid. Sulfate itself appears to trigger bronchoconstriction in persons with vulnerable airways and it is a major constituent of ultrafine particulates.

3.4.2   Particulate matter (PM)

PM is a collective name for fine solid or liquid particles added to the atmosphere by processing at the earth's surface. Particulate matter includes dust, smoke, soot, pollen, and soil particles. The natural sources include volcanoes, forest fires, and desert land. The significant amounts of particulates occur due to human activities, such as burning of fossil fuels in vehicles, power plants, and various industrial processes. It consists of a complex mixture of solid and liquid particles of organic and inorganic substances suspended in the air or aerosol. The major components of PM are sulfate, nitrates, ammonia, sodium chloride, carbon, mineral dust, and water.

PM is divided and nominated by their aerodynamic diameter, including total suspended particle (TSP), coarse particle, fine particle, ultrafine particle, and nanoparticle. The size of particles is directly linked to their potential for causing health problems. Larger particles carry much more substance but are much less likely to have an effect on the body because they do not penetrate into the lower respiratory tract. The largest particles, visible to the naked eye as specks of dust, are mostly filtered out in the nose. Particles above 100 μm may be sources of irritation to the mucous membranes of the eyes, nose, and throat but they do not get much further. Those particles smaller than 100 μm make up the inhalable fraction because they can be inhaled into the respiratory tract. Particles larger than about 20 μm generally do not enter the lower respiratory tract, below the throat. Those particles below 20 μm comprise the thoracic fraction because a high proportion can penetrate into the lungs. Particles below 10 μm enter the airways with greatest efficiency and may be deposited in the alveoli, or airspaces, that are the deepest structures of the lungs. Particles between 10 μm and 2.5 μm are called coarse particles. Particles below 2.5 μm are deposited in the alveoli with very high efficiency and are called "fine particles". Particles below 0.1 μm are called "ultra fine particles". Particulates are the deadliest form of air pollution due to their ability to penetrate deep into the lungs and blood streams unfiltered. Particulates pollution is predominantly anthropogenic source.

The effects of PM on health occur at levels of exposure currently being experienced by most urban and rural populations in both developed and developing countries. Numerous scientific studies have linked particulates pollution exposure to a variety of health problems, including increased respiratory symptoms (e.g., irritation of the airways, coughing, or difficulty breathing); decreased lung function; aggravated asthma; development of chronic bronchitis; arhythmia; and nonfatal heart attacks. Chronic exposure to particles contributes to the risk of premature death in people with heart or lung disease. The IARC and WHO designate airborne particulates as Group 1 carcinogen. An increase in the incidence of respiratory diseases and gastric cancer has been linked to the increase in particulate exposure level.

3.4.3 Nitrogen compounds

Nitrogen compounds, especially nitrogen oxides, are involved in the formation of ground-level ozone. Nitrogen oxides is the generic term for a group of highly reactive gases, all of which contain nitrogen and oxygen in varying amounts. Nitrogen oxide pollution mainly comes from vehicle engines and power plants, and plays an important role in the formation of acid rain and smog. Nitrogen oxides are highly reactive gases when nitrogen in fuel or combustion air to produce ozone and other pollutants. The initial product, nitric oxide (NO) is further oxidized in the atmosphere to form nitrogen dioxide (NO_2), a reddish brown gas that gives photochemical smog. Because of their inter-convertibility, the general term NO_X is used to describe the gases.

Nitrogen oxides can trigger serious respiratory problems. NO_2 is brown-red in color and is of greatest concern. Epidemiological studies have shown that the severity of symptoms of bronchitis in asthmatic children is associated with long-term exposure to NO_2. Reduced lung function development is also linked to NO_2 at the concentrations currently observed in cities of Europe and North America.

3.4.4 Carbon oxides

The predominant form of carbon oxides in the air is CO_2. It is usually considered as nontoxic and innocuous, but increasing atmospheric levels due to human activities appear to be causing a global climate warming that may have disastrous effects. Carbon dioxides emissions have increased significantly during 19th century because of the use of coal, oil and natural gas. It is used as a refrigerant in fire extinguishers and in beverage carbonation. Higher concentrations can affect respiratory function and cause excitation followed by depression of the central nervous system. Contact with liquefied CO_2 can cause frostbite. Briefly exposed to very high concentrations may damage the retina, leading to increased sensitivity to light (photophobia), abnormal eye movements, constriction of visual fields, and enlargement of blind spots.

Carbon monoxides(CO) is a colorless, odorless, nonirritating but highly toxic gas produced by incomplete combustion of fuel (coal, oil, charcoal, or gas), incineration of biomass or solid waste, or partially anaerobic decomposition of organic material. About 1 billion metric tons of CO are released to the atmosphere each year, half of them were from human activities. About 90% of the CO in the air is consumed in photochemical reaction that produces ozone. CO inhibits respiration in animals by binding irreversibly to hemoglobin. The gas reduces the ability of hemoglobin to carry oxygen to body tissue. The effects of carbon monoxides on health include headache, reduced mental alertness, and heart damage; it may even cause death.

3.4.5　Ozone

Ozone, the triatomic form of oxygen (O_3), is an odorless and colorless gas with high reactivity. Ozone occurs both in the earth's upper atmosphere and at ground level. It is not usually emitted directly into the air, but at ground-level it is created by a chemical reaction between NO_x and VOC emitted by vehicle, solvents, and industry in the presence of sunlight. It is the main gas found in photochemical smog. The highest levels of ozone pollution occur during periods of sunny weather.

Excessive ozone in the air can have a marked effect on human health, including chest pain, coughing, throat irritation, and congestion. It can worsen bronchitis, emphysema, and asthma. High ozone levels at the ground level also can reduce lung function and inflame the lung linings. Repeated exposure may permanently scar lung tissue.

3.4.6　Metals

Many toxic metals are mined and can be spread into the air either as toxic compounds or as aerosols in forms of exhaust fumes and fly ash (contaminated waste dust) by fuel combustion, ore smelting, and disposal of wastes.

Lead is fairly abundant naturally and has a wide spectrum of applications. The major sources of environmental lead exposure include: gasoline additives, lead-based paint, lead-soldered food containers, ceramic glazes, and industrial pollution. The amount of lead emissions worldwide is about 2 million metric tons per year, corresponding to two-thirds of all metallic air pollution. Depending on the level of exposure, lead can adversely affect the nervous system, kidney function, immune system, reproductive systems, as well as the cardiovascular system. Infants and young children are especially sensitive to even low levels of lead, which may contribute to behavioral problems, learning deficits, and lowered IQ.

Other toxic metals that occur in air pollution include mercury, nickel, cadmium, and manganese; all at very low concentrations.

3.4.7　Polycyclic aromatic hydrocarbons

Polycyclic aromatic hydrocarbons (PAHs) are a group of compounds formed during the incomplete combustion of coal, oil, gas, wood, garbage, or other organic substances. They can occur naturally from forest fires and volcanoes, and can also be manufactured. Other activities that released PAHs include driving, agricultural burning, roofing or working with coal tar products, sound-and water-proofing, coating pipes, steel-making, and paving with asphalt. Manufactured PAHs are colorless, white, or pale yellow solids. Some can take the form of needles, plates, crystals, or prisms. Due to widespread sources and persistent characteristics, PAHs disperse through atmospheric transport and exist almost everywhere. Human being is usually exposed to mixtures of PAHs in gaseous or particulate phases in ambient air.

The effects of PAHs on human health will depend mainly on the length and route of exposure, the amount or concentration of PAHs one is exposed to, and of course the innate toxicity of the PAHs. The effects of environmental exposure to low levels of PAHs on human health are not clear. Occupational exposure to high levels of pollutant mixtures containing PAHs have resulted in symptoms, such as eye irritation, nausea, vomiting, diarrhea, and confusion. Health effects from chronic or long-term exposure to PAHs may include decreased immune function, cataracts, kidney and liver damage, breathing problems, asthma-like symptoms, and lung function abnormalities, and repeated contact with skin may induce redness and skin inflammation. Naphthalene, a specific PAH, can cause the breakdown of red blood cells if inhaled or ingested in large amounts. Some PAHs have been demonstrated to be carcinogenic in humans and animals, and thus classified as carcinogenic materials.

3.4.8 Dioxins

Dioxins are a class of chemical contaminants that share certain chemical structures and biological characteristics. They are formed during combustion processes, such as waste incineration, forest fires, and trash burning, as well as during some industrial processes, such as paper pulp bleaching and herbicide manufacturing. As dioxins break down very slowly, past releases of dioxins from both man-made and natural sources are still present in the environment. Several hundred of these chemicals exist and are members of three closely related families: Polychlorinated chlorinated dibenzo-p-dioxins (PCDDs), Polychlorinated chlorinated dibenzofurans (PCDFs), and certain polychlorinated biphenyls (PCBs). 2,3,7,8-tetrachlorodibenzo-para-dioxin (TCDD), usually called dioxin, is known as the most toxic congener among PCDDs.

Dioxins belong to a group of compounds referred to as persistent organic pollutants or POPs. These POPs are very persistent in the environment and can travel long distances. Dioxin accumulates in the fatty tissues, where they may persist for months or years. Short-term exposure to high levels of dioxins may result in skin lesions, such as chloracne and patchy darkening of the skin, and altered liver function in humans. Long-term exposure is linked to impairment in the immune system, the nervous system, the endocrine system, and reproductive functions. Several types of cancer in animals have been linked to chronic exposure of dioxins. Based on evidence from animal studies and human epidemiological studies, TCDD was classified as a "known human carcinogen" by IARC in 1997.

Huang Hui

3.5   Indoor air pollution

Although many researches have been driven by outdoor air pollution, it is actually the indoor exposures which are often of greater magnitude and concern. Indoor air pollution poses many challenges to the health professional. According to a five-year survey conducted by the U. S. Environmental Protection Agency (EPA), the air pollution in many residential and commercial buildings is much more serious than that of outdoor air. There are three reasons. Firstly, the indoor environment is one of the most contactable environments for people, the quality of indoor air is directly related to the health of everyone, especially the elderly, children, and pregnant women. Secondly, types and sources of indoor air pollutants are increasing with development of economic and improvement of living standards, the types and quantities of indoor chemicals and new construction materials are increasing significantly than ever before. Thirdly, in the aftermath of the 1970s fuel crisis, "energy-efficient" office buildings tended to be relatively airtight, and fuel conservation programs greatly reduced the amount of fresh air added to air conditioning. Inadequate ventilation can increase indoor pollutant levels by not bringing in enough outdoor air to dilute emissions from indoor sources and by not carrying indoor air pollutants out of the home. High temperature and humidity levels can also increase concentrations of some pollutants.

Compared with developed countries, indoor air pollution in China is even more serious. According to statistics, China's deaths caused by indoor air pollution amounts to 111,000 people each year. Serious indoor environmental pollution also caused tremendous economic losses. The economic loss caused by the pollution of indoor environment in China was as high as 10.7 billion dollars.

"Indoor" indicates interior environment of home and office building. Nowadays, indoor air pollution problem has been an important part of public health worldwide.

3.5.1　Sources of indoor air pollution

There are many sources of indoor pollutants. According to the causes of pollutants and the approaches into the room, the main indoor air pollution sources can be divided into outdoor sources and indoor sources.

3.5.1.1　Indoor sources

(1) Combustion pollutants

Combustion products of fuels from cuisine and heater have become a major source of indoor air pollution. Combustion pollutants include fuel burning stoves, furnaces, fireplaces, heaters, and water heaters, using gas, oil, coal, wood, or other fuel. These fuels generate many kinds of hazardous air pollutants during combustion, including SO_2, NO_X, CO, CO_2, hydro carbons, and particulate matters. Smoke and oil from Chinese cuisine constitute a major source to indoor air pollution. The most dangerous combustion pollutants are carbon monoxide (CO) and nitrogen oxide (NO_X).

(2) Human activities

Metabolic wastes of human are eliminated from the body through expiration, excretory, and perspiration. Expiratory gas includes CO_2, water vapor, and some nitrogen compounds. Pathogenic microorganisms in the surface of the respiratory mucosa are eliminated along with droplets to contaminate indoor air when people chat, cough, and sneeze. Person's skin, clothes, and hygiene products became useless fragments, which could influence indoor air quality. Person's walk or other movements could transfer dust and microorganisms from floor and wall to air. Smoke fog through the use of tobacco, which contain more than 3,800 kinds of injurious ingredients and more than 14 kinds of carcinogens, is also a major source of indoor air pollution. Patients with respiratory infectious disease and carriers of the virus will release the flu virus, mycobacterium tuberculosis, streptococcus, and other pathogens through splash to pollute the indoor air. In addition, domestic pet activities are also an important source of indoor harmful substances and pathogenic microorganisms.

(3) Building materials and furnishings

Building and decorative materials can be divided into three types: natural building materials, recycled materials, and chemical products. The latter two materials contain various additives in their process of production, most of which are toxic and volatile materials. There are pollutants including asbestos-containing insulation, wet or damp carpet, and cabinetry or furniture made of certain pressed wood products in building materials and furniture.

(4) Indoor biological contamination

The good indoor air tightness, stable indoor microclimate, suitable temperature, high humidity, and poor ventilation provide a good breeding environment for biological allergens, such as fungi and dust mites. Mites are often hidden in beds, furniture, and floors, and are one of the most important media for spread of diseases at home. These biological allergens can cause allergic reactions in humans, act on biological organisms, and result in numerous harmful gases, such as carbon dioxide, ammonia, and hydrogen sulfide.

(5) Household chemicals

With the development of economy and the improvement of living standards, people's demands for household chemicals have also been increased. Household chemicals include detergents, clearing agents, adhesives, walls and furniture coatings, and household pesticides. These household chemicals contain volatile or non-volatile components, including poisonous organic compounds and inorganic toxic materials. Improper storage, usage, and management, as well as various factors, such as change of room temperature, will promote pollutants emission of household chemicals, including benzene, phenols, aldehydes, and alkanes, into indoor air.

(6) Household appliances

In recent years, household appliances, such as televisions, combination audio systems, microwave ovens, electric blankets, and air conditioners have entered into society and home. The resulting air pollution, noise pollution, electromagnetic waves, and mute interference have an undeniable impact on people's health.

3.5.1.2 Outdoor sources

Some pollutants are mainly present in outdoor or other indoor environments and can enter the room through gaps in doors, windows and other pipe work, as follows:

(1) Outdoor air

The industries and vehicles produce and exhaust gases, which will enter the home through doors, windows, and various pipe network. During summer time, SO_2, NO_X, particulate matters, and other toxic pollutants enter the indoor air through open windows, which cause higher pollutant concentration in indoor air than in outdoor air. In 1984, Methyl isocyanate leak occurred at Pesticide Plant in Bhopal, India. The coverage of the city's toxic gas affected residents of the city's housing. A total of more than 2,500 people were killed and more than 200,000 people were poisoned. It is by far the worst and the most typical poisoning incident in human history that outdoor air pollution sources affect indoor and outdoor residents. In addition, plant pollen, animal dander, and other allergenic substances can also easily enter the room to pollute indoor air.

(2) Building materials

Some buildings contain certain materials that can release hazardous substances. One of them is chemicals added in of the process of the construction, such as antifreeze added in winter construction. The other one is radon, a decay product from naturally occurring uranium in soil, occurs in gaseous form and emits alpha particles that cause harmful effect on human health. Radon can enter the home through cracks in the foundation floor and walls, drains, and other openings. According to a survey conducted by the U. S. Environmental Protection Agency, more than 14,000 deaths in the United States are related to radon pollution.

(3) Outdoor materials pollution

People get in and out of their home every day, can easily take contaminants from outdoors or indoor work environment to their home. Such pollutants are mainly atmospheric particulates and benzene, lead and asbestos in the working environment.

(4) Adjacent residential pollution

Adjacent residential pollutants are mainly indoor toxicants and fumigated insecticides from the exhaust duct of neighboring homes. The main pollutants include carbon monoxide and phosphine.

(5) Domestic water pollution

Unqualified domestic water contains pathogenic bacterium and chemical pollutants, such as Legionella and benzene, which are discharged into indoor air through water spray of shower system, air conditioners, and humidifiers. Such pollutants are mainly legionella, benzene, and motor oil.

3.5.2　Characteristics of indoor air pollution

Indoor air pollution has various sources and complex composition, the characteristics are as follows.

3.5.2.1　Outdoor pollutants and indoor air pollution

The concentrations of indoor pollutants are lower than outdoors. For example, the most common outdoor sulfur dioxide in the outdoor atmosphere is easily absorbed by materials, such as lime and wall paper on the surface of the building. Particulate matters are partially blocked by doors or screens in the indoor process and are adsorbed by the walls in the room.

3.5.2.2　Indoor and outdoor coexisting pollutants and indoor air pollution

The concentrations of indoor pollutants are often higher than outdoor of indoor and outdoor coexisting pollutants. For example, households using coal-fired stoves have higher concentrations of indoor air sulfur dioxide, nitrogen dioxide, particulate matter, carbon monoxide, and other combustion products than outdoors, especially households that using coal-fired stoves to cook and heat.

3.5.2.3　Smoking and the indoor air pollution

When cigarette is burning, the local temperature can reach as high as $900-1,000$ ℃, resulting in a large amount of harmful chemicals. Among them, 90% are the cigarette smoke, mainly nitrogen, carbon dioxide, carbon monoxide, cyanide, volatile nitrosamines, hydrocarbons, ammonia, volatile sulfur compounds, and phenols; 8% are particulate matter, mainly cigarette smoke and smoke Alkali (nicotine); and the rests are cadmium and other harmful radioactive materials. Smoking has become an important factor that cannot be ignored in aggravating indoor air pollution. Indoor air pollution caused by smoking has become a serious pollution problem in China.

3.5.2.4　Indoor air pollution from building materials and decorative objects

Building materials and decorative objects contain large amounts of organic pollutants and radioactive contaminants, which are extremely harmful to human beings. There are traditional natural materials, waste or recycled materials, and modern chemical products. Especially, many of the raw materials used for interior construction and decoration are added by a variety of additives, many of which have volatile additives, such as formaldehyde, benzene, toluene, xylene, trichlorethylene, chloroform, diisocyanates, toluene esters, naphthalene, and other substances. These materials will be released indoors to pollute the air. At present, the problem of indoor air pollution caused by volatile organic compounds, such as formaldehyde and radon, has become a widespread concern in China and around the world.

3.5.2.5　Indoor air pollution caused by air conditioning

Air conditioning can be divided into three systems: closed, straight-flow, and hybrid systems. Pollutants in the outdoor air can enter room through the air outlet of air conditioning. In addition, pollutants that are present in the room are not easily removed; and failure of the filter can lead to serious indoor air pollution. Due to the irrational air flow, a local dead space is formed. Besides, Legionella in cooling water can be spread through the air.

3.5.3 Variety, source and adverse health effect of indoor air pollutants

There are many types of indoor air pollutants, including chemical, biological, and radioactive pollutants. These three types of pollutants are often related to each other and co-existing. For example, cooking food or water and the use of air conditioning process can bring biological contaminants to the interior; the use of radium-containing building materials can cause indoor radon contamination.

Sources and hazards of common indoor air pollutants are shown in the Table 3-1.

Table 3-1　Sources and adverse health effect of common indoor air pollutants

Pollutants	Sources	Adverse health effect
Carbon Dioxide	Fuel combustion, smoking, human metabolism and so on	Respiratory center, entire body
Carbon Monoxide	Fuel combustion, smoking and so on	Central nervous system, cardiovascular system, entire body
Nitrogen Dioxide	Fuel combustion at high temperature, smoking, the introduction of outdoor air pollution and so on	Respiratory tract, entire body
Sulfur Dioxide	Sulfur fuel combustion, smoking and so on	Mucosa irritation, respiratory symptom; allergization, carcinogenesis and so on
Respirable Particulate Matter (PM_{10})	Wood and briquettes burning, smoking, the introduction of outdoor air pollution and so on	Mucosa irritation, respiratory symptom and so on
Formaldehyde	Fuel combustion, smoking, building decoration materials, household chemical products and so on	Olfactory stimuli, skin irritation, mucosa irritation, respiratory irritation, entire body
Total Volatile Organic Compounds	Building materials, decorative materials, household chemical products, fuel combustion, fumes, smoking and so on	Olfactory stimuli, mucosa irritation, allergization, respiratory symptoms, neurotoxic effects, entire body
Microorganism	Dust mites, fungi and pollen in dust, skins, hairs, shavings of human and animal	Allergization, respiratory symptoms and so on
Radon	Housing foundation, building materials and so on	Lung cancer and so on

3.5.3.1　Chemical indoor air pollutants

(1) Carbon dioxide (CO_2)

Source: In normal air, the concentration of CO_2 is 0.03% -0.04%. The main sources of indoor CO_2 are fuel combustion, plant and animal metabolism, and human respiration.

Adverse health effects: When the concentration of CO_2 is lower than 0.07%, people feel comfortable; when the concentration is 0.1%, individuals start to have discomfort feeling; when it reaches 3%, people breathe deeply and quickly; when it is 8%, a series of symptoms began to appear, including expiratory dyspnea, pulse quicken, general weakness, muscle twitches and cramps, and delirious consciousness; when it is as high as 30%, CO_2 can cause death. Increased CO_2 concentration results in anoxia, which is the main cause of death.

(2) Combustion products

Combustion products have long been a contributor to indoor air pollution. Women and young children are at risk because of women's gender roles, household responsibilities, behaviors—cooking, and young children spending a lot of time indoors, resulting in high exposure to indoor air pollution.

Sources: Combustion pollutants include fuel burning stoves, furnaces, fireplaces, heaters, and water heaters, using gas, oil, coal, wood, or other fuel. These fuels generate hazardous air pollutants during combustion. There are various sources of such pollutants. First, incineration products contain impurities, including coal sulfur, fluorine, arsenic, cadmium, ash, and so on. Second, as the solid fuel is burned, a large amount of SO_2, particulate matter, CO, CO_2, NO_X, and many organic components, such as PAHs, are generated. Third, cigarette smoking constitutes a major source of indoor air pollution.

Adverse health effects: Due to the different types of fuels, the types, quantities and hazards of their combustion products are also different.

Polycyclic aromatic hydrocarbons (PAHs) in combustion products have cancerogenic effect. Lung cancer rate is high in Xuanwei City, Yunnan Province, in which lung cancer mortality have positive correlation with benzoapyrene (BaP) concentration in local indoor air.

Unqualified coal, such as high fluorine coal and high arsenic coal, can cause indoor fluorine or arsenic exposure and result in fluorine or arsenic poisoning.

SO_2 is highly soluble in water and most inhaled SO_2 is absorbed by the mucous of the upper airways with little reaching the lung. SO_2 exposure has been related to reduced lung function, hospitalizations from cardiovascular and respiratory diseases, eye irritation, adverse pregnancy outcomes, and mortality.

NO_2 is nearly insoluble in water and can reach the lower respiratory tract. Health effects of NO_2 include irritation of the eyes, nose, and throat at higher concentrations. The main short—term effect is decreasing in lung function. Besides, NO_2 may increase respiratory infections and symptoms in children.

Carbon monoxide (CO) levels are closely related to the occurrence of atherosclerosis, myocardial infarction, and angina pectoris. When CO is inhaled, it binds to hemoglobin, with over 200 times the affinity of oxygen, to form carboxyhemoglobin (COHb). An increased level of COHb reduces the transport of oxygen to tissues and inhibits the release of oxygen. The levels of indoor CO have been associated with the increasing COHb levels in the blood. The brain and heart are sensitive to low oxygen conditions. Thus, individuals with cardiovascular and respiratory diseases are particularly susceptible to CO. Health response to CO include impairment, fatigue, decreased dexterity, dizziness, and nausea. Extremely high CO levels can result in mortality and severe neurological damage.

Particulate matter (PM) can enter the pulmonary tissue and has been associated with health effects, including respiratory symptoms, decline in pulmonary function, exacerbation of chronic respiratory, and cardiovascular diseases, as well as premature mortality.

Tobacco combustion products have the damage effect on respiratory system, nervous system, circulatory system, endocrine system, reproductive system, and immune system. Tobacco smoking is the main cause of lung cancer. Besides, it is associated with laryngeal cancer, pharynx cancer, oral cancer esophageal cancer, kidney cancer, pancreatic cancer, bladder cancer, and uterine cancer. In addition, the harm caused by passive smoking is particularly serious, which emerges as a hot research topic at present.

(3) Cooking fume

Source: While cooking, edible oil can produce cooking fumes, which is a mixed pollutant containing more than 200 kinds of components. Cooking fumes is ubiquitous in indoor air pollutants in China.

Adverse health effects: Cooking fumes is genotoxic, the genotoxicity comes mainly from the high temperature oxidation and polymerization of unsaturated fatty acids in oils and fats. Cooking soot is a risk factor for lung cancer. Research shows that cooking fume is one of the major contributors for lung cancer in Chinese women. Toxicity of cooking fume is related to the processing technologies of edible oil.

(4) Formaldehyde

Source: Formaldehyde is a volatile organic compound with a strong irritant, existing not only in a large number of decoration supplies, but also in building materials. Formaldehyde can also come from cosmetics, detergents, pesticides, disinfectants, preservatives, printing inks, paper, textile fibers, and so on. When room temperature exceeds 19 ℃, the formaldehyde in the product is easily released.

Adverse health effects: When indoor air formaldehyde concentration exceeds 0. 15 mg/m^3, its stimulation effect on eye conjunctiva and respiratory mucosa will occur. Symptoms include eye irritation, photophobia, dry throat, cough, sneezing, chest stuffy, xeroderma, and pruritus. Formaldehyde can cause allergic reactions, including allergic asthma and Henoch-Schonlein purpura. Individuals who are long-term exposed to high concentration of formaldehyde will suffer from neurotic symptoms and abnormal liver function. In lung function studies, exposure to high concentration of formaldehyde is relative to exhalation dysfunction. Genotoxicity studies have found that formaldehyde can cause genetic mutations and chromosomal damage. In 2006, International Agency for Research on Cancer (IARC) confirmed that formaldehyde is a human carcinogen that causes human nasopharyngeal cancer.

(5) Volatile organic compounds (VOCs)

Sources: VOCs come from building materials, decorative materials, household chemical products, fuel combustion, fumes, smoking, and so on.

Adverse health effects: VOCs mainly affect the central nervous system and digestive system; in severe cases it can cause damage to the liver and hematopoietic system and result in allergic reaction. Symptoms include dizziness, headache, drowsiness, weakness, chest stuffy, loss of appetite, and nausea. Benzene, as an organic solvent and diluent, can be used for residential decoration and handicrafts production. Benzene can damage the nervous and hematopoietic systems and is one of the confirmed carcinogens. Polyurethane foaming plastics discharge toluene diisocyanate (TDI) and can cause bronchial asthma.

3.5.3.2　Biological indoor air pollutants

Sources: Biological pollutants include molds, bacteria, viruses, pollen, animal dander, and particles from dust mites and cockroaches. Dust mites are commonly found in environments where people live and work, such as mattresses, pillows, futons, curtains, and so on, especially in humid indoor environment with poor ventilation.

Adverse health effects: Dust mites have strong allergenicity. Metamorphosis not only exists in dust mites itself, but also in its secretions and excretions. Dust mites are the major indoor bio-allergens that can enter the human body through air and cause sensitization due to repeated exposure, which can cause skin irritation, allergic asthma, and allergic rhinitis. In many homes of patients with allergic disease, a large number of dust mites can be detected.

3.5.3.3　Radioactive indoor air pollutants

Sources: Another indoor source is radon, which may concentrate in indoor air due to building location or be released from concrete and other building materials.

Adverse health effects: The human health hazards of large exposure to radon products are well known for the miners of Schneeberg, Germany and Jacymov, Czechoslovakia. Indoor radon exposure is estimated to be the second leading cause of lung cancer.

3.5.4   Diseases caused by indoor air pollution

The diseases caused by indoor air pollution include sick building syndrome (SBS), building-related illness (BRI), and multiple chemical sensitivity (MCS).

(1) Sick building syndrome (SBS)

Sick building syndrome is a syndrome caused by the combined effects of many factors in the interior of modern houses. Its exact reason is not yet clear. Due to air exchange rate is so low that a group of people who are active in the building have a series of non-specific symptoms. Symptoms include irritation of eyes, nose, throat, and upper respiratory tract, as well as headache, fatigue, lack of energy, forgetfulness, lethargy, general malaise, and poor work efficiency.

The characteristics of SBS are fast onset and affect a large number of patients. The cause is difficult to identify. The symptoms can be relieved or disappeared once the patient leaves the contaminated building.

(2) Building-related illness (BRI)

Building-related illness are diseases caused by the harmful effects of exposure to buildings. Harmful factors include bacteria, fungi, dust mites, carbon monoxide, formaldehyde, and so on. Such diseases include respiratory infections, asthma, atopic dermatitis, Legionnaires' disease, cardiovascular diseases, lung cancer, and so on. BRI and SBS obviously differ mainly in three aspects: the patient's symptoms can be clearly clinically diagnosed; the cause can be identified; the symptoms will not disappear soon even when patients leave the scene, and patients must be treated to restore health. All illnesses caused by Legionella, such as Legionnaires disease, radon-induced lung cancer, and indoor allergen-induced asthma are all belong to BRI.

(3) Multiple chemical sensitivity (MCS)

MCS is a disputed chronic condition attributes to low-level exposures to a variety of chemicals that act on a variety of human organ systems and cause a variety of symptoms. In the interior, long-term exposure to only a trace amount of chemical substances may also affect nervous system, respiratory system, digestive system, circulatory system, reproductive system, and immune system, resulting in eye irritation, sore throat, fatigue, movement disorders, insomnia, nausea, asthma, dermatitis, and other symptoms.

MCS is characterized by the recurrent, chronic process, and low concentrations of chemical contaminants exposure. Patients can have a variety of chemical allergies and multiple organ disease at the same time, and the symptoms will be improved or dissipated after elimination of pathogenic factors.

3.6   Assessment of air quality

3.6.1   Health assessment of ambient air pollution

Ambient air pollution is often a combination of multiple air pollutants. Environmental quality standards (EQSs) have been established as desirable levels to be maintained for protection of human health and the conservation of the living environment by Basic Environment Law. China recently revised its ambient air quality standards that were promulgated in 1996 (GB3095—1996) and promulgated a new standard in 2012 (GB3095—2012) by adjusting some pollutant limits and adding $PM_{2.5}$ and Daily maximum 8-hour average ozone concentration limits.

(1) The division of environmental air function zones: Group I areas are nature reserves, scenic spots, and other areas that need special protection; Group II areas are residential areas, commercial and traffic

mixed areas, cultural areas, industrial areas, and rural areas. Class 1 standard is imposed for Group Ⅰ areas; Class 2 standard is imposed for Group Ⅱ areas. The concentration limits of the basic items of ambient air pollutants are shown in Table 3-2.

Table 3-2　Concentration limits for various pollutants

Pollutant	Sampling time	Concentration limit		Unit of concentration
		Class 1 standard	Class 2 standard	
1　Sulfur Dioxide SO$_2$	Annual Average	20	60	$\mu g/m^3$
	Daily Average	50	150	
	Hourly Average	150	500	
2　Nitrogen Dioxide NO$_2$	Annual Average	40	40	$\mu g/m^3$
	Daily Average	80	80	
	Hourly Average	200	200	
3　Carbon Monoxide CO	Daily Average	4	4	$\mu g/m^3$
	Hourly Average	10	10	
4　Ozone O$_3$	Daily Maximum Of 8 Hours Average	100	160	$\mu g/m^3$
	Hourly Average	160	200	
5　Breathable Particles PM$_{10}$	Annual Average	40	70	$\mu g/m^3$
	Daily Average	50	150	
6　Fine Particulate Matter PM$_{2.5}$	Annual Average	15	35	$\mu g/m^3$
	Daily Average	35	75	

(2) An air quality index (AQI) is a number used by government agencies to communicate to the public how polluted the air is currently or how polluted it would be. The AQI level is based on the highest level among the 6 atmospheric pollutants, including SO$_2$, NO$_2$, PM$_{10}$, PM$_{2.5}$, CO and O$_3$. AQI is divided into six levels (Table 3-3), the higher the AQI value, the more serious the air pollution and the greater health hazard to the human body.

Table 3-3　AQI and health implications in China

Index value	AQI level	Air pollution level	Colors	Cautionary statements
0-50	Ⅰ	Good	Green	No health implication. Enjoy your usual outdoor activities
51-100	Ⅱ	Moderate	Yellow	Members of sensitive groups should reduce outdoor activities
101-150	Ⅲ	Lighty Polluted	Orange	Slightly irritations may occur. Children, elders and people with heart or breathing problems should restrict strenuous outdoor activities
151-200	Ⅳ	Moderately Polluted	Red	Slightly irritations may occur. Children, elders and people with heart or breathing problems should restrict strenuous outdoor activities. The general population should moderately reduce outdoor sports

Continue to Table 3-3

Index value	AQI level	Air pollution level	Colors	Cautionary statements
201-300	V	Heavily Polluted	Purple	Healthy people will be noticeably affected. Children, elders and people with heart and breathing problems remain indoors. Healthy individuals should reduce outdoor activities
>300	VI	Severely Polluted	Maroom	Healthy people will experience reduced endurance in activities. There may be strong irritations and symptoms and may trigger other illness. Children, elders and the sick ones should remain indoors and avoid exercise. Healthy individuals should avoid outdoor activities

3.6.2   Health assessment of indoor air pollution

Common indoor air quality evaluation indicators can be divided into the following categories: reactive air cleanliness (e. g. , CO_2); the total number of colonies; chemical reaction pollution indicators (e. g. , hemolytic streptococcus); and reaction radionuclide pollution indicators (e. g. , radon). The hygiene standards for controlling indoor pollution are shown in Table 3-4.

Table 3-4   Standards and guidelines for common indoor contaminants

Index category	Index	Standard limit	Comment
Air Cleanliness	CO_2	0.1%	Daily Average
	The Total Number Of Colonies	2,500 cfu/m³	Impacting Method Limit
	SO_2	0.50 mg/m³	Hourly Average
	CO	10 mg/m³	Hourly Average
	NO_2	0.24 mg/m³	Hourly Average
Chemical Pollution	Formaldehyde	0.10 mg/m³	Hourly Average
	Benzene	0.11 mg/m³	Hourly Average
	Benzoapyrene	1.0 mg/m³	Daily Average
	PM_{10}	0.15 mg/m³	Daily Average
	TVOCs	0.60 mg/m³	Daily Maximum of 8 Hours Average
Pathogenic Microbial Contamination	Hemolytic Streptococcus	36 cfu/m³	Impacting Method Limit
Radionuclide Contamination	Radon (^{222}Rn)	400 Bq/m³	Annual Average

Zhao Ran

3.7   Air pollution prevention and control

3.7.1   Atmospheric health protection measures

The extent of atmospheric pollution is influenced by natural and social factors, such as energy structure, industrial layout, traffic management, population density, topography, meteorology, and vegetation cover. Therefore, air pollution must adhere to the principle of comprehensive prevention and control. The total amount of pollutants discharged is the fundamental issue that determines the environmental quality. In order to solve the air pollution problem fundamentally, we must start from the control of the pollution source, and strictly implement the whole control process.

3.7.1.1   Arranging industrial layout rationally

Industrial construction should be located in small towns and industrial areas, especially heavy pollution smelting, oil, chemical, and other enterprises must be built in the outer suburbs. Local long−term wind direction and wind speed data should be taken into consideration to allocate the industrial zone, which should be located on the lower−side of wind direction, so that the least amount of harmful substances emitted from industrial enterprises will be blown to residential areas. Due to the frequent changes in wind direction, accidental discharges may also occur in the production process of industrial enterprises. Therefore, a certain distance of sanitation protection should be set up between industrial enterprises and residential areas.

3.7.1.2   Improving the urban greening system

Urban green system is an important part of urban ecosystem. It not only beautifies the environment but also plays an important role in the quality of the city's atmospheric environment. Perfect urban green system can adjust the city's microclimate by blocking, filtering, and adsorpting sand, dust, and harmful gases. In addition, the green system can make the air humidification and cooling, ease urban heat island effect.

3.7.1.3   Managing pollution sources in residential areas

The management of pollution sources that may pollute the indoor and outdoor air, such as restaurants, waste dumps, and bins in residential areas, should be strengthened to control the air pollution and protect citizens from health hazards.

3.7.1.4   Improving the energy structure to save energy

In the city, people should try to choose low sulfur and low ash coal. Compared with decentralized heating, central heating save energy and reduce smoke and sulfur dioxide generation. Gaseous fuel combustion can reduce atmospheric pollution and be used easily. Therefore, in cities, we should vigorously develop and popularize gaseous energy, such as natural gas and coal gas. In addition, new resources, such as hydropower, geothermal energy, wind energy, and solar energy should also be developed and implemented according to local conditions.

3.7.1.5   Controlling motor vehicle exhaust pollution

Measures to control the vehicle exhaust emissions include purification inside the vehicle, purification outside the vehicle, fuel improvements, and alternatives. Purification within the vehicle includes improvement in the engine structure and combustion in the design and production of motor vehicle, so that the new vehicle emissions meet the requirements of the country. Purification outside the vehicle is usually installed by exhaust catalytic purification device to make emissions of motor vehicles eligible. Vehicle fuel combustion is the main source of pollutants. Therefore, the improvement and replacement of fuels is one of the important measures to reduce the air pollution of motor vehicle.

3.7.1.6   Improving the production process to reduce emissions

Pollutant emissions can be reduced through the production process reform to replace the toxic raw materials with non−toxic or low−toxic raw materials. The method of separating particulate matter from exhaust gas through a dust collector can be used to control the particulate matter. The methods of adhesion, catalysis, condensation, and combustion can be used to treat gaseous pollutants.

3.7.2　Health measures to ensure room air cleanliness

(1) Reasonable choice of residential land

Residential place should be selected in the area that has clean air, fine sunshine, and well-ventilation system, no pollution source around the environment, and are far away from pollution area.

(2) Selection of building materials and decorative materials

People should choose materials without releasing harmful substances. In order to reduce and avoid the radon escape from building materials, we should pay attention to the material selection, and paint the surface of construction materials to reduce the indoor radon concentration. Low TVOC building materials and decorative materials should be used to reduce indoor formaldehyde and other volatile organic compounds concentration. We should avoid the use of fur carpet or tapestry and other decorations to reduce indoor dust and dust mites.

(3) Use measures to improve air quality

Gaseous fuels, such as gas or natural gas, should be used. The kitchen should be equipped with an exhaust fan or hood. Pay attention to ventilation when using gas or natural gas to make the fuel burn completely and avoid the generation of carbon monoxide.

(4) Improve personal hygiene

Change cooking habits and reduce frying to decrease fume. Regular cleaning and replacing bed linen are helpful to remove dust mites.

(5) Rational use and maintenance of various facilities

Air conditioning filter should be cleaned or replaced regularly. Similarly, all kinds of hygienic facilities, such as exhaust hoods, need to be regularly cleaned and repaired in time to ensure that clean air is circulated into the room.

Wang Meilin

Chapter 4

Water and Health

Water is essential to life. All living organisms are composed of cells that contain at least 60% water. Furthermore, their metabolic activities take place in a water solution. Organisms can exist only when they have access to adequate supplies of water. Water is involved in almost all human activities. Personal use of water includes drinking, cooking, bathing, laundering, and excreta disposal. Water is also necessity for many industrial operations as well as for transport. Another major use is for agriculture. An estimated 7% of the total consumption of water worldwide is for irrigating agricultural crops.

The total amount of water on Earth is estimated to be 1.38 billion km^3. Of this, about 97% is present as saltwater in the oceans, and only about 3% is present as freshwater. Nearly 70% of the freshwater is locked in glaciers and icebergs. Freshwater which can be easily developed and used is only about 1.05 million km^3. Some areas of the world have abundant freshwater resources while others have few. The total amount of freshwater resource in China ranks fourth in the world. However, it is only 28% of the world average in term of per capita, and China is one of the countries in the world which lacks the most water resource.

Water is considered to be a renewable resource, but it does not mean that it is inexhaustible. We have begun to understand only in recent years that we will probably exhaust our useable water supplies in some areas of the world because of the increases in human populations and the limited available supplies. In addition, freshwater demand is increasing for industrial, agricultural, and personal needs. Shortages of potable freshwater throughout the world can also be directly attributed to human abuse in the form of pollution. Water pollution has negatively affected water supplies throughout the world. Even in the economically advanced regions of the world, water quality is a major issue of concern.

4.1 Water resources

Water resources are sources of water that are potentially useful, and mainly refer to the freshwater which can be updated year by year. Natural water resources include three types: precipitation, surface water, and groundwater. Broadly speaking, the basic source of all water on Earth is precipitation: rain, snow, and sleet. Only about 30% of this, however, falls on land areas and that is not evenly distributed. About 70% of the precipitation that reaches land is evaporated or transpired (after uptake by vegetation) back into the atmosphere, 10% soaks into the ground and becomes groundwater, and 20% runs off into lakes, streams, and rivers, most of which ultimately flows into the oceans. The overall movement of water from precipitation through various pathways on Earth and back into the atmosphere is called the hydrologic cycle.

4.1.1　Precipitation

Precipitation has good water quality, low mineral content, but unstable water quantity as it comes from rain, snow and sleet. There are significant variations both geographically and seasonally within China and worldwide. In general, the annual average precipitation decreases progressively from the southeast coast to the northwest inland. Water quality of precipitation mainly depends on quality of atmosphere and local environmental conditions. Atmospheric pollutants are contained in precipitation of air polluted area. In the coastal area there is more salt and iodine in the precipitation. Some other areas where atmosphere is polluted by sulfur dioxide, nitrogen oxide, and other pollutants, will suffer from acid rain due to sulphuric acid and nitric acid in precipitation.

4.1.2　Surface water

Surface water is formed by the collection of rainfall runoff when precipitation landed on the ground. It includes water in the seas, rivers, lakes, and reservoirs. Surface water complements with groundwater and precipitation is the main supplementary source of surface water. In general, compared with groundwater, the hygienic features of surface water are large quantity, more pollution opportunities (high turbidity, higher bacteria content), less mineral salt content and softer water quality, more dissolved oxygen, and strong self-purification ability.

The quantity of surface water is influenced by climate and geological condition. The amount of water varies greatly with seasons. When precipitation largely gets into streams and rivers, and the water reaches the maximum is called the wet season, whereas the dry season is a yearly period of low rainfall and low water level.

Surface water is generally soft, with less mineral salt. The quality of surface water is mainly influenced by human activities, especially man-made pollution. Geological environment is also an important factor that affects the quality of surface water. For example, due to long-term contact with local soil, materials in soil can be dissolved in surface water, such as selenium-rich geological conditions which will result in high level of selenium in local surface water, namely selenium-rich water.

Self-purification ability of surface water varies greatly with the characteristics of water source. Enclosed water bodies, such as lakes and reservoirs, have poor self-purification ability due to low velocity of flow, and is known as "dead water"; while open water bodies, such as rivers, have strong self-purification capacity, and so called "living water". In some parts of China, attempt is being made to transform enclosed bodies, such as lakes, that suffering from eutrophication into open water bodies by connecting them with rivers.

4.1.3　Groundwater

Groundwater is the water hidden below the surface layer of the earth. Some groundwater is derived directly from precipitation. Other sources of groundwater include water that infiltrates from surface waters, including lakes and rivers. Permeable layer is composed of loose sand with large gaps, gravel, and sandy soil. It can not only permeate water, but also store water. Impermeable layer which is composed of clay and rock, cannot permeate water.

Groundwater can be divided into shallow groundwater, deep groundwater, and spring water. Shallow groundwater is the groundwater above the first impermeable layer. It can be easily accessed through wells dug beneath the ground surface, and commonly available at the point of need at relatively little cost, and reservoirs and long pipelines are not necessary. In rural areas of China, shallow groundwater is the major drinking water supply. Groundwater under the first impermeable layer is called deep groundwater. Due to the high quality and stable quantity, deep groundwater is often used as the source of centralized water supply. Springs occur where the water table intersects with the land surface. Sometimes groundwater is forced into a spring because a low permeable layer of rock or clay keeps the water from percolating deeper. A spring may also occur where subsurface pressure forces water to the surface through a fracture or fault zone that acts as a conduit for water movement from a confined aquifer.

The quality of groundwater is usually better than that of the surface water. There is less chance of pollution in groundwater as the soil and rocks that groundwater pass through can act as natural filters. Under the right conditions, this filtering system cleanses the water, trapping disease-causing microorganisms and particulates which contain toxic compounds. Unless it contains contaminants introduced by human activities, groundwater is normally free of suspended solids, bacteria, and other disease-causing organisms. On the other hand, groundwater exchanges material with the soil and rocks. Most often, the groundwater dissolves a mixture of minerals and the hardness of groundwater is usually higher than surface water. If the soil or rock surface is already highly contaminated or contains naturally toxic elements, the groundwater may be rendered toxic by these natural processes. Furthermore, groundwater has poor self-purification ability and relatively less dissolved oxygen, which is consumed by the biochemical process in soil.

4.2 Parameters of water quality

Pure water contains only H_2O. Natural water dissolves and carries substances ranging from nutrients to industrial and domestic wastes, which can be divided into: soluble matters (such as salts or compounds of calcium, magnesium, sodium, manganese, and oxygen, carbon dioxide and other gases); colloids substances (such as humus); and suspended matters (include clay, sand, algae, bacteria and protozoa). Natural water reacts with the substances in it and forms certain characteristics together with these substances. Water quality changes with the composition of natural water. The following water quality parameters (Table 4-1) can help us to detect water characteristics, study water pollution, and evaluate the safety of water.

Table 4-1　Parameters of water quality and significance of determination

Classification	Parameters	Hygienic significance
Physical parameters	Temperature	Suggesting whether water suffered from physical pollution or not
	Color	Evaluating sensory properties of water
	Smell and taste	Evaluating sensory properties of water and speculating on the harmful components in the water
	Turbidity	Judging whether water suffer from pollution or not
Chemical parameters	pH	Suggesting whether water polluted by acid wastewater or not
	Total solid	The less total solids content it is, the cleaner the water is
	Hardness	Hardness of groundwater is generally higher than that of surface water, and the hardness of surface water also increases when polluted by industrial high-hardness wastewater

Continue to Table 4-1

Classification	Parameters	Hygienic significance
Microbiological parameters	Nitrogen-containing compounds	Reflecting organic pollution and self-purification of water
	Dissolved oxygen	Indirect indicator for evaluating organic pollution and self-purification of water
	Chemical oxygen demand	Indirect indicator for evaluating organic pollution of water
	Biochemical oxygen demand	Indirect indicator for evaluating organic pollution of water, reflecting the actual situation of decomposition of organic matter by microorganisms in water
	Total organic carbon and total oxygen demand	Comprehensive indicators for evaluating organic pollution of water
	Toxicants	Reflecting pollution of water by toxic substances
	Bacteria count	Reflecting microbial pollution of water, the more serious the water polluted, the more bacteria count
	Fecal coliform	Directly reflecting the feces pollution in water and suggesting the possibility of contamination by pathogenic bacteria

4.2.1　Physical parameters

4.2.1.1　Temperature

Temperature is an important physical characteristic of water, which has effects on survival of aquatic life, water self-purification, and water use. Temperature of surface water changes with seasons and climates, ranging from 0.1 ℃ to 30 ℃. While temperature of groundwater remains 8-12 ℃, the sudden increase of groundwater temperature may suggest large amounts of heated water leaching from surface water. The release of heated water from industrial and power plants into rivers changes the average water temperature and causes thermal pollution. There are several problems with heated water. Warmer water holds less oxygen and favors different species than cooler water and may increase growth rates of undesirable organisms, including certain water plants and fish. Thus heating the water can disturb the aquatic ecosystem from its original conditions.

4.2.1.2　Color

Pure water is colorless. Color of natural water can be and is often caused by organic substances, such as algae or humic compounds. Too much humic compounds make water tawny. Different kinds of algae can make different colors of water, for example, Chlorella colors water green and Diatom colors water brown. Water exhibits special color when multicolored industrial wastes are discharged into water.

4.2.1.3　Odor

Pure water is odor-free. The odor of natural water is mainly from reproduction and death of aquatic life or microorganism; decomposition of organism; dissolved gases; and dissolved mineral salts. Many of the alga growth in lakes produce fishy odor, too much ferric salts give water astringency, and hydrogen sulphide produces a "rotten egg" odor. Water has special odor when taking up domestic sewage or industrial wastewater.

4.2.1.4　Turbidity

Water which is not clear but "dirty", in the sense that light transmission is inhibited, is known as turbid water. Turbidity can be caused by many materials, such as suspended particles and tiny colloidal particulates. Turbidity depends on the size, shape, content, kinds, and refractive index of particulates. The standard turbidity unit is turbidity formed by 1 mg SiO_2 in 1 L water, which is 1 unit of turbidity. Turbidity can be used to determine whether water is polluted. Turbidity of surface water changes with the geological conditions of the area that runoff pass through. Due to the natural filtering of soil and rocks, groundwater usually has low turbidity. But it must be emphasized that low turbidity does not mean there is no pollution in water.

4.2.2　Chemical parameters

4.2.2.1　pH

pH value of pure water is equal to 7, and the corresponding value of natural water is ranging from 6.5 to 8.5. pH value of water is one of the major indicators of water quality, defining the character of the chemical and biological processes occurring in water. Too much organic matters in water, which are oxidized and decomposed to produce free carbon dioxide, may reduce the pH value of water. When a large amount of acidic or alkaline wastewater is discharged into the water body, the pH value of water also changes obviously. In addition, acid rain can result in acidification of surface water.

4.2.2.2　Total solids

Total solids refer to residues from water sample as a result of extensive evaporation at certain temperatures, usually at 103－105 ℃ (slightly higher than the boiling point of water). Total solids can be divided into two fractions: the dissolved solids and the suspended solids, which are composed of organic matter, inorganic matter and various organisms. The less total solids content, the cleaner the water. Total solids content increases once water is polluted. The dissolved solids are the residues after evaporation of the filtrate from filtration of the water sample. The content of the dissolved solids mainly depends on the mineral salts and organic matters dissolved in the water. The suspended solids are the solids that cannot pass through the filter. When total solids are burned, minerals are left behind, while the organic matters are completely oxidized and volatilized. The loss of weight after burning can roughly indicate the content of organic matters in water.

4.2.2.3　Hardness

In general, hardness can be divided into carbonate hardness (bicarbonate and carbonate of calcium/magnesium) and non－carbonate hardness (sulfate and chloride of calcium/magnesium).

Hardness can also be divided into temporary hardness and permanent hardness. Hardness which can be removed after boiling the water is known as temporary hardness. Permanent hardness is the hardness that cannot be removed after boiling. In boiling water, bicarbonate decomposes into carbonate and precipitates, thus removed from water, so carbonate hardness is often considered to be equal to temporary hardness. But precipitation of calcium/magnesium carbonate is not completely, so temporary hardness is often less than carbonate hardness.

The hardness of natural water is very different due to different geological conditions. Hardness of groundwater is generally higher than that of surface water, because in the process of penetration groundwater absorbed carbon dioxide released from decomposition of organic matter in the soil, which can dissolve calcium carbonate and magnesium carbonate in stratum, as a result, hardness of groundwater increases. In surface water, only riverbed and lake bottom contact with the land surface. In addition, the content of carbon dioxide is low, so surface water often has low hardness. However, when polluted by industrial high－hardness wastewater, or solubility increased due to carbon dioxide released from decomposition of the organic pollutants, the hardness of surface water also increases.

4.2.2.4　Nitrogen－containing compounds

Nitrogen－containing compounds contain organic nitrogen, ammonia nitrogen, nitrite nitrogen, and nitrate nitrogen. Nitrogen is an important element in biological reactions. Nitrogen can be tied up in compounds such as amino acids and amines. In this form the nitrogen is known as organic nitrogen, which mainly comes from plants and animals, such as animal feces, decomposition of plants, algae, and protozoans. One of the intermediate compounds formed during biological metabolism is ammonia. Together with organic nitrogen, ammonia is considered to be an indicator of recent pollution by human and animal feces. It should be pointed out that surface water flowing through swamps has more ammonia nitrogen content, and the nitrate in soil can be reduced to nitrite and ammonia by anaerobic microorganism, which can also increase the concentration of ammonia nitrogen in water. Aerobic decomposition of ammonia eventually leads to the nitrite (NO_2^-) and nitrate (NO_3^-) nitrogen forms. Nitrogen goes through a series of increasingly stable compounds, finally ending up as nitrate. Nitrite is the intermediate product of ammonia nitrification. A high nitrite indicates that the inorganic process of organic matter in the water has not been completed, and the pollution still exists. Nitrate nitrogen is the final product of nitrogen oxidative decomposition of organic matter. High content of nitrate nitrogen and low content of ammonia nitrogen and nitrite nitrogen in water say the water is polluted by organic in the past, and now self-purification process has been complete. If ammonia nitrogen, nitrite nitrogen, and nitrate nitrogen all increase, it is suggested that water is suffering from persistent pollution or the pollution occurred in the past, and self-purification is now in progress. We can analyze the content of ammonia nitrogen, nitrite nitrogen, and nitrate nitrogen in the water and judge the pollution status of water quality.

4.2.2.5　Dissolved oxygen

Dissolved oxygen (DO) is the content of oxygen dissolved in water, which is related to oxygen partial pressure in the air and water temperature. Generally speaking, the oxygen partial pressure in the air is relatively constant in the same area, so the water temperature is the main influence factor of dissolved oxygen. The lower the water temperature, the higher the dissolved oxygen. The dissolved oxygen content of clean surface water is close to saturation. The deeper the water layer, the lower the dissolved oxygen. Oxygen released by photosynthesis of aquatic plant can cause the dissolved oxygen in water to be oversaturated. When water is polluted by organic matters or a large number of algae dies, dissolved oxygen can be consumed and decrease if the rate of consumption is greater than the rate of oxygen supplement from the atmosphere, thus the water body will appear anaerobic condition. At this time, anaerobic bacteria in water will decompose organic matters and produce ammonia, hydrogen sulfide, and methane, and make water black and smelly. Therefore, dissolved oxygen can be used as an indirect index to evaluate the organic pollution and self-purification of water body. It should be pointed out that the content of dissolved oxygen in groundwater is usually very low, so DO is not suitable to evaluate water quality of groundwater.

4.2.2.6　Biochemical oxygen demand

Biological oxygen demand (BOD) is the amount of oxygen necessary to decompose organic materials by aerobic microorganism in a unit volume of water. As the amount of organic waste in water increases, more oxygen is used, resulting in a higher BOD. Temperature, time, and light are three very important variables in the process of biological oxidation. In practical work, BOD test was standardized by requiring the test to be run in the dark at 20 ℃ for five days. This is defined as five-day BOD, or BOD_5^{20}.

It is important to understand that BOD is not a measure of any specific pollutant. Rather, it is a measure of the amount of oxygen required by bacteria and other microorganisms while stabilizing decomposable organic matter. It is a commonly used parameter in water quality management. BOD of most domestic sewage is about 250 mg/L, while BOD is usually below 1 mg/L in clean water.

4.2.2.7　Chemical oxygen demand

BOD can reflect the actual situation of decomposition of organic matter by microorganisms in water, but BOD test takes five days to run, and for samples containing more pollutants, dilution of the sample is necessary. If the organics were oxidized chemically instead of biologically, the test could be shortened considerably. Such oxidation is accomplished with the chemical oxygen demand test. Chemical oxygen demand (COD) refers to the consumption of oxygen during the process of oxidation of organic matters in water by highly efficient oxidants. Potassium dichromate and potassium permanganate are generally used as oxidizing agents. So COD is also called potassium dichromate index or potassium permanganate index. COD is an indirect index to evaluate the organic pollution of water body. Because nearly all organics and reductive inorganic matters are oxidized in the COD test and only some of them are decomposed during the BOD test, COD values are always higher than BOD values.

4.2.2.8　Total organic carbon and total oxygen demand

Total organic carbon (TOC) refers to the total carbon content of all organic matters in per liter of water sample. It is one of the comprehensive indexes to evaluate the degree of organic pollution in water body, although it cannot reflect properties of organic contaminants. Total oxygen demand (TOD) is the consumption of oxygen during the process of oxidation of reducing matters in water under certain condition. It can reflect the pollution degree of reducing matter in water. The higher the value of TOD, the more serious the pollution. Test of either TOC or TOD has significant advantages over the BOD and COD tests, and has been widely used in rapid automatic detection of water samples.

4.2.2.9　Toxicants

Toxicants mainly refer to heavy metals and organic matters which are difficult to be decomposed in water, such as mercury, cadmium, arsenic, chromium, lead, phenol, cyanide, and organic chlorine, etc. These harmful substances, except for fluorine and arsenic, which are related to geological environment, are mainly due to pollution from industrial, domestic, and agricultural waste water.

4.2.3　Microbiological parameters

Disease-carrying microorganisms are important biological pollutants. From the public health standpoint the microbiological quality of water is as important as the chemical quality of water. A number of diseases can be transmitted by water. However, there are many pathogens, and each has a specific detection procedure and must be screened individually. The concentration of these organisms can be so small as to make their detection impossible. It is a perfect example of the proverbial needle in a haystack. And yet only one or two organisms in the water might be sufficient to cause an infection. How then can we measure the bacteriological quality? The answer lies in the concept of indicator organisms. Bacteria count and fecal coliforms are chosen as the indicator of the microbiological quality in surface water.

When surface water is polluted by feces, domestic sewage, or industrial waste water, bacteria in water can increase in large quantities. Therefore, bacteria count and fecal coliforms can be used as direct indicators of water pollution by feces, and to indirectly evaluate water microbial pollution.

4.2.3.1　Bacteria count

Bacteria count refers to colonies in 1 mL water grow after incubated at agar medium under 37 ℃ for 24 hours. This parameter can reflect microbial pollution of water, the more serious the water polluted, the more bacteria count. It must be point out that bacteria count only indicates the count of bacteria which can grow under the incubation conditions instead of all bacteria, not to mention the presence of pathogens.

4.2.3.2　Fecal coliform

Total coliform refers to aerobic or facultative anaerobic gram−negative budless bacillus which could ferment lactose and produce acids and CO_2 after incubated within 24 hours under 37 ℃. If a large number of coliform is the present, there is a high chance of recent pollution by wastes from warm−blooded animals, and therefore the water may contain pathogenic organisms. There are two kinds of coliform in water, the fecal coliform is the organism normal to the digestive tracts of warm−blooded animals, and the other kind of coliform can survive in soil, water, and other natural environments. In practical work, it could be often used to distinguish fecal coliform from total coliform by rising incubation temperature up to 44.5 ℃ ±0.2 ℃, at which temperature, the coliform from natural environment, instead of digestive tracts of warm−blooded animals, cannot survive and grow. Therefore, compared with total coliform, fecal coliform can directly reflect the feces pollution in water.

This last point should be emphasized. The presence of coliform does not mean that there are pathogens in the water. It simply means that there might be. On the other hand, due to the fact that the resistance of some enterovirus to chlorine is often stronger than that of coliform, enterovirus can also be detected when value of coliform matches the hygiene standard.

4.3　Water pollution and pollutants outcome

Water pollution is the contamination of water bodies. It occurs when pollutants are directly or indirectly discharged into water bodies, exceeding the water self−purification capacity. It changes physicochemical properties of water and sediment, biological characteristics, and composition in aquatic environment, thus affecting the value of water, causing water quality deterioration, and even endangering human health or damaging the ecological environment. The pollutants that cause water pollution come mainly from human activities. In addition, natural factors can cause changes in certain components of water, such as endemic fluorosis induced by excessive fluorine content in local water, which can harm human body.

4.3.1　Sources of water pollution

There are three major types of water pollutants: physical pollutants (such as waste heat and radioactive substances), biological pollutants (such as disease−causing microorganisms and algae), and chemical pollutants (including a large number of inorganic and organic compounds). The sources of these pollutants can be summarized as follows.

4.3.1.1　Industrial wastewater

Industrial wastewater is the worldwide main source of water pollution. Each aspect of industrial production can produce wastewater, such as cooling water, washing wastewater, hydraulic mineral processing wastewater, leaching liquid and so on. The quality and quantity of industrial wastewater varies according to the products, procedure, and scale of production. For enterprises produce similar products, the quality and quantity of the wastewater are also different because of the different technological process, raw materials, and quality of production water supply. Steel plant discharges wastewater containing phenol and cyanide. Chemical plant and fertilizer plant discharge wastewater containing arsenic, mercury, chromium, pesticides, and other harmful substances. Wastewater containing a large number of organic compounds could be eliminated from paper mill. High temperature cooling water which can cause thermal pollution may be discharged from power plant. Wastewater with great influence on water pollution is mainly from metallurgy, chemical industry, electroplating, paper making, dyeing, leather making, and other enterprises.

4.3.1.2 Domestic sewage

Domestic sewage is mainly washing wastewater and fecal sewage, which contains a lot of organic matters, such as cellulose, starch, sugar, protein, fat, and microorganism including intestinal pathogens. There are also a large number of inorganic substances in domestic swage, such as chloride, sulfate, phosphate, ammonium salt, nitrite, nitrates, etc. In recent years, due to the extensive use of synthetic detergents, the phosphorus content in sewage has increased significantly. The enhance of wastewater enriched with nitrogen and phosphorus into water results in algae blooms, increase of organic matter, decrease of dissolved oxygen, and deterioration of water quality, this is so-called eutrophication. Nutrient enrichment and eutrophication can be greatly accelerated by human activities. In fact, many lakes have been shown to have been rapidly enriched with nutrients over the last 100 years due to pollution. Discharges, especially domestic sewage and agricultural wastewater, contain plant nutrients that often lead to nutrient enrichment and accelerated eutrophication. In China eutrophication has become the most important type of pollution of freshwater lakes, so that limit of high phosphorus synthetic detergent pollution is particularly urgent.

The urban surface runoff formed by precipitation which contacts with air pollutants and washes buildings, ground, and garbage is also a component of domestic sewage. In addition, sewage from hospital, including the domestic wastewater from patients and medical wastewater, which contains a large number of pathogens is a special kind of domestic sewage.

4.3.1.3 Agricultural wastewater

Agricultural wastewater is irrigation water that flows through farmland or agricultural sewage. Agricultural wastewater contains plenty of fertilizers, which contribute to eutrophication, highly residual and toxic pesticides, forming a worldwide water pollution and antibiotics.

4.3.1.4 Others

Industrial solid waste and urban garbage are increasing. This waste often contains a large number of soluble inorganic and organic compounds, and pathogenic microorganism, etc. which are washed by the rain, enter runoff and cause water pollution. Offshore oil exploitation and oil spill from large oil tanker are also important sources of pollution.

4.3.2 Pollution characteristics of water

4.3.2.1 Rivers

Under the circumstance of the same amount of pollutant discharges, the degree of rivers pollution depends on the dilution ratio (the ratio of volume of runoff and amount of sewage discharged into rivers). Rivers with high dilution ratios have strong dilution ability, thus the possibility and degree of pollution are comparatively low. When rivers have strong mixing capacity, together with thrust of water flow, the upstream pollution can quickly affect the downstream. The volume of rivers can affect the diffusion mode of pollutants. In small or medium-sized rivers, pollutants can disperse vertically and horizontally. As a result, pollution not only occurs in drain outlet, it can affect tens of kilometers of downstream. The mixing of the pollutants in vertical and horizontal directions allows the pollutants to be evenly distributed throughout the whole section. In rivers with large flow, pollutants are not easy to be mixed with water in the whole section, pollution belt with high concentration of pollutants only forms near the bank, and affects water quality of local waters' downstream. So the range of river pollution is not limited to sewage outlet, but often affects the downstream areas, even can affect the ocean.

4.3.2.2   Lakes and reservoirs

Lakes and reservoirs are characterized by wide water surface, low velocity of flow, strong capability of precipitation, poor mixing ability, and slow water exchange. The pollutants in these places are not easy to be diluted by water, and it is also difficult to be transferred to downstream by water flow. In addition, the low velocity of flow reduces reaeration (O_2 dissolved into the water from the atmosphere), thus weakening self-purification ability of lakes.

When accepting sewage containing high concentration of nitrogen and phosphorus, lakes and reservoirs are vulnerable to eutrophication. This kind of phenomenon is called "water bloom" in freshwater such as rivers and lakes, and "red tide" in the ocean. Because the colors of the dominant planktonic algae are different, the surface often appears blue, red, brown, ivory, and so on. An increase in the populations of plants can lead to a decrease in the dissolved oxygen content of the water from plant death and decomposition. This decreases the suitability of the area as a habitat for many species of fish and other organisms. The increase in turbidity and color, which occurs during eutrophication, renders the water unsuitable for domestic use or difficult tobe treated to a suitable standard for this purpose. Meanwhile, the anaerobic bacteria reproduce intensively, decompose organics, produce harmful gases (such as ammonia, methane, and hydrogen sulfide), worsen the sensory properties of water, and reduce value of water. Furthermore, toxin produced by algae leads to the death of fish, other aquatic organisms, and also of terrestrial organisms using the water.

4.3.2.3   Groundwater

Pollutants in surface waters can migrate downward. Furthermore, underground storage leakage is also a source of groundwater pollution. Due to the filtering and adsorption capability of soil and the protection of surface layer, groundwater has less chance to be polluted, and pollution processes are slow. But once groundwater is polluted obviously, it is hard to clean up. Groundwater pollution differs in several ways from surface water pollution. Firstly, groundwater systems are complicated and the contaminants are invisible to naked eyes. This makes it more difficult to find contaminants and to design a treatment system that either destroys the contaminants in the ground or takes them to the surface for cleanup. Furthermore, groundwater often has low content of dissolved oxygen, and bacterial degradation of pollutants does not occur readily in groundwater due to the lack of microorganism. In addition, the opportunity for dispersion and dilution of the pollutants in groundwater is very limited. So groundwater has poor self-purification ability.

4.3.2.4   Seas and oceans

The sources of pollution in seas and oceans are numerous and complicated. All kinds of industrial wastewater and domestic sewage enter into the ocean and the pollutants are hard to be moved out. As a result, pollutants that are difficult to be degraded accumulate in the ocean or in marine organisms, and form persistent marine pollution. Other sources of oil pollution are offshore vessels and large oil tanker accidents, as well as offshore oil drilling operations. Serious oil pollution in local water can affect the survival of marine life, such as fish and birds. Furthermore, as the world's oceans are interlinked, a spill from an oil tanker creates an oil slick that can affect a vast area of the ocean. Pollutants spread to every corner of the ocean through tidal action and ocean current. So another feature of marine pollution is the wide range of pollution.

4.3.3   Water pollutants outcomes

4.3.3.1   Self-purification

Self-purification refers to the process that after water bodies are contaminated, pollutants in water are diluted, dispersed, decomposed, or sank to the bottom under the physical, chemical, and biological action.

Thus, concentration of pollutants in water gradually reduces, and finally water quality recovers to the initial status.

There are many factors which can affect water self-purification process, such as topography and hydrological conditions of the water body, species and quantity of microorganism in water, temperature and reaeration capacity (related to wind speed, wind direction, and turbulent flow, etc.), as well as the property and the concentration of pollutants. Mechanisms of self-purification include physical, chemical, and biological purification. These effects can interact with each other and occur at the same time. The initial stage of self-purification is mainly physical and chemical, while the later stage is mainly biological.

Physical purification includes dilution, mixing, precipitation, and absorption. Pollutants discharged to water can be mixed and diluted by the clean water. Obviously, the faster the water flow, the better the dilution effect. The suspended particles in water are gradually sinking under gravity, and are involved in the formation of sediment. However, the pollutants settled to the bottom can be re-suspended in water when water flow increases or sediment is stirred, which results in secondary pollution. In addition, the pollutants in the water can also be absorbed by solid (such as suspended minerals, clay), and migrated to or settled in the solid. The physical purification process of water body is also related to the velocity of flow, the shape of river bed, and the position of discharge outlet. For lakes, reservoirs, and oceans, there are more factors affecting water dilution, such as the direction of flow, wind direction, wind speed, water temperature, and tide. Although the process of physical purification only changes the distribution of pollutants instead of the absolute amount of pollutants, it is helpful for the subsequent chemical and biological purification process.

Chemical purification refers to the phenomenon that the concentration and toxicity of pollutants in water reduce due to chemical actions, such as oxidation-reduction reaction, combination reaction, decomposition reaction, and neutralization. Pollutants, such as phenol and cyanide, are prone to participation in decomposition and combination reactions in water. Oxidation-reduction reaction is the main action in chemical purification. Heavy metal ions such as manganese can be oxidized to insoluble manganese hydroxide, and then precipitate. Other reactions in chemical purification are photolytic reaction and photochemical oxidation reaction. Chemical purification process changes the absolute quantity of pollutants, but it is important to note that pollutant's toxicity may be either reduced or increased by chemical reactions, especially the latter should be attached great importance.

Biological purification is that pollutants are decomposed by metabolism of organisms in water, such as bacteria, fungi, algae, aquatic plants, protozoa, shellfish, insect larvae, and fish, thus, the pollutants reduce, or even disappear. Biological purification is the most important and active action in self-purification of surface water. Some special microbial population and hydrophytes (such as duckweed, water hyacinth, and reed) can absorb, decompose, or concentrate synthetic organic compounds. Heavy metals, such as mercury, chromium and zinc are difficult to be degraded.

When dissolved oxygen is abundant in water, suspended and dissolved organic matter can be decomposed into simple inorganic substances (such as carbon dioxide, water, sulfate, and nitrate) by aerobic microorganism, so that the water can be cleaned up. Dissolved oxygen in the water is consumed during decomposition of organic matter by aerobic microorganism. At the same time, oxygen from the atmosphere is continuously dissolved into the water. In addition, oxygen released by photosynthesis of aquatic plant is also added to the water, this is the process of reoxygenation. During biological purification of organic matters, the content of dissolved oxygen is the result of the interaction between oxygen consumption and reoxygenation. If the water is loaded with organic material, the simultaneous action of deoxygenation and reoxygenation forms the dissolved oxygen sag curve (Figure 4-1). When organic matters are discharged to the water, a number of changes occur downstream from the point of discharge. As the organics are decomposed, oxygen is used at a greater rate than before the occurrence of the pollution, and the dissolved oxygen level drops. The rate of reaeration also increases, but this is often not strong enough to prevent a total depletion of oxygen in water. When this happens, the water becomes anaerobic. Often, however, the dissolved oxygen does not drop to zero, and the water recovers without experiencing a period of anaerobiosis. The most serious concern of water quality is the point in the curve where the dissolved oxygen concentration is the least, which is so-called C_p point. After this point, when the rate of reaeration overwhelms deoxygenation, dissolved oxygen increases gradually and water is cleaned up. Environmental quality standard for surface water defines the threshold for a water pollution alert (dissolved oxygen content at C_p point) as a dissolved oxygen content of less than 4 mg/L. It indicates that the organic matters discharged into water have not exceeded the self-purification capacity of the water body. If too much organic matters enter into water, dissolved oxygen at the C_p point is lower than the threshold, even drops to zero at certain stream segment downstream of the sewage outlet. Anaerobic bacteria decompose organic matters at this time, and produce hydrogen sulfide and methane, thus cause the water black and smelly, and deteriorate water quality.

4.3.3.2   Pollutants migration

Migration of pollutants refers to the transfer of pollutants from one location to another, from one medium to another. After entering the flowing water body, the pollutants are dispersed rapidly from the vertical and horizontal, and along the directions of water flow, moved downstream. Pollutants can be transferred or settled by absorption and coagulation of solid particles and colloid material. Some pollutants, such as volatile phenol, hydrocyanic acid, and ammonia can be volatilized into atmosphere.

Pollutants, such as toxic metals and organic compounds that are difficult to be decomposed, can also be transferred by bioenrichment and biomagnifications. Bioenrichment is the uptake and retention of a pollutant by an organism results in the development of elevated concentration, which may have deleterious effects. Biomagnifications is the process whereby pollutants are passed from one trophic level to another and exhibit increasing concentrations in organisms related to their trophic status. That is the tendency for some substances to concentrate with each trophic level. Thus, a sequential increase in concentration could be expected in a food chain, with organisms at the highest levels exhibiting the highest concentrations.

Biomagnifications has been used to explain the high concentrations of some pollutants, such as DDT, in top carnivores, such as eagles. DDT is a kind of organochlorine pesticide with stable chemical properties. It is poorly soluble in water, but quite soluble in fats and organic oils, and its biological half-life is up to 25 years. DDT can be taken up by aquatic organisms and stored in their fatty tissues. When these aquatic organisms or plants were eaten, the metabolism of the predators tended to favor the retention of DDT in the body fat, and the predators concentrated it in their own bodies. Each step in the food chain results in an increased concentration of DDT. Finally, the carnivorous birds at the top of the food chain seem to have concentrations sufficient to cause toxic effects. As an example of DDT illustrates, fat-soluble organic compounds can have subtle, hidden, but important environmental effects. They do undergo trophic-level concentration or biomagnifications, and thus negative effects can take place when the compound appears to be only a trace substance in the environment, and human who is at the highest levels of food chain will be the worst victim. The discovery of biomagnifications has led to a better understanding of the pathways of pollutants in the environment.

4.3.3.3   Pollutants transformation

Aquatic transformation processes include physical and chemical actions, photolysis, and biodegradation. Physical transformation is realized mainly by volatilization, adsorption, and decay of radioactive elements, while chemical transformation is realized mainly by hydrolysis, combination reaction, and oxidation-reduction reaction. Photolysis refers to decomposition of organic compounds by absorption of energy of certain solar radiation (wavelength is more than 290 nm). The photolysis of pollutants depends upon the energy of incident sunlight, the absorption spectrum of the molecule, and the presence of photosensitizers in water. Biodegradation of pollutants by aquatic organisms (bacteria, fungi, protozoa, and algae) are important removal and transformation processes in water. Many organisms possess metabolic pathways capable of deactivation and/or activation of pollutants.

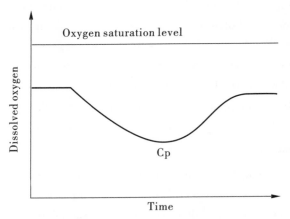

Figure 4-1   Dissolved oxygen sag curve

4.4   Water pollution hazard and diseases

4.4.1   Water pollution hazards

Water is a major part of the human body, and is needed in the process of all physiological activities, such as nutrition convey, temperature regulation, and waste excreting. Groundwater around the world is threatened by pollutions from agricultural and industrial sources, such as solid waste, on-site wastewater treatment, oil and gas extraction and refining, mining, and manufacturing. Consumption of the contaminated water in our daily life is harmful to human health.

4.4.1.1   Biological water pollution

Biological pollution can cause the occurrence of waterborne diseases through drinking and contacting the contaminated water, even the outbreak of epidemic, which will lead to serious health problem. The most common waterborne diseases are intestinal infectious diseases (e. g. , cholera, typhoid, bacterial dysentery, hepatitis A, and cryptosporidiosis) and parasitic diseases (e. g. , schistosomiasis and giardiasis).

Intestinal infectious diseases and parasitic diseases: Intestinal infectious diseases are still occurring occasionally in developing countries, even outbreak in some cases. Therefore, the hazard of pathogenic microorganism water pollution is still a prominent problem in developing countries. According to the World Health Organization(WHO), about 1. 2 billion people in developing countries suffer from unsafe drinking water each year, and more than 4 million children die from waterborne diseases. Approximately 0. 5-1. 8 million children die from diarrhoea globally each year, about 40% -50% of which due to rotavirus infection. Using domestic sewage collection and treatment as a proxy, microbial contamination has decreased significantly in most developed countries. In contrast, microbial pathogens are the most pressing water quality issue in many developing countries.

The harm of algae toxins in water: Water bloom and red tide occur in many countries. The pollution of algae is another important hazard to the biological contamination of water. The harm of algae toxin to human health has become a global environmental problem. Breeding and overriding the surface of water, the algae worsen the physical properties of the water and endanger the survival of aquatic organisms. Biological toxins of metabolism or harmful substances secreted by some algae can damage the ecological environment of water, and lead to the abnormal biological community structure. Some algae toxins can also cause human poisoning and even death. In December 1986, shellfishes contaminated with the red tide toxin poisoned 135 people and killed one in Fujian province, China. Cyanobacteria in eutrophicated lake water is a major toxin-producing species. There are more than 40 known toxin-producing species. Among them, the microcystin and the nodularin produced by microcystis aeruginosa and spumigena, respectively, are the two kinds of the most abundant and harmful toxin in eutrophic water. Microcystin is one kind of widely distributed hepatic toxin with bioactive cyclic peptides and a verified tumor promoter. The number of reported outbreaks of paralytic shellfish poison, a harmful algal toxin found in eutrophic waters, increased from fewer than 20 in 1970, to more than 100 in 2009 (Anderson, et al. 2010).

4.4.1.2   Chemical water pollution

In contaminated water, poisonous and harmful chemicals include mercury, arsenic, chromium, phenol, cyanide, polychlorinated biphenyls (PCBs), pesticide and their by-products, such as dichlorodiphenyltrichloroethane (DDT). The pollutants of greatest concern are persistent, toxic and bioaccumulative. Organisms can accumulate contaminants from water, sediment, and food, acquiring contaminant levels in the tissue much higher than those in the surrounding environment, causing the acute and chronic poisoning of human body.

(1) Mercury and methyl mercury

Mercury exists in the form of metallic mercury, inorganic mercury and organic mercury in natural environment. Some microorganisms can convert inorganic mercury into more toxic organic mercury, including methyl mercury, dimethyl mercury, phenyl mercury and ethyl mercury. The amount of mercury in uncontaminated natural water is generally low. The mercury content in water of river and lake in China is generally under 1.0 μg/L. For example, the concentration of mercury is 0.1 - 0.4 μg/L in the Yellow River, 0.14 μg/L in the Yangtze River, and 0.025 μg/L in the Dongting Lake. The main source of mercury pollutants in water are from industrial enterprises, such as smelting, chlorine-alkali, chemical, instrument, electron, pigments, and mercury pesticides. Mercury in surface water can be partially volatilizes into the atmosphere, but most of it is deposited in sediment. Mercury in sediment can be converted to methyl mercury or dimethyl mercury in the presence of anaerobic bacteria (e.g., methanogens). Methyl mercury is soluble in water and can be gradually accumulated in aquatic organisms through the food chain to reach a higher concentration. For instance, the methyl mercury concentration in fish can be tens of thousands of times higher than in water. Thus, the main hazard of mercury in water is chronic methyl-mercury poisoning caused by intaking fish and shellfish accumulated with high concentration of methyl mercury. There have been many reports of methyl mercury poisoning around the world, the most notable one of which is about minamata in Japan.

(2) Arsenic

Both naturally occurring arsenic and the arsenic mobilized by human activities threaten the quality of drinking water in many countries. Groundwater contaminated with arsenic from natural geologic sources affects 35−75 million people. Surface water pollution in some regions has led to the development of groundwater as a source of drinking water, resulting in inadvertently exposing people to these natural sources of arsenic (Schwarzenbach et al. 2010; Brunt et al. 2004).

(3) Polychlorinated biphenyls

PCBs are chlorine−containing organic compounds, having the properties of acid−resistance, alkali−resistance, corrosion−resistance, insulation, heat resistance and non−flammability. PCBs are hard to be broken down in water because of their low water−solubility, but soluble in organic solvents and fats, thus, they can be easily enriched in adipose tissue of organisms. PCBs are widely used in industry as insulating liquids for transformers and additives in paints, and enter water with industrial and urban wastewater prevailingly. PCBs are extremely stable in water and are considered as a kind of widespread persistent organic pollutants (POPs). The average concentration of PCBs is 0.013 μg/L in the Second Songhua River, 0.62 μg/kg in sediment, and 6.4−214 μg/kg in fish. PCBs can be bio−enriched into the food chain by ingestion of aquatic organisms. In consideration of the toxic and low degradability of PCBs, the toxic chemicals control agency announced restrictions of PCBs in 1976. In the same year the United States Environmental Protection Agency (EPA) set a water quality standard for PCBs. In 1977, the US EPA began to restrict the use of PCBs, and by 1979 all production, sales and use of PCBs were banned. Although being banned for several decades in many developed countries, the widespread use of PCBs has caused global pollution, from arctic sea mammals to birds' eggs at the South Pole, and has still been found in water, sediments, organisms, and even in milk.

Although conventional toxic contaminants are declining in many industrialized areas, new−type pollutants are raising mounting concerns. Polybrominated diphenyl ethers (PBDEs), for example, a type of POPs used as a flame retardant has increased exponentially over the past three decades in North America, Europe and Japan (Schwarzenbach et al. 2010). There are also increasingly concerns about pharmaceuticals and personal care products that are not removed by most sewage treatment systems, and thus enter the environment, the long−term negative effects of which on aquatic organisms and humans are largely unknown.

4.4.1.3 Physical water pollution thermal pollution and radioactive pollution

(1) Thermal pollution

The discharged hot water of circulation cooling system from thermal power plants, nuclear power plants, steel mills and the waste water from oil, chemical, foundry, paper and other industries contains a lot of "heat". After being discharged into surface water, the increasing water temperature leads to a series of physical, chemical and biological changes. The victims of thermal pollution are mainly aquatic organisms. They may be retarded or dead under anaerobic condition due to the hot temperature of water, thus affect the environmental and ecological balance. Meanwhile, the excessive growth of some aquatic plants can hinder water flow and navigation.

(2) Radioactive pollution

Radioactive pollution in water refers to the pollution caused by the human activities that release radioactive materials. Radioactive substances can be divided into natural and artificial radioactive sources. There are many paths for these radioactive substances to come into human body and harm health, such as through drinking water, contaminated food or even through breath. After the radioactive material enters the human body, the body will be continuously exposed by external or internal radiation until the radionuclide is transformed into a stable nuclide or totally expelled from the body. The radioactive substances absorbed into the blood can be evenly distributed, and some of them are relatively concentrated in certain organs or tissues, for instance, ^{131}I and ^{222}Rn are mainly gathered in thyroid and lung, respectively, while ^{235}U is stored in kidney predominantly.

4.4.2　Water–related diseases

Same as the case with food, there are multiple diseases that can be transmitted through contaminated drinking water. Diseases caused by microorganisms and chemicals in drinking water are defined as water–related diseases by WHO. These diseases include malaria with water–related vectors and schistosomiasis whose vector spends part of its life cycle in water, and minamata disease due to methylmercury poisoning, etc.

Epidemiological study of cholera in London conducted by John Snow in 1854 was considered to be the first positive evidence that public water supplies could be a source of infection. Nowadays, water–related diseases are still a continuing public health problem in developing countries because of lack of access to adequate drinking water and sanitation, this is further evidenced by the cholera epidemic in Haiti following the 2010 earthquake (Walton and Ivers, 2011). Contaminated water can be a source of infection in humans through several distinct avenues. In general, there are four principal pathways of exposure that water can have effects on human health: waterborne diseases, water–contact diseases, water–insect–related diseases, and water–wash diseases.

4.4.2.1　Waterborne communicable diseases

The quality of water is the most important concern in waterborne diseases. The pathogens involved include a wide variety of viruses, bacteria and protozoan parasites. According to the WHO data, the consumption of contaminated water accounts for an estimated 1.2 billion illnesses in the developing countries of the world. The pathogens of waterborne diseases mainly include: bacteria, such as salmonella typhi, vibrio cholera, and dysentery bacillus; viruses, such as hepatitis virus, poliovirus, and adenovirus; and parasites, such as giardia and soluble amoeba. The contaminated water may cause mild bowel diseases or serious diseases such as dysentery, typhoid, and cholera.

Major epidemics of cholera and other waterborne diseases broke out periodically in the US until the end of the nineteenth century (Introduction to Public Health, 5th Edition, 2011). Although outbreaks of disease due to drinking water are uncommon in the US, they do still occur and can lead to serious acute, chronic, or sometimes fatal health consequences, particularly in those sensitive populations, such as the aged and pregnant women (Reynolds et al. 2007).

Such diseases are a major public health concern, especially in Africa. Global health statistics indicated that Africa and South Asia were the most severely affected areas by waterborne disease (WHO, 2004). In 2009, 221,226 cases of cholera were reported by 45 countries from all continents (Global Environment Outlook 5, 2012). For decades, there have been hundreds of outbreaks of waterborne diseases in China and millions of people were affected. For example, an outbreak of hepatitis taking place in the city of Shanghai, Jiangsu and Zhejiang province in the spring of 1988 affected more than 400 thousand people. In Shanghai, 31,076 hepatitis cases were reported from January to April in 1988, with an average morbidity rate of 4,082 per 100 thousand people. The pandemic of hepatitis was caused by intaking the raw scapharcasubcrenata from Qidong area of Jiangsu province, where the aquaculture water was severely polluted by the hepatitis virus.

The impacts of waterborne diseases are divided into ingestion and recreational exposures for the purposes of assessing. In US, the more common waterborne diseases that result from the ingestion of water are caused by bacteria, viruses, and parasites (Table 4–2) (Environmental Health, 3rd Edition, 2005). A typical waterborne bacteria–related disease outbreak owing to recreational exposure occurred in Illinois, US in

1998. At present, waterborne diseases have not been fully controlled, either in developed or in developing countries and are still a serious health problem (Environmental Health, 3rd Edition, 2005).

Table 4-2   Diseases transmitted through contaminated drinking water

Disease	Causative agent	Source
Bacterial infections		
Salmonellosis	Salmonella sp.	Animal and human feces
Typhoid fever	Salmonella typhi.	
Paratyphoid fever	Salmonella paratyphi-A.	
Shigellosis(bacillic dysentery)	Shigella sp.	Human feces
Cholera	Vibrio cholerae	Human feces
Leptospirosis	Leptospira sp.	Human feces
Gastroenteritis	Escherichia coli	Animal and human feces
Diarrhea	Campylobacter jejuni	Human feces
Viral infections		
Viral hepatitis	Hepatitis A	Human feces
Acute gastronenteritis	Norwalk-like virus	Human feces
Waterborne parasites		
Amebiasis(amebic dysentery)	Entamocba histolytica	Human feces
Diarrhea	Cyclospora cayetanensis	Human feces
Gastroenteritis	Cryptosporidium parvum	Animal and human feces
Giardiasis	Giardia lamblia	Animal and human feces

Note: Reproduced with permission from Environmental Health, 3rd Edition, 2005. chapter 7, p168.

4.4.2.2   Chemical pollution poisoning

Water pollutants generally include, in addition to microbial pathogens, a wide range of chemicals that may not merely be toxic in drinking water but have harmful effects on fish, clams and other wildlife. People may be poisoned as a result of consuming the fish that have accumulated these toxins in their flesh (Introduction to Public Health, 2011). Chemicals in drinking water have been a concern for decades, ranging from mercury, arsenic, and led to fluoride (preventing dental caries) and chlorine (disinfectants) (Environmental Health, 4th Edition, 2011).

The health damages caused by chemical pollution of drinking water mainly include the following aspects.

(1) Acute and chronic poisoning

Water polluted by industrial wastewater and urban sewage containing various hazardous chemicals can lead to poisoning and diseases, such as hydrogen sulfide, pesticide, mercury, phenol and PCBs poisoning via consuming contaminated water or food. Minamata disease, for example, is methylmercury poisoning that occurred in humans who ingested fish and shellfish contaminated by methylmercury (Chisso Co. Ltd.). In May 1956, Minamata disease was first officially reported in Minamata City, south-west region of Japan's Kyushu Island. The marine products in Minamata Bay displayed high levels of Hg contamination (5.61-35.7 ppm). The Hg contents in the hair of patients, their family members and inhabitants of the Shiranui Sea coastline were also detected at extremely high levels (max. 705 ppm) (Masazumi Harada, 1995). The most typical example of PCBs' harm to people is the "rice bran oil poisoning incident" in Japan in 1968.

After taking the rice bran oil contaminated with PCBs (2,000 mg/kg and 3,000 mg/kg), victims exhibited intoxication with cardinal symptoms, such as rash, pigmentation, eyelid edema, eye secretion and gastrointestinal symptoms etc. Severe cases showed serious liver damage with symptoms like jaundice and liver coma, and even death.

(2) Carcinogenesis

Some carcinogenic chemicals, such as arsenic, chromium, cadmium, nickel, benzene, nitrite, asbestos, and polycyclic aromatic hydrocarbons (PAHs) can accumulate in suspension, sediment, and aquatic organisms via contaminated water. Long-term consumption of those water or biological product with such accumulated carcinogenic chemicals may lead to cancer. For example, a large number of animal experiments have been confirmed that nitrosamine is a strong carcinogen and can cause tumors in offspring through placenta and induction. The effects of teratogenesis and mutagenesis can also be caused by nitrosamine. Epidemiological studies have shown that certain cancers, such as gastric cancer, esophageal cancer, liver cancer, colon cancer, and bladder cancer, may be related with the intake of nitrosamine.

(3) Harm of chlorinated disinfection by-products of drinking water

Chlorination of drinking water plays a key role in controlling the spread of pathogens and the epidemic of infectious diseases. Nevertheless, with the deepening of research, the problems caused by chlorine disinfection are gradually attractive. In the process of chlorination, various organic pollutants in water may react with the disinfectant to produce chlorinated disinfection by-products, such as chloroform and chloroacetic acid. There have been many epidemiological studies supporting the relationship between chlorinated disinfection by-products and human cancer, although there have been opposite views. Therefore, whether the chlorinated disinfection by-products can cause cancer remains uncertain.

4.4.2.3　Other health problems

Besides biological and chemical pollutants, there are many other reasons for the adverse health effects caused by contaminated drinking water, such as, biogeochemical diseases caused by higher or lower elements in natural water, eutrophication of lake water caused by algal and toxin pollution, and health damages caused by secondary water supply pollution of high buildings. Among them, the pollution of algae toxin to water body has been a global environmental problem and attracted more and more attention, especially the harm to human health. Cyanobacteria (blue-green algae) in eutrophic freshwater lakes are the main toxic species. Microcystin produced by microcystis aeruginosa and nodularin does the greatest harm to human health. Studies have shown that microcystin can not only cause poisoning and death of animals, but also significantly enhance the malignant transformation of cells initiated by 3-methylcholanthane and organic pollutants, activate ras oncogene, and induce the persistent high expression of early response genes c-fos and c-jun, which promote cell proliferation. These are considered to be one of the possible mechanisms of carcinogenesis of microcystin.

4.5　Standards for drinking water quality

About 80% of the world's population lives in areas with high threat of water security, and the most severe category encompassing 3.4 billion people. Although significant progress in access to improved drinking water has been achieved in many regions of the world since 1990, several regions, including most of Africa and other rural areas in developing countries, still lack access to improved drinking water sources (UNDESA 2010).

4.5.1   Guidelines for drinking water quality

The primary purpose of the guidelines for drinking water quality is the protection of public health. Recommendations in the guidelines for managing the risk are not only from hazards that may compromise the safety of drinking water but also from other sources of exposure to these hazards, such as waste, air, food and consumer products. According to WHO Guidelines for drinking-water quality, safe drinking water does not represent any significant risk to health over a lifetime of consumption, including different sensitivities that may occur across the life stages (Guidelines for Drinking-water Quality, 4th Edition, WHO, 2011).

4.5.2   Standards for drinking water quality

The development of standards for drinking water quality is based on the water security of people's lifetime. The factors that should be considered include good sensory properties, without pathogens, harmless chemicals, and radioactive substances, as well as economic and technological feasibility, etc. Different counties formulate their own standards refering to Guidelines for Drinking-water Quality, 4th Edition (WHO, 2011), which is a minimum recommended by WHO to ensure a safe water supply.

4.5.2.1   WHO standards

WHO released the fourth edition of Drinking-water Quality on July 4, 2011, calling on governments worldwide to think the priority of prevention, the intensity of drinking water quality and the risk management of drinking water contamination. The guidelines, based on WHO's 50 years of work on drinking water quality, have been updated significantly, including the guidelines for new emerging pollutants. It also made some valuable recommendations for the first time, covering factors from rainwater harvesting to storage, government decision-making, and even global climate change. Significant changes were made in this edition comparing to the previous one to clarify and elaborate on the implementation of methods to identify hazards and manage risk. This includes identifying health-based goals, developing water safety plans from the catchment area to consumers, and conducting independent monitoring. There are four parts and 12 chapters in the "guidelines", including the main consideration "principles", the framework of drinking water safety, the assurance of drinking water safety and the application of "guidelines" in special circumstances, and a specific introduction of supporting information (Guidelines for Drinking-water Quality, 4th Edition, WHO, 2011).

4.5.2.2   Chinese standards

Standards for Drinking Water Quality (GB5749-2006, China), the national current standards, cover a total of 106 enforced index and 28 reference index. The enforced index is made up of 42 items of regular indices and limitations and 64 items of non-regular indices and limitations.

Regular indices and limitations. The regular indices include sensory and general chemical index, toxicological index, radioactive index, and microbiological index. The sensory properties and general chemical indexes are mainly to ensure good sensory properties when consuming. Toxicological indexes are designed to ensure that the drinking water quality is not toxic and does no potential harm to human health. Microbiological index are designed to ensure the safety of drinking water quality in epidemiology. Comparisons of regular indices and limitations among China, America and European Union can be found in Table 4-3.

Table 4-3　Regular indices and limitations' comparison of water quality

Indexes	Limitations		
	China GB5749-2006	America MCL(MCLG)	the European Union DWD
1. Microbiological indexes			
Total coliform group(MPN/100 mL or CFU/100 mL)	Negative	5	
Thermotolerant coliforms(MPN/100 mL or CFU/100 mL)	Negative		
Escherichia coli(MPN/100 mL or CFU/100 mL)	Negative		0
Total colony(CFU/mL)	100		
2. Toxicological indexes			
Arsenic(mg/L)	0.01	0.01	0.01
Cadmium(mg/L)	0.005	0.005	0.005
Chromium(hexavalent [Cr(Ⅵ)])(mg/L)	0.05	0.1	0.05
Lead(mg/L)	0.01	0.015	0.01
Mercury(mg/L)	0.001	0.002	0.001
Selenium(mg/L)	0.01	0.05	0.01
Cyanide(mg/L)	0.05		0.05
Fluoride(mg/L)	1.0	4.0	1.5
Nitrate(calculated as N)(mg/L)	Groundwater source limit is 20	10	50
Trichloromethane(mg/L)	0.06		
Carbon tetrachloride(mg/L)	0.002	0.005	
Bromate(when using ozone, mg/L)	0.01		0.01
Formaldehyde(when using ozone, mg/L)	0.9		
Chlorite(when using chlorine dioxide to disinfect, mg/L)	0.7		
Chlorate(when using chlorine dioxide disinfection, mg/L)	0.7		
3. Sensory properties and general chemical indexes			
Chromaticity(platinum cobalt chromaticity unit)	15	15	User acceptable and no smell
Turbidity/NTU	1	N/A	User acceptable and no smell
Smell and taste	Odorless odor		User acceptable and no smell
Visible to the naked eye	Nothing		
pH	6.5-8.5	6.5-8.5	6.5-9.5
Aluminum(mg/L)	0.2	0.05-0.2	0.2
Iron(mg/L)	0.3	0.3	0.2
Manganese(mg/L)	0.1	0.05	0.05
Copper(mg/L)	1.0	1.3	2.0
Zinc(mg/L)	1.0	5	

Continue to Table 4-3

Indexes	Limitations		
	China GB5749-2006	America MCL(MCLG)	the European Union DWD
Chloride(mg/L)	250	250	250
Nitrate(mg/L)	250	250	250
Total dissolved solid(mg/L)	1,000	500	
Total hardness(with $CaCO_3$, mg/L)	450		
Oxygen consumption(calculated as O_2, mg/L)	3		5
Volatile phenols(calculated as phenol, mg/L)	0.002		
Anionic detergent(mg/L)	0.3		
4. Radioactivity index			
Total α radioactivity(Bq/L)	0.5		
Total β radioactivity(Bq/L)	1		

Non-regular indices and limitations: In addition to regular indices, Standards for Drinking Water Quality (GB5749-2006, China) also provide 64 Non-regular indices and limitations, including two microbial indices, 39 toxicological indices and 3 sensory and general chemical indices. Among them, microbial index increased the detection of microorganisms such as giardia and cryptosporidium, which are difficult to kill completely by general disinfection methods. Unlike the previous standards that were applied only to centralized drinking water supply in city, this standard can also be applied in rural areas and non-centralized way of drinking water supply. Comparisons of non-regular indices and limitations among China, America and European Union can be found in Table 4-4.

Table 4-4   Non-regular indices and limitaions' comparison of water quality

Indexes	Limitations		
	China GB574(CJ94)	America MCL(MCLG)	the European Union DWD
1. Microbiological indexes			
Giardia (PCS/10L)	< 1	0	
Cryptosporidium (PCS/10L)	< 1		
2. Toxicological indexes			
Antimony (mg/L)	0.005	0.006	0.005
Barium (mg/L)	0.7	2	
Beryllium (mg/L)	0.002	0.004	
Boron (mg/L)	0.5		1.0
Molybdenum (mg/L)	0.07		
Nickel (mg/L)	0.02		0.02
Silver (mg/L)	0.05	0.1	
Thallium (mg/L)	0.000,1	0.000,5	

Continue to Table 4－4

Indexes	Limitations		
	China GB574(CJ94)	America MCL(MCLG)	the European Union DWD
Cyanide chloride (in CN) (mg/L)	0.07		
Monochlorodibromomethane (mg/L)	0.1		
Dichloro-bromomethane (mg/L)	0.06		
Dichloroacetic acid (mg/L)	0.05		
1,2-dichloroethane (mg/L)	0.03	0.005	0.003
Dichloromethane (mg/L)	0.02	0.005	
Total trihalomethane (mg/L)	The sum of the measured values and their respective limits is less than 1	0.1	0.1
1,1,1-trichloroethane (mg/L)	2	0.2	
Trichloroacetic acid (mg/L)	0.01		
Trichloroacetaldehyde (mg/L)	0.1		
2,4,6-trichlorophenol (mg/L)	0.2		
Tribromomethane (mg/L)	0.1		
Heptachlor (mg/L)	0.000,4	0.000,4	
Malathion (mg/L)	0.25		
Pentachlorophenol (mg/L)	0.009		
Hexachlorocyclohexane (total amount) (mg/L)	0.005		
Hexachlorobenzene (mg/L)	0.001	0.001	
Dimethoate (mg/L)	0.08		
Phosphorus parathion (mg/L)	0.003		
Chloramphenicol (mg/L)	0.3		
Methyl parathion (mg/L)	0.02		
Methyl parathion (mg/L)	0.01		
Carbofuran (mg/L)	0.007	0.04	
Lindan (mg/L)	0.002	0.002	
Chlorpyrifos (mg/L)	0.03		
Glyphosate (mg/L)	0.7		
Dichlorvos (mg/L)	0.001		
Atrazine (mg/L)	0.002	0.003	
Deltamethrin (mg/L)	0.02		
2,4-D (mg/L)	0.03	0.07	
DDT (mg/L)	0.001		
Ethyl benzene (mg/L)	0.3	0.7	

Continue to Table 4−4

Indexes	Limitations		
	China GB574(CJ94)	America MCL(MCLG)	the European Union DWD
Xylene (total amount) (mg/L)	0.5	10	
1,1−dichloroethylene (mg/L)	0.03		
1,2−dichloroethylene (mg/L)	0.05	0.17	
1,2−dichlorobenzene (mg/L)	1	0.075	
1,4−dichlorobenzene (mg/L)	0.3	0.6	
Trichloroethylene (mg/L)	0.07	0	a
Trichlorobenzene (total amount) (mg/L)	0.02		
Hexachloroprene (mg/L)	0.000,6		
Acrylamide (mg/L)	0.000,5	0	0.000,1
Tetrachloroethylene (mg/L)	0.04	0.005	b (a+b⩽0.01)
Toluene (mg/L)	0.7	1	
Dimethyl phthalate (2−ethyl hexyl) ester (mg/L)	0.008	0.006	
Epichlorohydrin (mg/L)	0.000,4	0	
Benzene (mg/L)	0.01	0.005	
Styrene (mg/L)	0.02	0.1	
Benzopyrene (mg/L)	0.000,01	0.000,2	
Vinyl chloride (mg/L)	0.005		0.000,5
Chlorobenzene (mg/L)	0.3	0.1	
Microcystis toxin−LR (mg/L)	0.001		
3. Sensory properties and general chemical indexes			
Ammonia nitrogen (in N) (mg/L)	0.5		
Sulfide (mg/L)	0.02		
Sodium (mg/L)	200		

4.5.2.3 American standards

As one of the earliest countries in the world to set the standards of drinking water quality, the US has revised the standards for more than 10 times since 1914. In the 1974 Safe Drinking Water Act, the basic U. S. federal law required drinking water and its sources, such as rivers, lakes, reservoirs, springs, and ground water wells to be protected. Accordingly, the EPA has developed a series of primary standards and secondary standards. Designed to protect human health from both naturally occurring and human−made contaminants, the primary standards include maximum contaminant level goals (MCLGs) for selected inorganic contaminants, volatile organic chemicals, and radioactive materials, as well as limits for the presence of coliform organisms (Environmental Health, 4th Edition, 2011). Designed to ensure that drinking water is aesthetically pleasing in terms of temperature, color, taste, and odor, the secondary standards include limits for iron, which can discolor clothes during laundering; sulfates and dissolved solids, which can have the same effect as a laxative; and minerals that can, for example, interfere with the taste of beverages.

4.5.2.4   The European Union standards

Drinking water quality standards of the European Union (EU), also called Drinking Water Directive, set in 1980. The standards covered a total of 61 items including microbiological index, index of poisonous and harmful substances, sensory index and physiochemical index. In 1998, the EU revised its Drinking Water Directive (DWD) (98/83/EC), which concerns the quality of water intended for human consumption and is required for all the EU number states to comply with. Its objective is to protect human health from adverse effects of any contamination of water intended for human consumption by ensuring that it is wholesome and clean. In 2000, the EU passed the Water Framework Directive, an overarching piece of legislation that brings together all existing EU legislations on water resources.

4.5.3   Water quality monitoring

Water quality monitoring is the process of measuring various index data, which can reflect the environmental quality of water body. The purpose of water quality monitoring is to determine whether the environmental quality of water is consistent with the corresponding environmental quality standards and to provide basic data for rational use and protection of water resources. The possible water pollution degree, its impact on human health, and the evaluation of the practical effects of control measures can be judged by water quality monitoring, which can provide a scientific basis for formulating the pollutants discharge standard.

4.5.3.1   Types of water supply

The demand for public water is made up of authorized consumption by domestic and non-domestic consumers and water losses. Domestic consumers use water within the household for drinking, personal hygiene, cooking and cleaning, and outside the dwelling for cleaning patios, irrigating gardens, filling ponds and swimming pools, and washing cars. Non-domestic consumption comprises industrial, commercial, institutional and agricultural demand legitimately drawn from the distribution mains. This category also includes legitimate public use for irrigating public parks and green areas, street cleaning, flushing water mains and sewers, and for fire-fighting (Water Supply, 6th Edition, 2009).

No matter what kind of demand for public water, there are usually two ways for consumers to get water: central water supply and separate water supply. Water from central water supply is collected from the water source and sent to the consumers through the water pipe and water distribution network after disinfection and purification. This method is favorable for the selection and protection of water source and convenient for water consumption and supervision. However, once water quality is polluted, it is more widespread. Separate water supply is the user draws water directly from the water source without any facilities or only simple facilities, such as well water, spring water, river water, and pond water. The water quality of separate water supply is hard to be guaranteed(Figure 4-2).

4.5.3.2   Water quality monitoring methods

The range of water monitoring is extensive, including uncontaminated and contaminated natural water (river, lake, sea and groundwater) and various industrial drains. Since the latter is not the source of drinking water, it is not included in this section. Main monitoring items can be divided into two categories: one is a comprehensive index reflecting the status of water quality, such as temperature, chromaticity and turbidity, pH, conductivity, suspended solids, dissolved oxygen, chemical oxygen demand (COD), and biochemical oxygen demand (BOD), etc.; the other is toxic substances, such as phenol, cyanide, arsenic, lead, chromium, cadmium, mercury, and organic pesticides. Water quality monitoring can provide data and information for environmental management, providing a basis for assessing the quality of surface water and ground water. The rules and regulations of the spots-setting, sampling, monitoring methods, and data processing of surface/wastewater or groundwater monitoring are set according to<Technical Specifications Requirements for Monitoring of Surface Water and Waste Water> (HJ/T 91-2002, China) and<Technical Specifications for Environmental Monitoring of Groundwater> (HJ/T 164-2004, China), respectively. The specification is suitable for groundwater monitoring, but not suitable for underground hot water, mineral water, and brine.

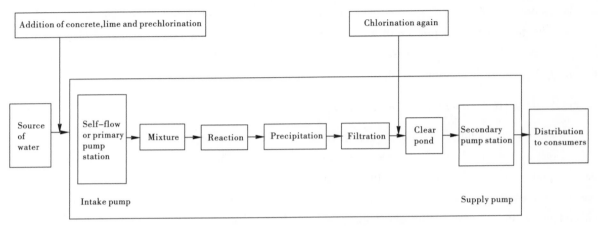

Figure 4-2　Principal steps in central water supply

4.6　Purification and treatment of water

For the protection of water, especially the sanitary condition of urban drinking water sources, a series water protection measures should be adopted. The implementation of "clearer production" and "energy conservation and emission reduction" and prevention from the source are the fundamental measures to prevent water pollution.

4.6.1　Industrial wastewater treatment

The treatment of industrial wastewater can be divided into three levels: Primary treatment to remove the floating substance and most suspended state pollutants, secondary treatment to remove the organic pollutants, and tertiary treatment to further remove the pollutants that left after the secondary treatment, including organic matter of failure microbial degradation, as well as phosphorus, nitrogen, and soluble inorganic substances. As might be anticipated, wastewater from industrial operations contain a wide range of contaminants. For this reason, treatment methods, either singly or in combination, should include physical, chemical, physical-chemical, and biological treatments(Figure 4-3).

4.6.1.1　Physical treatment

Physical treatment technology includes mechanical retention devices, oil removal tank, sedimentation tank, and membrane treatment, etc. Mechanical retention devices (such as grille, screen cloth) are used to maintain the larger suspended matter and floater resistance by the wastewater flows through the mechanical retention equipment of the pore. The oil removal tank is used to block the grease floats on the water surface by the baffle in the oil tank. There are many kinds of sedimentation tank, such as horizontal-flow, vertical-flow, and so on, which remove the suspended matter in wastewater into the sludge hopper at the bottom of the tank by gravity sedimentation. Physical treatment is generally used for primary treatment of sewage.

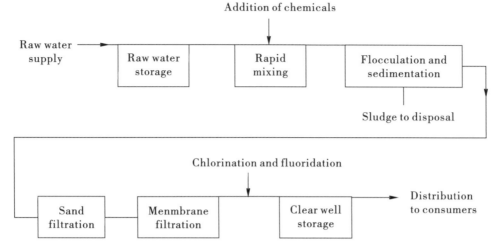

Figure 4-3   **Principal steps in the water purification process**

Note: Reproduced from Environmental Health, 4th Edition, 2011. chapter 7, p155.

4.6.1.2   Chemical treatment

Chemical treatment is used to remove dissolved or colloidal substances in industrial wastewater, including coagulation sedimentation, acid−base neutralization, oxidation reduction, and so on.

(1) Coagulation sedimentation

All the wastewater containing colloidal substances, tiny suspended solids, and emulsified oil can be treated by coagulating sedimentation using a mixed reaction tank facility.

(2) Acid−base neutralization

According to the theory of the formation of salt and water by the reaction of acid and base, acid and base wastewater are introduced into a special tank or drainage ditch to react.

(3) Oxidation reduction

To achieve the purpose of wastewater treatment, some oxidants or reducing agents are used to transform hazardous substances in wastewater into non−toxic or slightly toxic chemicals.

4.6.1.3   Physical−chemical treatment

Physical−chemical treatment is used to purify industrial wastewater through the combined action of physics and chemistry, such as adsorption, extraction, ion exchange, electro−dialysis, and other treatment technology.

(1) Adsorption method

Purify the wastewater using porous solid to adsorb pollutants in wastewater. The commonly used adsorbents include activated carbon, sulphonated coal, cinder, and so on. This method can remove organic compounds, such as phenols, benzene, synthetic dyes, petroleum and their products, which are difficult to be degraded by microorganisms or destroyed by general oxidation methods.

(2) Extraction method

Since certain dissolved substances in different liquid have different phase distribution coefficients, the industrial wastewater can be purified by isolating the pollutants from the extractant, while the extraction agent is difficult to dissolve in water, the pollutants in water can easily enter the extractant. Extraction treatment is usually used to treat wastewater containing high concentration of phenol, aniline, benzene, and acetic acid.

(3) Ion exchange method

The ion exchange is used to exchange the ion from the resin and the pollutant ion in waste water, so as to purify the industrial wastewater. This method is suitable for the recovery of heavy metals, such as mercury, cadmium, chromium, and copper in wastewater.

(4) Electrodialysis method

Electrodialysis refers to the directional process of ions migration to separate the anion and cation in the wastewater by selectively passing through ion exchange membrane under the action of electric field. Ion exchange membrane is usually made of polymer material.

4.6.1.4 Biological treatment

The organic pollutants in wastewater can be transformed into stable and harmless substances via the metabolism of microorganisms, according to which, biological treatment is divided into aerobic biological treatment and anaerobic biological treatment.

(1) Aerobic biological treatment

Organic materials containing carbon and nitrogen in wastewater can be decomposed into carbon dioxide, nitrogen, organic matter, carbon dioxide, nitrate, sulfate, and water by aerobic microorganisms, when there is sufficient dissolved oxygen in water. Aerobic biological treatment can be further divided into activated sludge process (aeration) and biofilm process. A method to purify sewage is aeration, it uses activated sludge that contains a large number of aerobic microorganisms under strong aeration conditions, which is commonly used in the treatment of wastewater from synthetic resin industry containing formaldehyde, electroplating industry of cyanide and textile printing and dyeing, wood corrosion, pesticides and other production. A method to degrade the organic substance in wastewater is called biofilm, it works by biofilm flowing on the surface of the fixed support and the microorganism. Biofilm has large surface area to adsorb many organic substances in wastewater and has strong oxidation capacity to decompose organic substances, thus to promote the purification of wastewater.

(2) Anaerobic biological treatment

The anaerobic microorganism is used to decompose organic matter under hypoxia. The products of anaerobic decomposition are methane, hydrogen sulfide, ammonia, hydrogen, and carbon dioxide. Anaerobic biological treatment is mainly used for the treatment of sludge in wastewater, and also of high concentrations of organic wastewater (such as meat, food processing plant wastewater, slaughterhouse wastewater). The sludge after anaerobic treatment is easier to dewater than the original one, it contains less pathogenic bacteria and parasite eggs, smells better, and is easy for crops to absorb nutrients.

4.6.2 Sanitary sewage treatment

The main components of domestic sewage are water and solid substance, the latter is mainly composed of cellulose, oil, protein, and its decomposition products. Domestic sewage is suitable for the reproduction of a variety of microorganisms, it often contains a large number of bacteria and pathogens (such as intestinal pathogens, parasites, and eggs). Domestic sewage usually enters the municipal wastewater treatment plant and can be discharged into the water after treatment. Its treatment methods commonly include physical treatment (grid, screen mesh, sedimentation tank, etc.) and biological treatment (activated sludge process, biological filter method), the principle and equipment of which are the same as industrial wastewater treatment. For towns without sewage treatment plants, septic tanks should be constructed outside the building to accommodate fecal, sewage, and other domestic sewage from the flush toilets.

Domestic sewage usually contains a certain amount of nitrogen, phosphorus, potassium, and other fertilizer ingredients. Under suitable natural conditions, the treated domestic sewage can be used for farmland irrigation to increase soil fertility and water content, increase crop yield, and purify sewage by biological oxidation. However, the quality of domestic sewage must meet the standards of irrigation water quality or fishery water quality (Figure 4−4).

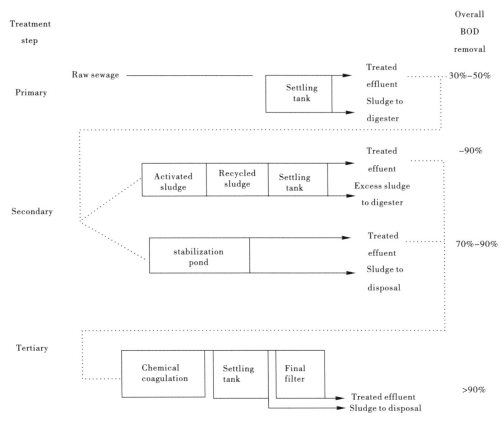

Figure 4−4   Primary, secondary, and tertiary stages in the treatment of municipal sewage

Note: Reproduced from Environmental Health, 4th Edition, 2011. chapter 8, p181.

4.6.3   Approaches to wastewater treatment

In recent years, additional technologies have been developed and applied in the purification of water not only for the efficiency of treatment but also for environmental protection. Three of these are polymer coagulants, ultraviolet radiation, and membrane filtration. UV radiation is effective against bacteria, viruses, and parasites, it is now being applied in more than 2,000 wastewater−treatment installations in the US. Since turbidity can severely reduce the effectiveness of UV radiation, it is often used to filter the sewage prior to applying the UV process (Environmental Health, 4th Edition, 2011). Membrane bioreactor technology, developed in the late 20th century, is a new technology that combines membrane separation technology and biological technology. It can improve active sludge concentration and control hydraulic retention time (HRT) and sludge retention time (SRT) respectively by using membrane separation device to activate sludge and macromolecular substance in the biochemical reaction tank. Most of the bacteria, microorganisms, heat source, the carriers of the virus can be trapped in sewage for further disinfection. Some tertiary treatment processes such as advanced oxidation and activated carbon filtration have been shown to be rather effective in micropollutant removal in drinking water, but in many cases these techniques are cost−prohibitive and not sustainable. To some extent, bioaugmentation is a viable alternative for micropollutant removal in drinking water and further studies are warranted to fill knowledge gaps and bring the concept to practical implementation (Jessica Benner et al. 2013). Magnetic separation technology, an efficient, cost-effective, high separation efficiency, non-secondary pollution, and easy operation, green and economic separation technology, also shows potential in the field of water treatment. Due to these advantages, the magnetic separation technology is being paid more and more attention in the research and application in water treatment, especially the high gradient magnetic separation (HGMS) and superconducting magnetic separation (SMS). In addition, on the basis of continuous improvement of the new type filler and equipment, research and development of high mass transfer biological packing and equipment will also improve the efficiency of biological membrane method sewage treatment process.

Zhao Ran

Chapter 5

Soil and Health

5.1　Endemic fluorosis

Endemic fluorosis is a chronic systemic disease characterized by skeletal fluorosis and dental fluorosis. This disease is mainly caused by excessive fluoride content in the environment of certain areas, and the local residents have long-term excessive fluoride intake through drinking water, food and air.

5.1.1　The epidemiological characteristics of endemic fluorosis

5.1.1.1　Type and distribution of disease areas

Endemic fluorosis is an ancient endemic disease that has beenendangering human health since ancient times. It has occurred in all regions of the world and is endemic in more than 50 countries and regions. Asia is one of the most serious areas of fluorosis, and China is one of the countries with the most widespread endemic fluorosis, the most affected population and the most serious disease. Except for Shanghai, endemic fluorosis occurs and prevails in all provinces, cities and autonomous regions of China. By the end of 2014, 28 provinces and autonomous regions exist drinking-water type disease area, 12 provinces and cities have coal-burning pollution type disease area, 7 provinces and cities, especially in minority areas have brick tea type fluorosis disease area, mainly distributed in rural areas. About 110 million people are exposed to excessive fluoride, which are distributed in 127,006 natural villages.

（1）Drinking-water type disease area

The fluorosis area caused by drinking water with high fluorine content isdrinking-water type disease area, which is main disease area. Generally, it is characterized by high fluorine content in groundwater, which is mainly affected by arid and semi-arid climate. The accumulation law of ion leaching leads to the lower fluoride content in water in mountainous areas with high terrain, and the fluorine content in water in sloping plain and plain area increases gradually, forming plain disease area. Drinking water type disease areas are mainly distributed in plain, piedmont inclined plain and basin, in the vast area to the north of Huaihe-Qinling-Kunlun mountain line, such as the western Northeast Plain, the North China Plain, the East China Plain, the Central Plains, the Hexi Corridor, Tarim Basin and Junggar basin. Thus, a vast area of fluorosis area is formed from Shandong Peninsula in the east to South Tianshan Mountain in Xinjiang in the west. In addition, some areas are affected by fluorine-bearing mineral deposits to form local high-fluoride areas such as fluorite ore or apatite ore in Zhejiang, Henan, Yunnan, Liaoning and Sichuan. Hot springs often have high fluorine content, which can cause disease if used as drinking water. This kind of disease area is mainly scattered in the northern region, and the scope of these disease areas is generally small.

Drinking-water type disease area is the most widely distributed. Its characteristic is that the fluorine content in drinking water is higher than the national drinking water standard 1.0 mg/L, and the highest is even 17 mg/L. The prevalence of fluorosis is significantly positively correlated with the fluoride content in drinking water. According to the "Twelfth-Five Year Plan" endemic disease assessment report, the population of drinking-water type disease areas is 87.28 million, and the number of patients with skeletal fluorosis is about 15.25-16.67 million in China.

(2) Coal-burning pollution type disease area

Indoor air and food are seriously polluted because residents use local coal with high fluorine content for cooking, heating, and burning coal in open stoves without chimneys, and baking grain and pepper with coal fire. Endemic fluorosis caused by inhalation of polluted air and ingesting contaminated food is a type of disease confirmed by China in 1970s. The disease areas are mainly distributed in Shananxi, Sichuan, Hubei, Guizhou, Yunnan, Hunan and Jiangxi provinces. Among them, the disease in Southwest China is the most severe, and there are also several small disease areas in the north of China. The average concentration of fluorine in coal is 80 mg/kg in worldwide, while the average concentration of fluorine in coal-burning type fluorosis areas in China is 1,590-2,158 mg/kg, the highest is 3,263 mg/kg. In these areas, the fluorine content in the indoor air is 0.018-0.039 mg/m^3, the highest is 0.5 mg/m^3. The fluorine content in corn and pepper (dry weight) roasted by coal fire reaches 84.2 mg/kg and 565 mg/kg, respectively. By the end of 2014, the population of the coal-burning pollution type fluorosis areas in China was about 32.65 million, involving 173 counties, 33,376 villages, and 8.05 million households.

(3) Drinking brick tea type disease area

Drinking brick tea type disease area is a type of fluorosis caused by drinking brick tea powder with high fluorine content for a long time. Drinking brick tea type fluorosis has been discovered in China in recent years. The fluorine content in drinking water and food is not high in the locality. In 1981, Bai Xuexin first reported fluorosis caused by drinking brick-tea for a long time in Rangtang County, Aba Tibetan Autonomous Prefecture, Sichuan Province. Drinking brick tea disease areas are mainly distributed in Inner Mongolia, Tibet, Sichuan, Qinghai, Gansu and Xinjiang and other ethnic minority areas where brick tea is used to drink, such as Tibetan, Kazak, Mongolian inhabited areas. Local residents have the habit of drinking milk tea, and the teas used for brewing milk tea is brick tea. Brick tea is the daily necessities of these nomadic minorities. There is a saying among local residents, "it is better to have no food for three days than to have no tea for one day." This kind of eating and living habits inherited for generations has created a unique fluorosis area of drinking brick tea type in the world. According to the WHO report, the average fluorine content in tea is 97 mg/kg in the world. The average fluorine content in black tea, green tea and scented tea in China is about 125 mg/kg, while that in brick tea is as high as 493 mg/kg and the highest is 1, 175 mg/kg. At present, there are 230 counties and 14,912 villages in drinking brick tea type disease area with a population of 16 million. The epidemiological characteristics are that the conditions of adults are more serious than that of children; the conditions of Tibetans are more severe than that of Mongolians; X-ray examination confirms the prevalence rate of skeletal fluorosis is higher. The National Center for Endemic Disease Control and Prevention organized experts to carry on epidemiological study on drinking brick tea type fluorosis areas. Based on the study, the hygienic standard for fluorine content of brick tea in China was put forward. And the fluorine content of brick tea should be $\leqslant$ 300mg/kg. It is estimated that there are about 10 million people drinking brick tea in China. The daily fluorine intake of adults and children in disease areas ranges from 8. 05 to 14. 77 mg, and more than 90% of fluorine comes from brick tea. The distribution of fluorosis areas in China is characterized by drinking–water type in the north and coal–burning pollution type in the south. The intersection areas are roughly at north of the Yangtze River and south of Qinling and Huaihe River. Drinking brick tea type disease areas are mainly located in the Midwest and Inner Mongolia.

5.1.1.2　Population distribution

The occurrence of endemic fluorosis is related to quantity and duration of fluorine intake, the individual 's ability to excrete fluoride, individual sensitivity to fluorine, fluorine accumulation, as well as physical growth and development. The incidence of fluorosis is associated with the exposure level to fluoride. The incubation period of skeletal fluorosis is short in patients with high fluoride content exposure. The patients with a long onset time of the patients can last as long as 10–30 years, while those in the seriously ill areas can suffer from fluorosis within 2–3 years. In drinking–water type and coal–burning pollution type disease area, the incidence of patients is not related to nationality or occupation, but mainly related to the amount of fluoride exposure, such as the living conditions and living habits of residents which can affect the intake of fluoride. Generally, Herdsmen drink more tea than farmers, so the incidence of fluorosis in Herdsmen is higher. In the coal–burning pollution type disease area, the fluorine intake of farmers is more than that of the cadres and workers who consume commodity grain, thus leading to difference in pathogenesis. In the case of drinking brick tea type fluorosis, the ethnic group who like to drink high–fluorine brick tea are more likely to suffer from the disease than those who drink less tea. Therefore, the local Han people are seldom affected by fluorosis. For dental fluorosis and skeletal fluorosis, their incidence and disease condition are positively correlated with fluoride intake. Although different types of disease may vary in severity, but this pattern is consistent. Taking drinking–water type disease area as an example, when the fluoride content in water is above 0. 5 mg/L, dental fluorosis begins to appear. At 1. 0 mg/L, the incidence rate of dental fluorosis can reach 20% –30% . When it is higher than 1. 5 mg/L, the number of dental fluorosis increases obviously. More than 10. 0 mg/L, severe skeletal fluorosis appears.

(1)Age

Endemic fluorosis is closely related to age. Dental fluorosis mainly occurs in the growing permanent teeth, and deciduous teeth generally do not develop dental fluorosis. People who move to areas with high fluoride after permanent teeth are formed do not suffer from dental fluorosis. The incidence of skeletal fluorosis is mainly in adults. With increase of age, the incidence rate of skeletal fluorosis increases, and the condition is serious.

(2)Gender

There was no significant gender difference in the incidence of endemic fluorosis. However, due to the influence ofprocreation, lactation and other factors, women´s condition is often more serious, especially prone to osteoporosis and softening, while men are mainly osteosclerosis.

(3)Residence time

After eruption of permanent teeth, dental fluorosis will not occur again in immigrants, but they are more sensitive to skeletal fluorosis than the local residents. The longer people live in the disease area, the higher prevalence of skeletal fluorosis, and the more serious the condition. In general, the onset time of immigrants from non–endemic areas was shorter than that of residents in endemic areas. People who move to the serious disease area can get sick within 1–2 years, and the condition is serious.

(4) Other factors

The occurrence of endemic fluorosis is also affected by other factors, mainly diet and nutrition factors. Protein, vitamin, calcium, selenium and antioxidants have antagonistic effects on fluorine toxicity. Under the condition of the same exposure concentration of fluoride, the prevalence of fluorosis is low and the condition is mild in the economically developed areas with good nutritional status. On the contrary, the prevalence of fluorosis is high and the disease is serious in areas with poor nutritional status, and dental fluorosis occurs even when the fluoride content in drinking water is less than 1mg/L. Secondly, the absorption of fluoride can be promoted at conditions of low calcium concentration, low hardness and high pH in drinking water. The patient's condition is generally mild in the drinking−water type disease area with high contents of calcium and iron ions in water. Climate factors affect water consumption, thus affecting the incidence of disease. In the humid area with lower temperature, the water consumption is less and the disease is light. However, in arid and hot summer Shache area, the incidence rate of dental fluorosis is more than 30% , while the fluoride content in water is only about 0.6 mg/L. There were individual differences in the incidence of fluorosis. In the same disease area, even in the same family, there are differences in incidence and non−incidence or the severity of disease.

5.1.1.3   Determination and division of the disease area

Division of endemic fluorosis areas (GB 17018−2011) stipulates the determination of endemic fluorosis areas and the division of endemic fluorosis severity in China.

(1) Determination of disease areas

1) Drinking water type disease area

The fluorine content in drinking water is more than 1.2 mg/L, and the prevalence of dental fluorosis in children aged 8−12 years old and lived in the local area is more than 30% .

2) Coal−burning pollution type disease area

Residents are used to burn coal in open stoves, and the prevalence of dental fluorosis in local children aged 8−12 years old born locally is greater than 30% .

3) Drinking brick tea type disease area

The average daily intake of fluoride in tea is more than 3.5 mg by the population over 16 years old, and there are patients with skeletal fluorosis confirmed by X−ray examination.

(2) Severity division of disease area

1) The endemic fluorosis area of drinking water type and coal−burning pollution type:

● Mild disease area: the prevalence rate of moderate or higher dental fluorosis in children aged 8−12 years old born in the local area is ≤ 20% , or X−ray examination confirms that there are mild skeletal fluorosis patients, but there are no patients with moderate or severe skeletal fluorosis.

● Moderate disease area: the prevalence rate of moderate and severe dental fluorosis in local children aged 8−12 years old is more than 20% and less than 40% , or X−ray examination confirm there are patients with moderate and severe skeletal fluorosis, but the prevalence of severe skeletal fluorosis is no more than 2% .

● Severe disease area: the prevalence rate of moderate and severe dental fluorosis in local children aged 8−12 years old was more than 40% , or the prevalence rate of severe skeletal fluorosis confirmed by X−ray examination is more than 2% .

2) The endemic fluorosis area of drinking brick tea type:

● Mild disease area: X−ray examination confirms that there is no moderate or severe skeletal fluorosis in the population aged 36 to 45 years.

• Moderate disease area: according to X-ray examination, the prevalence rate of moderate or severe skeletal fluorosis in the population aged 36-45 years is no more than 10%.

• Severe disease area: the prevalence of moderate and severe skeletal fluorosis is more than 10% in the population aged 36 to 45 years old.

5.1.2 Preventive measures and treatment principles

The etiology of endemic fluorosis is clear, mainly due to excessive intake of fluoride, and is also related to the specific natural geological environment and bad living habits. Therefore, the fundamental preventive measure of endemic fluorosis is to reduce the intake of fluoride. Since 1978, China has invested a large amount of money to improve water in endemic fluorosis areas. By the end of 2010, the improvement rate of water quality in endemic villages reached 81. 89%; In coal-burning endemic fluorosis areas, 7. 42 million stoves were improved and the improvement rate was 92. 60%; The detection rate of dental fluorosis in children dropped from 65. 5% in 2004 to 49. 5% in whole China. The prevention and treatment effect are obvious. However, the operation of water defluoridation projects and the use of improved stoves are not optimistic. According to the survey data, the qualified rate of fluoride content in water of the national defluoridation and water improvement project in 2011 was 79. 26%. In 2012, the qualified rate of the improved furnace in the national monitoring points of coal-burning pollution type endemic fluorosis was 87. 81%. Therefore, the prevention and control of endemic fluorosis in China still needs to be strengthened, and the preventive measures such as improving water and changing stoves should be further implemented.

5.1.2.1 Drinking water type endemic fluorosis

(1)Changing water source

If the water source with low fluorine content can be used in the disease area, the water source should be changed first. ① In most arid areas of China, the fluorine content in shallow groundwater is high, while that in the deep groundwater is low. Therefore, the deep groundwater is suitable for drinking and meets the requirements of disease prevention. ② Introducing surface water with low fluorine content: the surface water such as rivers, lakes and springs near the disease area is introduced into the disease area as water source. ③ Collecting precipitation: in water deficient areas, small reservoirs or water cellars are built to store natural precipitation.

(2)Defluorination of drinking water

This method is applicable to the disease area without low-fluoride water source. Physical and chemical methods are used to reduce fluoride content. These methods include electrodialysis, reverse osmosis, activated alumina adsorption, aluminum salt or phosphate coagulation precipitation, bone carbon adsorption and so on. In areas where the fluorine content in drinking water is not high, measures should be taken to reduce the fluorine content in food. In areas with high fluorine content, crops with low fluorine content are selected to be planted, while fertilizers (such as Phosphate Rock) and pesticides (such as Fluoroamide) with high fluorine content are avoided.

5.1.2.2 Coal-burning pollution type fluorosis

(1)Improve the stove

The backward coal burning methods are transformed. The stove should have a good furnace structure and be equipped with smoke exhaust facilities to discharge fluorine-containing smoke and dust out of the room.

(2)Reduce food fluoride pollution

Food should be prevented from being polluted by fluorine. The preservation method of baked corn and peppers should be changed. The grain can be dried under natural conditions or on heated Kang. Direct contact of smoke with food should be avoided.

(3) No or less use of high fluorine coal

Fuel should be replaced or coal consumptionshould be reduced to minimize the fluorine content in the air.

5.1.2.3 Drinking brick tea type fluorosis

New brick tea with low fluorine content should be developed, and the content of fluorine in present brick tea should be reduced. And other kinds of low fluorine tea species should be afforded to replace brick tea in the fluorosis areas.

5.1.3 Treatment principles

At present, there is no specific treatment for endemic fluorosis. The principle of treatment is to reduce the intake and absorption of fluoride, promote the excretion of fluoride, antagonize the toxicity of fluoride, enhance the body resistance andtreat symptom appropriately.

5.1.3.1 Adjust diet reasonably and promote balanced diet

The nutritional status of patients should be strengthened and improved, which can enhance the body´s resistance and reduce the original condition. A diet rich in protein, calcium, magnesium and vitamins is advocated, and food should contain enough calories. Special attention should be paid to the nutritional supplement of children and pregnant women. High calcium, protein and vitamin A, vitamin C and vitamin D in diet are particularly important.

5.1.3.2 Drug therapy

Calcium and vitamin D, aluminium hydroxide gel, serpentine, etc. can be used for treatment. The patients with nerve injury should be given B vitamins (vitamin B_1, vitamin B_6 and vitamin B_{12}), adenosine triphosphate and coenzyme A to improve the normal metabolism of nerve cells and reduce the toxic effect of fluoride.

5.1.3.3 Dental fluorosis treatment

The treatment of dental fluorosis can be treated by coating method, drug decolorization method (hydrogen peroxide or dilute hydrochloric acid, etc.) and restoration method. The fluoride toothpaste also has a certaincurative effect.

5.1.3.4 Others

Patients with skeletal fluorosis who have spinal stenosis and compression of spinal cord or cauda equina should undergo laminectomy. For severe deformities, orthopedic surgery can be performed. The symptomatic treatment of skeletal fluorosis is mainly to relieve pain. Sedatives can be given to patients with symptoms such as numbness of hands and feet, convulsion.

5.2 Iodine deficiency disease

Iodine is an essential microelement for human beings, and its insufficient intake is harmful to health. Different levels of iodine deficiency are related to the degree of insufficiency of iodine intake, the period of occurrence and duration. However, excessive intake of iodine also has adverse effect on health, such as iodine-induced goiter and iodine poisoning.

Iodine deficiency diseases (IDD) refer to a series of diseases caused by deficiency of iodine intake in all life cycle, including endemic goiter, endemic cretinism, endemic subclinical cretinism, miscarriage, premature birth, stillbirth, etc. These forms of diseases are caused by iodine deficiency at different stages of human development, while goiter and cretinism are the most obvious manifestations of iodine deficiency disorders.

5.2.1   The epidemiological characteristics of iodine deficiency disease

5.2.1.1   Common characteristics

IDD is a worldwide endemic disease which is found in 110 countries around the world. There are about 2.2 billion people living in the areas suffering from IDD. China was one of the most serious iodine-deficiency epidemic countries in the world. Before taking the intervention measure of iodized salt, IDD existed all over in China except Shanghai. According to the statistical data in 1970s, there were 374 million people lived in the areas of endemic iodine deficiency, and nearly 35 million people suffered from endemic goiter and about 250,000 people with endemic cretinism in China. In 1979, comprehensive prevention and control measures with iodized salt were implemented in some serious iodine deficiency areas. By 1993, the case numbers of endemic goiter and cretinism had been reduced to about 8 million and about 180,000 respectively in China.

According to the survey, soil, water quality and weather conditions have an important impact on the prevalence of iodine deficiency disorders. The prevalence of IDD has geographical distribution features. The prevalence is higher in mountainous areas than that in the plain areas, higher in the inland than that in the coastal area, and higher in the countryside than that in the city.

5.2.1.2   Regional distribution of IDD

Obvious regional distribution is the main characteristic of the disease. The main epidemics are the areas far from the sea, especially the mountain and hilly ground. In the plains and coastal areas, cases are scattered. In the past, there was a varying degree of popularity around the world except Iceland. The Himalayan region of Asia, the Andean mountains in Latin America, and the Congo river basin in Africa are all well-known serious endemic areas. Common features of the endemic zones in the mountain areas include topographical slopes, severe flooding, concentrated rainfall, severe water erosion, and minimal iodine content. In addition to the mountains, some hilly ground and plain areas also have varying degrees of popularity.

5.2.1.3   Population distribution

People could suffer IDD at all age stages in the endemic area. The age of onset is generally in adolescence and earlier in girls than in boys. The earlier the IDD, the more severe the IDD. The prevalence of adults is higher in women than that in men, but there is no obvious gender difference in severe epidemic areas. The prevalence rates from severe to mild disease are 1:1 to 1:8 in men and women.

5.2.1.4   Time trends

The epidemic situation of iodine deficiency disease can be changed rapidly after iodine intervention. From 1995 to 2005, national monitoring of IDD showed that endemic goiter rates of children were 20.4% (1995), 10.9% (1997), 8.8% (1999), 5.8% (2002) and 5.0% (2005) respectively, and has dropped dramatically in China.

5.2.2   Factors affecting the prevalence of iodine deficiency diseases

5.2.2.1   Natural geographical factors

The level of iodine in the environment is affected by many factors such as topography, climate, soil, hydrology, vegetation, etc. So far from the ocean, steep mountains, barren land, sparse vegetation, concentrated rainfall and erosion of soil and water have extremely close relationship with the popularity of iodine deficiency disorders.

5.2.2.2 Iodine content in environment

The iodine needed by the body comes from food, soil and water in the environment. The iodine in the soil is absorbed by the plant which is then ingested by the human body. Iodine content in water not only reflects the level of iodine in the environment, but also reflects the level of iodine in human body, which is closely related to the prevalence of iodine deficiency disease.

5.2.2.3 Synergistic effect

Goitrogen is widespread in the environment, but usually does not cause goiter, because of its low content. However, if the environment is severely deficient in iodine and has high levels of goitrogen, the two factors can have a powerful synergistic effect, which is the main reason for the formation of serious goiter.

5.2.2.4 State of the economy

Nowadays, the endemic goiter is mainly distributed in developing countries, and the poorer the country, the more popular. Also, the poorer the families, the higher incidence rate. Most of the endemic areas are in remote mountainous areas and rural areas, where transportation is inconvenient and the economy is underdeveloped. Once the traffic conditions are improved, material exchanges are frequent and living standards are improved, the epidemic will be alleviated even without preventive measures such as introducing of iodized salt.

5.2.2.5 Malnutrition

Protein and energy malnutrition and vitamin deficiency could exacerbate iodine deficiency and the effect of goitrogen, promoting the prevalence of endemic goiter.

5.2.3 Criteria for definition of endemic area

The delimitation for the endemic areas of iodine deficiency diseases in China (GB 16005−2009) gives the determining criteria: ①The median concentration of water iodine is less than 10 μg/L. ②The median urine iodine concentration in children between 8 to 10 years old was is less than 100 μg/L and more than 20% of the samples have the median concentration less than 50μg/L. ③The thyroid enlargement rate of children between 8 to 10 is more than 5%. Fulfilled with all of the three indicators, it could be defined as IDD endemic area. In areas where iodized salt or other control measures have been taken, with the first and third indicators, it could be judged as IDD endemic area.

5.2.4 Prevention measures and treatment principles

5.2.4.1 Preventive measures

One of the most widely distributed and harmful endemic diseases is IDD in China, and the essential measure to prevent IDD is iodine supplementation. As early as 1956, the state made specific provisions on the prevention and treatment of endemic goiter. Since 1979, the comprehensive control measures of iodized salt have been implemented. In 1996, the comprehensive prevention and control measures for iodized salt were fully implemented in China. In 2000, China has basically achieved its phased goal of eliminating iodine deficiency disorders. The fifth national surveillance of iodine deficiency disorders in 2005 showed that the elimination of iodine deficiency disorders in China has entered the ranks of the most advanced countries in the world. The results of monitoring of the national iodine deficiency disorders in 2011 proved that China has achieved remarkable results in prevention and treatment of iodine deficiency disorders at the national level. However, at present, three provinces or autonomous regions (Tibet, Qinghai, and Xinjiang) have not yet achieved the goal of eliminating IDD. In particular, some crude salt-producing areas, ethnic minority areas and impoverished mountainous areas are still affected by the natural environment, economy, culture and life customs and other factors. The coverage of iodized salt has been low in the long term, and endemic cases have been reported in local these areas. The lack of iodine in the natural environment is an constant fact. Long-term iodine supplementation is the only effective way to continuously improve the iodine nutritional status of the population living in these areas.

(1) The preferred method for preventing iodine deficiency

It has been proved that iodized salt is the most reliable and effective measure, which is more convenient, economical and reliable than other methods, and cannot be replaced by other methods. According to the implementation experience of countries with universal salt iodization, the iodine nutrition of general population after taking iodized salt (the original actual daily iodine intake increased by 150 ~200 μg per day) will not have any adverse impact on health (except for people living in high iodine areas, even with thyroid diseases). National salt iodization is the best measure to eliminate iodine deficiency disorders, but in the past practice, it was found that the patient with a chronic deficiency presented certain side effects after the rapid or excessive intake of iodine, e. g. , elevated incidences of hyperthyroidism and autoimmune thyroid disease.

Considering the vast area of China, a large population, the difference of the iodine absorbed by the body, the economic levels of different regions, diets and habits, From March 2012, China began to implement the prevention and control strategy of 'local conditions, classified guidance, scientific iodine supplement'. Iodized salt is made of a large amount of salt mixed with a small amount of iodide (potassium iodide or potassium iodate). The WHO recommends the proportion of iodine adding to salt is one in 10,000. China's national standard for edible iodized salt content (GB 26878−2011) stipulates that after adding iodine to table salt, the iodine content (in terms of iodine) in the fortified salt products (iodized salt) is 20 ~30 mg/kg, with an average allowable range of +/−30%. Based on the actual level of iodine nutrition in the local population, the departments of health in all provinces, autonomous regions and municipalities directly under the Central Government should select the average level of iodine content suitable for the local conditions according to Table 5−1.

Table 5−1　Iodine content in iodized table salt

Ordinal number	The iodine levelto be selected (mg/kg)	Allowable iodine content range (mg/kg)
1	20	14−26
2	25	18−33
3	30	21−39

In order to prevent iodine loss, iodized salt should bekept dry and well protected. Pregnant women have a high demand for iodine, and the state of pregnancy has two effects on iodine metabolism in the body: ①Higher glomerular filtration rate and the higher urinary iodine excretion. ②The thyroid hormone synthesized by the fetus increases the demand for iodine. In addition, the intake of iodized salt during pregnancy is usually limited, so women's demand for iodine increases by 40% to 50% during pregnancy. The severe iodine deficiency can result in a series of serious consequences such as fetal neurodysplasia.

(2) Iodine oil made from vegetable oil and iodine compounds can be used as a substitute for unsupplied iodized salt in some remote areas. The infants under 12 months of age could receive 0. 5ml (237 μg)

of injection and individuals aged between 1 to 45 year old could be injected with 1. 0 ml. Follow up for 6 to 12 months and observe the hypothyroidism or hyperthyroidism for every three years. The dose of oral iodine oil is usually about 1. 5 times of the injection dose, which is repeated every two years. Although iodized oil is an effective way to prevent iodine deficiency, it cannot replace iodized salt. In the absence of the iodized salt, the iodine oil should be introduced.

(3)Other ways to provide iodine including iodine fortified bread, iodized drinking water, iodine−rich sea foods and so on. It is important to pay attention to the particularity of high iodine when carrying out the universal iodine. Use iodized salt and iodine oil should be moderate, if dosage is too high, iodine poisoning or high iodine induced goiter might be the consequence. The iodized salt should not be supplied to the population in high iodine area. The prevention of high iodized goiter is to remove the high iodine source and reduce the amount of iodine to the normal amount of iodine. The drinking water with high iodine can be replaced by the normal iodine drinking water. The epidemic area of iodine−deficient goiter should be further investigated for the prevention of specific causes. If the water source is polluted, pollution should be eliminated and water quality should be improved. If the water is not deficient in iodine, but its hardness is too high, the source of soft water or boiled water should be selected.

5.2.4.2　Principles of treatment

(1)Endemic goiter

Generally speaking, in iodine deficiency area, goiter with I and II degrees will get better without special treatment as long as iodine supplement persists.

1)Thyroid hormone therapy——In the case of the treatment of iodine, it is suspected that the hormone therapy can be used to promote the recovery of swollen glands. Thyroid tablets, l–t3 (a), l–t4 and other treatments can be used.

2)Surgical therapy——Patients with III degree nodular goiter, especially those with oppression symptoms or suspected cancer, may undergo surgery to remove enlarged thyroid tissue.

(2)Endemic cretinism

The earlier treatment of mucous edema is, the better treatment effect is. Once the treatment is implemented, it can control the development of the disease, reduce or avoid the neurological and intellectual damage later. The ideal therapeutic effect can be quickly received with a moderate dose of thyroid hormone, and a timely 'replacement therapy'. Varieties of vitamins such as vitamin A, vitamin D, vitamin B_1, vitamin B_2, vitamin B_6, vitamin C, other elements such as calcium, magnesium, zinc, iron, phosphorus, etc. , and other drugs such as ganoderma lucidum and other traditional Chinese medicines (TCM) could be used as the adjuvant treatment. Meanwhile, patients should keep a good nutritional status, improve their intelligence, receive live training and education, so that they could polish up their physical capacity, intelligence, and survival ability.

The fifth national survey of iodine deficiency disorders showed that the rate of thyromegaly in children was dropped from 20. 4% in 1995 to 5. 0% in 2005. By the end of 2010, China has achieved the goal of eliminating IDD in most provinces except Tibet, Xinjiang, and Qinghai.

Huang Bo

5.3   Soil pollution

5.3.1   Introduction

The thin layer of material that covers the earth's surface is known as soil. On the average, soil consists of 45% mineral, 25% water, 25% air, and 5% organic matter. Mature soils are arranged in a series of zones or soil horizons. A cross—sectional view of the horizons in a soil is soil profile (Figure 5–1). The top layer (or O horizon) and the topsoil layer (or A horizon) teem with bacteria, fungi, earthworms, and small insects that interact in complex food webs. The productive topsoil consists mostly of partially decomposed organic matter, called humus, and some inorganic mineral particles. The topsoil layer that covers much of the earth's terrestrial surface is the foundation of civilization. B horizon called as subsoil that is usually lighter in color, dense and low in organic matter. The layer of transition (C horizon) is almost completely void of organic matter and is made up of partially weathered parent material.

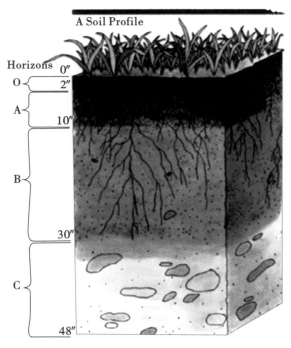

Figure 5–1   **The soil profile**

O horizon is organic layer andconsists of leaf litter and other organic material lying on the surface of the soil. A horizon is usually loose and crumbly with varying amounts of organic matter. B horizon is subsoils layer and C horizon is transition layer (Miller GT. Living in the Environment, 13th Edition).

Soils can have a beneficial or adverse effect on human health; likewise, human activity can improve or harm soil health. Both soil and humans must be in a state of well—being with respect to their physical, chemical, and biological characteristics. In the new anthropogenic era, several strategies have been suggested to improve human health by maintaining or improving soil health. Soil pollution is defined as the presence of toxic chemicals (pollutants or contaminants) from anthropogenic sources in soil, high enough concentrations pose a risk to human health and/or the ecosystem.

Soil pollution is an alarming issue. It has been identified as the third most important threat to soil functions in Europe and Eurasia, fourth in North Africa, fifth in Asia, seventh in the Northwest Pacific, eighth in North America, and ninth in sub-Saharan Africa and Latin America (FAO and ITPS, 2015). National attempts to estimate the extent of soil pollution have been undertaken mainly in developed countries. There are also approximately 3 million potentially polluted sites in the European Economic Area and cooperating countries in the West Balkans (EEA-39) (EEA, 2014) and more than 1,300 polluted or contaminated sites in the United States of America (USA) are included on the Superfund National Priorities List (US EPA, 2013). The total number of contaminated sites is estimated at 80,000 across Australia (DECA, 2010). According to the Chinese Environmental Protection Ministry, 16% of all Chinese soils and 19% of its agricultural soils are categorized as polluted (CCICED, 2015). In low-and middle income countries, the lack of data and information makes one of the world's biggest global problems invisible to the international community. It is evident that there is an urgent need to implement a global assessment of soil pollution (FAO, 2018).

5.3.1.1　Environmental background value

Trace elements in soils result from the weathering of rocks and minerals in the parent material of the soil. Soil environmental background value means the natural range in the concentration of an element that can be expected prior to contamination through human activity. This describes an ideal situation that almost no longer exists in most countries. This term can also be defined as the normal abundance of an element in barren earth material or a theoretical natural concentration of a substance in a specific environmental sample. Environmental background value for relevant soils is valuable and very important for establishing soil contamination criteria and health risk assessment of soil pollution.

5.3.1.2　Environmental capacity

The soil environmental capacity on pollutants is the maximum pollution acceptable capacity in a unit of soil within a limited time. It refers to the limit values of soil pollutants while maintaining the normal structure and function of the bio-and eco-system of soil, ensuring biological yield and quality of agricultural products without environmental pollution.

5.3.2　Source of soil pollution

There are two mainsources through which soil pollution is generated: anthropogenic sources and natural sources. Artificial contaminants are the main source of soil pollution and consist of a large variety of contaminants or chemicals, both organic and inorganic. Artificial soil pollution is usually caused by the improper disposal of waste from industrial or urban sources, industrial activities, and agricultural pesticides. Natural processes can also lead to an accumulation of toxic chemicals in the soil, however this type of pollution is recorded only in a few cases. Artificial soil pollution can occur either alone or in combination with natural soil contaminations.

Pollutants can get into the soil through different ways, for example, from the atmosphere with precipitation water, by wind or other types of soil disturbances, and from surface water bodies and shallow groundwater. In general, soil environment can be polluted through the following three common ways.

5.3.2.1　Deposition of air pollutants

Casting and manufacturing processes, including furnaces or other processes and construction activities may result in the dispersion of contaminants in the air; and transportation activities may release toxic vehicle emissions. All of these air pollutants may freely settle down or accompany with rain to contaminate the soil. This pollution is characterized by a circular or zonal distribution in the center of air pollution, and elongating along the main wind direction. The radius of contamination can reach 5−10 km or even further, mainly concentrated in the soil surface layer.

5.3.2.2 Irrigation of polluted water

Soil can also be polluted by water pollutants, such as waste water irrigation, industrial waste water, and domestic sewage. For instance, water body used for irrigation was contaminated by chemical waste dumping, either accidental or illegal dumps. This pollution is characterized by spreading from the surface to the deeper part of the soil, even reaching the depth of groundwater along the river or branch channels.

5.3.2.3 Solid wastes

Mining activities involving crushing and processing of raw materials emit toxic substances in soil. For the storage of waste in landfills, the waste products may leak into groundwater or generate toxic vapors. Other similar soil pollution includes agricultural activities involving diffusion of herbicides, pesticides and fertilizers, or accidental spills and leaks during storage. This kind of soil pollution is relatively limited and fixed, although some of them can be migrated further through diffusion and eluviation.

5.3.3 Main soil pollutants and their health effects

Heavy metals, such as lead (Pb), cadmium (Cd), mercury (Hg), chromium (Cr), copper (Cu), zinc (Zn) and nickel (Ni), refer to those metals with densities greater than 5 g/cm^3. Due to similarities in chemical properties and environmental behavior, metalloid arsenic (As) often falls into the heavy metal category. Heavy metal pollution pervaded many parts of the world, especially in China due to rapid urbanization and industrial development. The national survey that covers 6.3×10^6 km^2 land soil from 2005 to 2013 across China showed that 19.40% of the soil samples in the investigated farmland were polluted and the main pollutants were heavy metals (Bulletin of National Soil Pollution Survey, 2014).

The dominant sources of soil heavy metal pollution are mining, smelting operations, plating, battery manufacturing, sewage irrigation, and sludge application. The oral ingestion of heavy metals via soil−crop systems has been widely studied and considered as the predominant pathway for human exposure to soil heavy metals. Elevated concentrations of heavy metals in soil may not only result in potential environmental impacts on soil, water, air, and organisms, but also directly and in directly affect humans. At the same time, heavy metal pollutants in urban soils can be easily transferred into humans through non−dietary ingestion, inhalation, or dermal contact. Due to their high toxicity and persistence existence in the environment, lead (Pb), mercury (Hg), cadmium (Cd), chromium (Cr) and arsenic (As) are commonly considered as the priority heavy metals which should be controlled in China. Exposure to excess heavy metals may affect the digestive system, neurological system, cardiovascular system and immune system, or increase cancer risk in human. More detailed epidemiological studies on the potential risks of heavy metals are warranted.

5.3.3.1 Cadmium

Cadmium pollution in agricultural soils may be caused by the deposition of airborne cadmium particles, application of the cadmium content of phosphate fertilizers, and sewage sludge used for fertilization. Many crops, such as rice and tobacco leaves, can retain relatively high cadmium levels from the polluted soil. The average total daily intake of cadmium via food ranges from less than 10 to more than 50 μg/d according to different dietary habits.

About 2%−10% of oral intake of cadmium is transferred to the bloodstream. Metallothionein is induced by liver binds cadmium. When released to the blood, the complex is subsequently excreted through the kidney glomeruli, then mostly reabsorbed by the tubulus cells, and finally accumulated in the kidney cortex. The biological half-life of cadmium is 10-20 years; therefore, the accumulation in the body seems to continue during the major part of the life. The liver is the main storage organ for cadmium in the body, but the highest concentration of cadmium is eventually accumulated in the kidneys. In general, about one-half of the cadmium burden is located in liver and kidneys.

Acute cadmium poisoning most frequently occurs after inhalation of cadmium fume. After a latency of a few hours, the first symptoms may suggest metal fume fever, and then be followed by toxic pneumonitis. Recovery is often slow and may take months. After acute cadmium pneumonitis, progressive pulmonary fibrosis has been observed several years later. Oral cadmium exposure may cause acute poisoning too.

The chronic form of cadmium poisoning is a result of long-term accumulation in the body, where the kidney is the target organ. More details about chronic cadmium poisoning see "Itai-itai disease" in the next section. Long-term inhalation of cadmium can lead to emphysema, which may also be of importance in regard to cadmium retention in the lungs of smokers. Experimental animal studies showed that pulmonary exposure to cadmium compounds may cause lung cancer, and epidemiological evidence on cancer of the lung, prostate, and kidneys has confirmed that cadmium should be regarded as a carcinogenic metal. Additional animal experiments also suggested that this metal may be a teratogen.

5.3.3.2 Arsenic

Major sources of environmental arsenic pollution are primary metal smelters and coal burning. Dissolved arsenic compounds in groundwater can cause severe exposures, especially in certain parts of South America, West Bengal, and Taiwan in China. Easily soluble arsenic compounds may be absorbed rather efficiently through the respiratory and gastrointestinal tracts. As (V) seems to be partially converted to As (III). When exposure to inorganic arsenic compounds, after methylation in the liver, the methylated arsenic species are the main part of the urinary arsenic excretion. The average biological half-life for inorganic arsenic in the body is about four days. After an acute exposure to inorganic arsenic, the arsenic excretion in urine increases for a week or more. An additional, somewhat slower excretion occurs through hairs, nails, and skin cells. Both skin and lungs may constitute a "slow" arsenic compartment with a long biological half-time.

Acute intoxication due to ingestion of arsenic trioxide or lead arsenate first causes vomiting, colics, and diarrhea, followed by fever, cardiotoxicity, peripheral edema, and shock, which can lead to death within 12-48 hours. Patients who survive after an acute intoxication usually exhibit anemia and leukopenia and may experience peripheral nervous damage 1-2 weeks later. Late effects include loss of hair and nail deformities. Recovery from peripheral neurotoxicity is slow and may take several months.

Under chronic exposure conditions, neuropathy, mainly of sensorimotor type, may develop and cause neuralgic pain and paresthesia in the extremities, muscle weakness, especially in the fingers, and motor in coordination may also occur. These effects may occur as a late result of an acute exposure or a result of a long-term exposure to arsenic, where chronic skin symptoms may occur at the same time. Chronic skin symptoms include chronic eczema, hyperpigmentation of the skin, and hyperkeratosis, especially on foot soles and palms. Development of skin cancer may be seen later. For example squamous cell carcinomas mostly at the hyperkeratosis on the extremities, and basal cell carcinomas can be in any region. Vascular effects may result in Raynaud's phenomenon, acrocyanosis, and necrosis (Blackfoot disease). Some epidemiological studies in Chile and Argentina have shown increased incidences of bladder and lung cancers. In most studies, the exposures were mixed, thus the effects of As(III) and As(V) cannot be separated. Teratogenic effects of arsenic have also been reported.

5.3.3.3　Chromium

Chromium most commonly occurs as trivalent compounds. Divalent compounds are rather unstable, and hexavalent chromates are reduced to trivalent compounds in the presence of oxidizing substances. Soluble chromates likely predominate in food and drinking water. The gastrointestinal uptake of Cr(VI) is only a few percent, and the absorption of Cr(III) is even less. Organic complexes of chromium may be more easily absorbed. The fate of inhaled chromium particles and the transfer within the body depend on the particle size and solubility of the compounds. Excretion is mainly via the urine.

Chromium is an essential trace metal (as glucose tolerance factor) for humans. Glucose intolerance, weight loss, and peripheral neuropathy in patients undergoing long-term intravenous nutrition may be cured by Cr(III) supplements. Because of the different solubility, the toxicity of the chromium compounds varies. Trivalent chromium is less toxic, apparently due to the lower solubility and lower biological mobility. The major toxicity of chromium includes corrosion of skin and mucous membranes, allergic responses, and carcinogenicity. Long-term inhalation of Cr(VI) compounds in chromium-plating workshops has caused severe corrosion of the nasal mucous membranes with defects in the nasal septum in the past. These effects are now rarely seen. Chromate may cause circumscribed ulcers (chrome holes) at the knuckles, nail roots, or other exposed skin areas. Chromate is the most common cause of allergic contact dermatitis among males and has also been identified as a cause of asthma, probably mediated by a type I allergic reaction. Chromium is a well-documented human carcinogen, and occupational exposures resulting from the production of ferrochrome and of chromates have caused an increased frequency of cancer in the respiratory tract. Although trivalent chromium compounds may be involved in the carcinogenesis, exposure to such compounds has not been shown to cause cancer in epidemiological studies.

5.3.3.4　Thallium

Thallium has important uses in various industrial processes. Environmental thallium pollution occurs near mines and refineries because zinc, cadmium, and copper ores usually contain thallium. Cement production and coal burning also cause thallium emissions. Thallium compounds are tasteless and odorless. The lethal doses of thallium may be less than 1 g. Gastrointestinal absorption is almost complete, and uptake through the skin can also lead to several cases of intoxication. Excretion is mainly via the intestine and the kidney. The slow excretion takes place through hair and nails, which may provide a profile of recent thallium levels in the body. When an acute poisoning occurs, acute gastrointestinal effects are followed by peripheral neuropathy with muscle weakness and "burning feet syndrome" within a few days. The associated mental disturbances include irritability, concentration difficulties, and somnolence. Hair loss (alopecia) occurs about 1-3 weeks after the acute exposure. Thus, the characteristic triad, gastroenteritis, polyneuropathy, and hair loss are seen only at a rather late stage of the intoxication. In survivors of severe poisoning, some nervous system damages may remain after recovery. A large-scale study of the Germany residents near a thallium-polluting cement factory found that elevated urine-thallium concentrations were associated with polyneuritic symptoms, sleep disorders, headache, fatigue, and other nonspecific symptoms.

Minimization and elimination of heavy metals pollution are far more desirable compared to other pollution control strategies. These aims could be achieved by reducing the use of heavy metal-containing items or recycling them before discharging into environment.

5.3.3.5　Pesticides

Pesticides are chemicals used to kill unwanted pests that may diminish crops or affect human life. Pesticides are global contaminants found in air, rain, snow, soil, surface and groundwater, fog, and even in the Arctic ice pack. Common types of pesticides include insecticides (insect killers, e. g. , ants, aphids, beetles, bugs, caterpillars, cockroaches, mosquitoes, and termites), herbicides (weed killers, e. g. , weeds, grasses, algae, and woody plants), fungicides (fungus killers, e. g. , mildew, molds, rot, and plant diseases), nematocides (round worm killers), and rodenticides (rats and mouse killers). The EPA (Environmental Protection Agency) estimates that 84% of U. S. homes use pesticide products, such as bait boxes, pest strips, bug bombs, flea collars, pesticide pet shampoos, and weed killers for lawns and gardens.

Pesticides can be inhaled, ingested through food, water, or direct skin contact. Depending on the length of exposure and the concentration of the pollutants, they cause serious health concerns, particularly for children, but also for adults. Exposure to pesticides can trigger or exacerbate asthma, induce bronchospasm, or increase bronchial hyperreactivity. At high doses, certain pesticides can act as airway irritants. Low levels are insufficient to cause acute poisoning, but can trigger severe reactions in those without a previous diagnosis of asthma. Each year, more than 250,000 people in the United States become ill because of household pesticide use, and such pesticides are major source of accidental poisonings and deaths for children under age 5.

Besides, scientists are becoming increasingly concerned about the following possible harm of pesticide: genetic mutations, birth defects, nervous system disorders (especially behavioral disorders, e. g. , Parkinson disease), and negative effects on the immune and endocrine systems from long-term exposure to low levels of various pesticides. Many pesticides can be considered as potential endocrine disruptors based on animal findings. Questions have been raised about the relevance of the findings in wildlife to human populations. However human studies have conflicting findings in the role of pesticides attributed to endocrine disruptors, such as decreasing quantity and quality of sperm, increasing incidence of breast and prostate cancer, cryptorchidism and hypospadias. Epidemiological studies in populations with occupational and environmental exposure to pesticides showed increased risk of cancer, birth defects, adverse effects on reproduction and fertility, as well as neurological damage. Pesticide use in the home has consistently shown the increased risk of several childhood cancers in the United States and other countries. In conclusion, the possible toxicity of pesticides includes birth defects, endocrine disruption, reproductive problems, leukemia and other cancers, as well as diseases of the nervous and immune system.

5.3.3.6 Persistent organic pollutants

Persistent organic pollutants (POPs) are organic compounds that are resistant to environmental degradation through chemical, biological, and photolytic processes. A great concern has been drawn globally due to their persistent, bioaccumulative, high toxic nature and their propensity to travel long distances to affect even remote and uninhabited parts of the globe. POPs have diverse physical-chemical properties and are released in the environment from varied sources. Although some POPs arise naturally, most of them are synthetic. Many POPs are used as pesticides, solvents, pharmaceuticals, and industrial chemicals.

POPs may be deposited far from their sources because of their resistance in environment, leading to bioaccumulation through the food web. Concentrations of POPs can become higher and higher by bioaccumulation as they move up through the marine food chain and accumulate in the fatty tissues of living organisms at higher trophic levels. Marine mammals are found usually carrying high burdens of POPs worldwide. POPs can disrupt the endocrine, reproductive, and immune systems of human being. The developing nervous system and brain are most vulnerable, thus children are most susceptible to POPs from airborne dust, soil and food. Behavioral problems, cancer, diabetes, and thyroid problems can also be caused by POPs pollution. Even background concentrations can increase the risk of cancer, neurological and reproductive problems, as well as endocrine and immune diseases.

Although many countries have banned these chemicals, they remain stockpiled, produced or used illegally, or, they continue to exist in soil or other environmental media because of lengthy half-lives. The initial Stockholm Convention on POPs in 2001 recognized only twelve POPs (Aldrin, Chlordane, Dichlorodiphenyltrichloroethane (DDT), Dieldrin, Endrin, Heptachlor, Hexachlorobenzene (HCB), Mirex, Toxaphene, Polychlorinated biphenyls (PCBs), Dioxins, and Polychlorinated dibenzofurans). Because of their adverse effects on human health and the environment, the initial Stockholm Convention on POPs places a global ban on these particularly harmful and toxic compounds and requires its parties to take measures to eliminate or reduce the release of POPs in the environment. Since 2001, this list has been expanded to include some polycyclic aromatic hydrocarbons (PAHs), brominated flame retardants, and other compounds. The following POPs have been added to the initial list: Chlordecone, α-Hexachlorocyclohexane (α-HCH) and β-Hexachlorocyclohexane (β-HCH), Hexabromodiphenylether (hexaBDE) and heptabromodiphenylether (heptaBDE), Lindane, Pentachlorobenzene (PeCB), Tetrabromodiphenylether (tetraBDE), Perfluorooctanesulfonic acid (PFOS), Endosulfans, and Hexabromocyclododecane (HBCD). Until now, there are 23 POPs in the Stockholm Convention list.

DDT is probably the most infamous POP. It was widely used as insecticide during WWII to protect against malaria and typhus. After the war, DDT was used as an agricultural insecticide. In 1962, the American biologist Rachel Carson published Silent Spring, describing the impact of DDT spraying on the US environment and human health. DDT's persistence in the soil can reach up to 10-15 years after application. Although DDT has been banned or restricted in most of the world, persistent DDT residues are widespread throughout the world, including the arctic. DDT is toxic to many organisms, including birds, where it is detrimental to reproduction due to eggshell thinning. DDT can be detected in foods all over the world, food-borne DDT remains the greatest source of human exposure. Short-term acute effects of DDT on humans are limited. However long-term exposure has been associated with chronic health problems, including increased risk of cancer, diabetes, and neurological disease, as well as reduced success in reproduction.

5.3.3.7 Biologic pollutants

Fungi, protozoa, and bacteria are important biological agents for the degradation of soil pollution. However the risk of infection by organisms in the soil has been known for centuries. Pathogenic organisms in soil enter humans by three pathways: ingestion (e. g. , Clostridium botulinum), inhalation (Aspergillus fumigatus), through the skin (hook worm) and skin lesions (Clostridium tetani). Soil pathogens can be divided into three classes, geo-indigenous (biologic pollutants that can metabolize, grow, and reproduce in soil), geo-transportable (transport of pathogens can be enhanced by soil), and geo-treatable (e. g. , viruses, bacteria, protozoa, or helminths introduced into soil by humans and animals). Usually the third ones are inactivated rapidly in soil by biological and abiotic factors. Despite of the fact that geo-indigenous biologic pollutants are indigenous to soil, human and animal wastes, garbage, and waste water generate much geo-treatable biological soil pollution. There are three ways that soil biological pollutants can harm human health: human-soil-human, animal-soil-human, and soil-human.

In the human-soil-human way, most cases occur because of ingestion or contact with the food or soil that was polluted by pathogens from patients. Many viruses, bacteria, protozoa or helminths can be introduced into soil. For example, bacterial pathogens such as E. coli, Salmonella, Shigella, Campylobacter jejuni, and Listeria are commonly found in polluted soil. The protozoa Cryptosporidium and human pathogenic viruses are also found in soil. Deliberate introduction of the pathogens occurs through land application of animal manures and biosolids in developed countries, and raw human wastes ("night soil") in developing countries. Irrigation with sewage effluent is another potential source of introduced pathogens.

In the animal—soil—human way, most cases occur because of ingestion or contact the food or soil that was polluted by pathogens from suffered animals. Bacillus anthracis is a bacterial geo—indigenous pathogen that causes lethal disease in humans via pulmonary, gastrointestinal, or cutaneous modes of infection. The organism is found worldwide and can remain viable in soil for many years because it is a spore former. Fortunately, human infections from Bacillus anthracis occur only following amplification of Bacillus numbers in animal carcasses. Anthrax infections from soil alone are less common.

Geo—indigenous pathogens cause infection by the soil—human way. They are found in all soils and capable of metabolism growth and reproduction. The usual pathogens include Clostridium tetani (tetanus) and Clostridium botulinum. The spore—forming ones can survive in soil for a long time and have the most serious effects on human health. Once coming into anaerobic human tissues, Clostridium tetani spores revert to the vegetative form, multiply and produce a neurotoxin, named tetanospasmin. Clostridium botulinum is a gram—positive, anaerobic, spore—forming bacterium that can produce a neurotoxin known as botulinum. The botulinum toxin can cause a severe flaccid paralytic disease in humans and other animals.

There are other biological pollutants, such as antibiotic resistant bacteria, antibiotic resistant genes (ARGs), and related mobile genetic elements (MGEs). Studies showed that sewage sludge and animal slurries contained antibiotic resistant bacteria, ARGs and/or MGEs. The class 1 integron, the most popular MGEs found in environment, is a kind of genetic elements that carries antibiotic and quaternary ammonium compound resistance genes. Bacteria carrying class 1 integron in sewage sludge added to soil can increase the reservoir of antibiotic—resistant bacteria in humans. The antibiotic resistant bacteria, pathogens, mixed with antibiotic—producing bacteria in soil may lead to horizontal gene transfer that poses a direct threat to human health. Human may be exposed to antibiotics, antibiotic—resistant genes, or antibiotic—resistant bacteria through crops, water, and animal products. Their potential health risk needs to be assessed in detail.

5.4　Itai-itai disease

Itai—itai disease is a strange disease that appeared in the downstream basin of the Jinzu River around 1912 and it was called by locals as "itai—itaibyo", because of the way victims crying out "itai—itai" under the excruciating pain they endured.

5.4.1　Cause and mechanism of itai-itai disease

In 1968, the Ministry of Health and Welfare in Japan officially announced that the Itai—itai disease was chronic cadmium poisoning. Victims suffered from calcium deficiency are often at old age, with malnutrition, hormone imbalance or being pregnant or breast feeding.

Itai—itai disease is caused by cadmium poisoning due to mining in Toyama Prefecture. The earliest records of gold mining in the area date back to 1710. Regular silver mining started in 1589, and soon thereafter, mining for lead, copper, and zinc began. The causes of the poisoning were not well understood and, up to 1946, it was thought to be simply a regional disease or a type of bacterial infection. Medical tests started in the 1940s and 1950s to search for the cause of the disease. Initially, it was expected to be lead poisoning due to the lead mining up stream. In 1955, Dr. Hagino and his colleagues suspected that cadmium can be the cause of the disease. Until 1968, the Ministry of Health and Welfare in Japan issued a statement that itai—itai disease was caused by the cadmium poisoning.

The heavy metals discharged from the Kamioka Mines into the Jinzu River were deposited in the river bed, and accumulated especially at the bottom of Jinzu River Dams. The cadmium in the river bed was dissolved in river water and polluted the agricultural water where the disease broke out. The cadmium dissolved in the agricultural water was absorbed by the thereby soil where the rice grew. Of the heavy metals that contaminated the soil, cadmium absorbed by the rice is 3 times higher than zinc, lead, and copper, and it concentrated inside of the unpolished rice. The cadmium was introduced into the human body by eating rice with high concentration of cadmium for a long time.

5.4.2   Symptoms and clinical features

One of the main effects of cadmium poisoning is weak and brittle bones. Lumbar and leg pain is common, and a waddling gait often develops due to bone deformities caused by the cadmium. The pain eventually becomes debilitating, with fractures becoming more common as the bone weakens. Other complications include coughing, anemia, and kidney failure, even death. A remarkable prevalence in older adults and postmenopausal women has been observed. The cause of this phenomenon is not fully understood. Current research has pointed that general malnourishment, as well as poor calcium metabolism are related to the women's age.

Renal tubular dysfunction is a well-known clinical feature due to environmental cadmium exposure. The first sign of kidney dysfunction is usually an increased excretion of low-molecular proteins in the urine, notably β_2-microglobulin (β_2-MG), retinol binding protein (RBP), beta-N-acetyl-glucosaminidase (NAG), and metallothionein (MT). Another specific finding of itai-itai disease is osteomalacia. Subsequent losses of protein and minerals, and disturbances of vitamin D metabolism may lead to osteomalacia, and followed by skeletal changes and multi-fractures. Environmental cadmium exposures at low levels are associated with decreased bone mineral density and increased risk of bone fractures. Environmental cadmium pollution may accelerate age-related declines of both renal function and bone density.

The diagnostic criteria of mild cadmium poisoning include more than one year contact with cadmium and its compounds, double increased creatinine-corrected urinary cadmium concentration more than 5 μmol/mol creatinine (or 5 μg/g creatinine), other complications such as dizziness, debilitation, dysosmia, backache and pain in limbs, and at same time accompanying with any of the following: ①Creatinine-corrected urinary cadmium concentration exceeding 9.6 μmol/mol creatinine (or 1,000 μg/g creatinine); ②Creatinine-corrected urinary RBP concentration exceeding 5.1 mol/mol creatinine (or 1,000 μg/g creatinine). Beside all the clinical features of mild cadmium poisoning, patients suffering chronic renal insufficiency accompanied by osteoporosis or osteomalacia can be diagnosed as severe cadmium poisoning

The reduction of the levels of cadmium in the water supply reduced the number of new disease victims; no new victim has been recorded since 1946. Although improved nutrition and medical care has reduced the occurrence of itai-itai disease, the mines are still in operation and cadmium pollution levels remain high.

5.5   Soil pollution prevention and control

In view of the serious soil pollution in China, the legislation of soil pollution prevention and control is urgent. There are no specific laws or administrative regulations on soil pollution prevention and control in China. Over the past few decades, various soil survey and monitoring programs have been carried out to investigate the soil quality and provide a scientific basis for the environment policy making in China. In addition to soil surveys, soil monitoring is essential to control contaminants in soils. It is necessary to set up routine monitoring systems at various scales (national, provincial, and local scales). This is currently an important priority for the environmental protection administration of China.

5.5.1　Soil environmental standards

It is difficult to establish a definition of "normal concentrations" in soil environment. It can be easier to establish hazardous concentrations for human made substances that do not naturally occur in soils, but it can be challenging to do the same for heavy metals and metalloids, which can originate from the weathering of rocks and mining. In that case, the parent material, climate and weathering rate need to be taken into consideration before establishing thresholds. Additionally, land use and management practices can affect the background levels of substances occurring in soils. When referring to recommended levels, there are also many differences from country to country and among regions, not only about the value itself, but also about the name used to define it, including screening values, threshold values, acceptable concentrations, target values, intervention values, clean up values, and many others. For that reason, to carry out a global study on the actual state of soil pollution and to be able to make comparisons is extremely complex. However, this is one of the main challenges when making a regional or global assessment of soil pollution.

In 1995, China enacted the Environmental Quality Standards for Soils (GB15618-1995). Maximum allowable concentrations of ten pollutants and the corresponding monitoring methods were provided in this document. This standard has been the most important legal basis and criteria for soil quality protection and pollution prevention in China. In 2006 and 2007, the State Environmental Protection Administration of China issued Environmental Quality Evaluation Standards for Farmland of Edible Agricultural Products (HJ 332-2006), Environmental Quality Evaluation Standards for Farmland of Greenhouse Vegetable Production (HJ 333-2006), and Standard of Soil Quality Assessment for Exhibition Sites (HJ 350-2007). In 2010, the Ministry of Environmental Protection revised and issued Farmland Environmental Quality Evaluation Standards for Livestock and Poultry Production (HJ 568-2010). This standard regulates construction land and includes a soil quality index for As, Cd, Cr, Cu, Hg, Ni, Pb, zinc, HCH and DDT. Among them, As, Cd, Cr, Hg, and Pb are the most strictly controlled indicators.

The Soil Screening Guidance (SSG) from U.S. EPA presents a framework for developing risk-based, soil screening levels (SSLs) to protect human health. The screening levels are not national cleanup levels; instead, they are intended to be used to streamline the evaluation and cleanup of site soils by helping site managers eliminating areas, pathways and/or chemicals of concern at National Priority List sites.

5.5.2　Refuse disposal and contaminated soil remediation

Refuse disposal means the measures for soil pollution control, including decontamination of feces, hazard-free urban waste treatment, safe treatment of toxic and harmful disposal from industrial activities, and protection of waste water irrigation. Waste management or waste disposal includes collection, transport, treatment, and disposal of waste together with monitoring and regulation. It also encompasses the legal and regulatory framework that relate to waste management encompassing guidance on recycling. A large portion of waste management practices deal with municipal solid waste (MSW), which is caused by household, industrial, and commercial activities. There are mainly two ways of waste management, landfill and waste incineration. Despite incineration and other waste treatment techniques, landfill dominates waste disposal in low-income and middle-income countries. Without proper management, many landfills represent serious hazards as typified by the landslide in Shenzhen, China on 20 December 2015. Both of incineration and landfill may lead new pollution to the environment and harm human health. Reducing, reusing and recycling (the three Rs) are the ways that consumers can minimize the volume of waste they generate. Perhaps the entire world is in a need of changing lifestyle. For example, one doesn't need to purchase a new product (e. g. , car, cell phone, television, computer) simply because the old one is no longer in style.

Over the past 20 years, investigation and remediation have been done in many of the contaminated soil sites and areas in China. China is planning to invest billions of dollars in soil remediation in the coming years. The Ministry of Environmental Protection approved and passed the "soil pollution control action plan" in March 18, 2014. According to this action plan, remediation of contaminated soil will become the focus of soil environmental protection. Some remediation technologies in China are still at individual level and experimental stage. The development strategy of future remediation technologies focuses on green, environmental-friendly biological remediation, combining remediation, in-situ remediation, equipped completely quick remediation, and supplying technical support for agricultural soil contamination, industrial enterprises, brown field, mining sites, etc.

Zhu Jingyuan

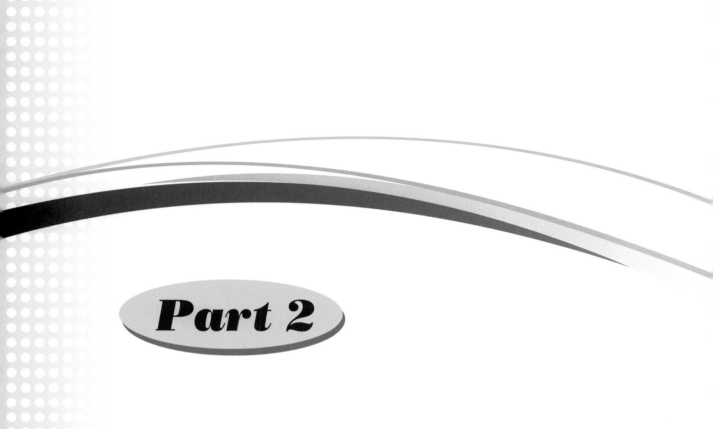

Part 2

Diet, Nutrition and Health

Chapter 6

Nutrition Basics

6.1 Energy

6.1.1 Source of energy

Energy is involved in most of the processes that sustain human life. The source of energy for human body includes carbohydrate, fat and protein (and alcohol if presented). Macronutrients, carbohydrate, fat and protein, from variety of foods, can be oxidized into water and carbon dioxide in human body finally. The energy will be released in the process of oxidizing. The international scientific community uses the joule (J) as the unit of energy. Traditionally, in food related context, the unit of energy is calorie, abbreviated Cal. The unit kilocalories (kcal), 1 kcal = 1,000 cal, is often used when the expression of higher calories values are encountered in nutrition. Calories can easily be converted to joules by the factor 4.18:1 cal = 4.18 J, or 1 kcal = 4.18 kJ. Based on the heats of combustion of protein, fat and carbohydrate, after corrections for losses in digestion, absorption and urinary excretion of urea, the energy values are 17 kJ/g (4.0 kcal/g) for protein, 37 kJ/g (9.0 kcal/g) for fat and 17 kJ/g (4.0 kcal/g) for carbohydrates, regardless of the food in which it is found. The rounded value for alcohol is 29 kJ/g (7.0 kcal/g).

6.1.2 Energy expenditure

Energy expenditure includes three defined components: basal metabolic rate (BMR), thermic effect of foods, and the effect of exercise or physical activity. The definition of BMR is the rate at which the body utilizes energy to sustain basic life processes such as heartbeat, breath, renal function, and blood circulation. Basal energy expenditure (BEE) is the presentation of BMR as units of kcal/24 hours. Energy exchanges happening in cells of human body form the basal metabolism. About 60%–75% of the daily energy expenditure is attributed by the basal metabolic rate. For adults, BMR declines with the increase of age and usually decreases by 1%–2% per decade after age 20, with the principal cause as the loss of lean body mass.

The second component of energy expenditure is the thermic effect of food, also known as diet−induced thermogenesis. During the processing of food in one's body, including digestion, absorption, transports, metabolism and the storage of energy from ingested food, there's an increase in energy expenditure associated with the body's processing of food, which is called the thermic effect. For the most of time, 10% of the caloric intake is the value used for the thermic effect of food when a mixed diet is consumed within 24 hours.

The most variable of the components of energy expenditure is that used for physical activity. Energy spent on physical activity is also the only component that is easily altered. It's reported that on average, physical activity explains for about 20% – 40% of total energy expenditure. A sedentary person may expend considerably less than 20% of total energy expenditure; on the contrary, a physical active person can expend much more than 40% of total energy expenditure. Not only the type of activity itself, but also the intensity, duration and the frequency with which the activity is performed; the body mass of the person; the gender of the person; the person's efficiency at performing the activity; and any extraneous movements that may accompany the activity are factors impinging on energy expenditure during exercise.

6.1.3　Energy balance

6.1.3.1　Concept of energy balance

Energy balance in human body is a condition when the energy input is equal to the energy expenditure. Result of consistent imbalance of energy is either a gain or a loss of body weight. If less energy is consumed than energy expended, the amount of tissue in human body will be reduced. Although an ideal goal of a weight loss is to lose adipose tissue, but in reality, other tissue such as muscle, which are essential to capacity of physical activity, can be lost as well. If the energy input is larger than energy expenditure, the adipose stores will be increased, leading to overweight and obesity.

6.1.3.2　Negative energy balance

Many people go on diet for losing weight. The ultimate goal of losing weight is to lose adipose tissue and to retain lean body mass. To achieve the goal of losing weight, preferably losing body fat, a negative energy balance over an extended period is required. The principle of negative energy balance is to design a dietary intervention that calories consumed should be less than the calories expended. The imbalance can be accomplished by either reducing energy intake, raising the energy expenditure through physical activity, or a combination of both. To what extent the composition of macronutrients of diets can have effects on the amount of weight loss is not clear. A study has been done to measure the caloric deficiency and the length of time that a person is exposed to negative life style factors shown to be a good indicator of weight loss. Several studies have disclosed that low carbohydrate diets with high fat and moderately high protein have resulted in greater weight loss over a six–month period. However most have shown that this advantage will be lost after a year, because of certain risk factors and chronic diseases such as, maintaining blood pressure and lipid profiles, certain amount of weight loss counts, regardless of the composition of diet driven.

6.1.3.3　Positive energy balance

Weight gain is brought about by a positive energy balance. As stated in previous part of this chapter, the metabolism of carbohydrate, protein, fat and alcohol are integrated. The primary nutrients contributing to energy producing are alcohol (when presented), carbohydrate and fat. In most cases, human body's energy comes from carbohydrate and fat under the circumstance that alcohol is not involved. Carbohydrate, also known as sugar, is first used for energy. As the human body's requirements of energy are reached, glucose is then used to synthesize glycogen. The process of glycogen synthesis stops when the stores are filled. If the storage of glycogen is filled, then the additional glucose presented will be converted to fatty acids. The amount of fatty acids that are oxidized for energy decreases with increased glucose being used for energy. If small amount of fatty acids are not being oxidized, it means fewer fatty acid are needed, so less lipolysis takes place.

The de novo synthesis of fatty acids occurs when the quantity of carbohydrate exceeds the total energy requirements. These newly synthesized fatty acids are made into triacylglycerols and will be transported from the liver by very low–density lipoprotein (VLDL). This is the process that extra fatty acids are taken up by the adipocyte. When the dietary fatty acids found in triacylglycerols are not used for energy, they are taken up and stored as triacylglycerides without using much metabolic energy in adipocytes. If the energy imbalance continues, the adipocytes in the human body increase and are capable of accepting the additional triacylglycerol. If a positive energy balance is maintained during the latter childhood and early puberty, one of the consequences is that the number of fat cells will be accelerated rapidly. In later life, under the condition of positive energy balance, the size of fat cells can enlarge while their numbers increase as well. If the body fat is losing, it's the result of the size of fat cells becoming smaller, rather than the number of fat cells decreasing.

6.2 Macronutrients

6.2.1 Protein

Protein, a complex biological compound composed of amino acids, is essential for the body. Proteins are the basic element of all life and are the most abundant and most versatile macromolecules in cell components. Whether in animal or plant sources, proteins will be found. Proteins are made from a combination of amino acids which always contain nitrogen. Through the process of digestion, proteins in food are broken down into amino acids, then reassembled into proteins by the liver. The digestion of proteins takes about 2 hours. The nitrogen found in proteins is what sets it apart from the other macronutrients. Nitrogen gives proteins their unique function of building and repairing the various body tissues, allowing the production of hormones and digestive enzymes, and a strong immune system. The continuous synthesis and the subsequent hydrolysis of protein within cells and organs enable the body to rebuild, repair tissue protein and adapt to internal/or external alterations. For example, red blood cells have a life of about 120 days; and the skin is shed and replaced continuously; proteins in the gut and bone marrow are renewed faster whereas the turnover rate of collagen is very slow and that of brain cells is negligible. In general, the rate of protein replacement of the entire body is greater than the usual dietary intake and may be as high as 400 g/day, or about 3.5% of the total body protein.

6.2.1.1 Amino acids

Proteins are biological macromolecules whose basic unit is an amino acid. Amino acids are connected by peptide bonds in a certain order. Due to the different arrangement order, lengths of the chains and spatial structures, numerous proteins with different functions are formed. Amino acids are organic compounds containing amine (—NH_2) and carboxyl (—COOH) functional groups, along with a side chain (R group) specific to each amino acid. For human beings, there are 22 basic amino acids. Amino acids are called the building blocks of proteins, because they are the foundation for the synthesis of a large number of proteins. They can be divided into three kinds from a nutritional point of view: essential amino acid, nonessential amino acids and conditionally essential amino acids.

(1) Essential amino acid

Essential amino acids mean that they cannot be synthesized in human body and must therefore be obtained from the diet, which includes lysine, tryptophan, phenylalanine, methionine, threonine, isoleucine, leucine and valine. In addition, histidine is required for infant. The amino acids that enter the free amino acid pool are: incorporated into proteins; converted to other physiologically important compounds such as nucleic acids, porphyrins, glutathione, and creatine or catabolized via transamination and oxidative reactions, then eliminated from the body as carbon dioxide, water, and nitrogen (principally as urea and ammonia) and provide energy for human body; converted to carbohydrates and fats. Therefore, essential amino acids are very important for growth, normal metabolism and life maintenance.

(2) Non-essential amino acids

Non-essential amino acids which can be synthesized by the body in adequate amounts include glycine, alanine, serine, aspartic acid, asparagine, glutamic acid, glutamine, proline and arginine. The nonessential amino acids are also critical for the organism since they may participate in diverse cellular reactions and functions, and provide precursors for the synthesis of many important cellular constituents.

(3) Conditionally essential amino acids

Cystine and tyrosine which are synthesized from methionine and phenylalanine, respectively are considered conditionally as essential amino acids. The requirements of methionine and phenylalanine are significantly reduced by the provision of cystine and tyrosine. Methionine is also synthesized into the nonessential amino acids taurine and homocysteine.

(4) Amino acid pattern and limiting amino acids

The quantity and proportion of essential amino acids are varied in both human body proteins and dietary proteins. The composition ratio of various essential amino acids in a certain protein is called amino acid pattern. The calculation method is to set the tryptophan content of the protein as 1, and then calculate the corresponding ratio of other essential amino acids. The series of ratios is the amino acid pattern of the protein. The more similar the amino acid pattern of food protein to human protein is, the easier essential amino acids can be used and the higher the nutritional value of the protein is. In general, the amino acid pattern of fish and eggs and other animal proteins is similar to human body protein. Therefore, they are known as complete protein and have higher nutritional values. In contrast, most plant proteins are semi-complete proteins. These relatively low levels of essential amino acids are called limiting amino acids, the lowest of which is called the first limiting amino acid, and the rest ones are named by analogy. Plant proteins tend to be relatively deficient in lysine, methionine, arginine and tryptophan. When soybeans and cereals are mixed, the two have a good "protein complementarity", which is also a better way to improve the nutritional value of protein.

6.2.1.2 Protein functions

The fundamental importance of proteins to the living cells and the human beings has long been appreciated. Proteins are important: in the composition of human tissues; for constituting a variety of important physiological active substances in the body and for providing energy.

(1) Composition of human tissues

Proteins are the main building blocks for tissue regeneration and repair as well as the material basis of all life. The lean mass of body, such as muscle, heart, liver, kidney and other organs, contain a lot of protein. Bone and teeth contain a lot of collagen; nails contain keratin; cells contain protein from the cell membrane to the various structures within the cells. Overall, protein is very important for human growth and development and is an indispensable structural component of the human body.

(2) Constituting a variety of important physiological active substances

Proteins constitute the body's essential catalytic and regulatory functions of various enzymes. There are thousands of enzymes in our body, each of them has specific task to regulate only one biochemical reaction. Hundreds of biochemical reactions happen per minute in human cells. The normal biological process and energy producing rely on sufficient corresponding enzyme, otherwise, the metabolic disorder or illness would be the consequence if the enzyme quantity or quality are poor.

Proteins are the main building material of hormones, which are important in the regulation of physiological function. The hormones, such as growth hormone, insulin, thyroid hormone and so on, regulate various physiological activities of organs in the body and maintain the homoeostasis of the internal environment.

Proteins are important carriers in the body and play critical roles in maintaining normal metabolism. The good examples of protein carriers are hemoglobin (delivery of oxygen), lipoproteins (fat transport), cell membrane receptors and transporters.

Proteins are crucial to maintain the body's osmotic pressure balance and the acid−base balance of body fluids.

In addition, proteins constitute the neurotransmitter, acetylcholine, serotonin and etc. Proteins are also important in blood coagulation, visual formation, immune regulation, body movement and so on.

(3) Energy providing

Protein can be hydrolyzed and release energy when the body needs. One gram of food protein produces about 16.7 kJ of energy in the body.

6.2.1.3   Digestion and absorption of protein

Digestion of food protein starts from stomach, where pepsin (produced from propepsin through gastric acid activation) as the major enzyme to digest the dietary protein into small peptides and free amino acids. However, the main site of protein digestion and absorption is in small intestine. Trypsin and chymotrypsin secreted by pancreas break protein down into oligopeptides and free amino acids, which are then absorbed by the small intestinal mucosal cells. In small intestinal mucosal cells, oligopeptidases ultimately hydrolyse oligopeptides into free amino acids, which are transported to the liver via the hepatic portal vein and utilized by liver and other organs. The liver is the key organ in the metabolism of proteins. It selectively removes amino acids from the portal vein circulation for the synthesis of its own proteins and for many of the specialized proteins such as lipoproteins, plasma albumins, globulins, and fibrinogen as well as nonprotein nitrogenous substances such as creatine. There are also protein macromolecules and peptides which can be directly absorbed.

Absorption of amino acids into the small intestinal mucosal cells is in an active transport manner. The neutral, acidic and basic amino acids are transported by their own specific active transport system, resulting in competition among amino acids with similar structures when they share the same transport system. As a result of such competition, amino acids with high contents are correspondingly absorbed more in order to ensure that intestine can absorb amino acids according to the proportion of which in food. Due to this competitive effect, the same type of amino acid absorption will be reduced if some certain amino acid level is too high in the dietary protein. For example, the absorption of isoleucine and valine will be reduced if excessive leucine is added, resulting in decreased nutritional value of the food protein.

The digested and absorbed protein in the intestine not only from food but also the sloughed mucosal cells and digestive juice. Non absorbent protein is excreted from the body.

6.2.1.4   Metabolism of protein

Absorbed amino acids are first stored in various organs, tissues and body fluids, which are referred as amino acids pool. These amino acids are mainly used to synthetize body proteins to ensure the body's protein being constantly updated and repaired. The amino acids might be transformed as glycogen and fat when they are not needed for protein synthesis, while the nitrogen leftover will be used for the formation of urea, ammonia, uric acid and creatinine.

The amino acids are transported throughout the body by the systemic circulation and are rapidly removed from the circulation by various tissue cells. Similarly, amino acids and products of amino acid metabolism constantly enter to the circulation from the tissues. The amino acid pool is available for any given tissue at any given time thus including exogenous (dietary sources) and endogenous (tissue breakdown) sources. These sources are indistinguishable.

In general, we will lose about 20 g of protein daily due to the fall of the skin, hair and mucous membranes, menstrual bleeding for women and sloughing of intestinal epithelial cells. This inevitable nitrogen discharge is known as the necessary nitrogen loss (obligatory nitrogen losses, ONL). When dietary carbohydrates and fats do not meet the body's energy needs or dietary protein intake is excessive, the proteins will be used as energy sources or converted into carbohydrates and fats, respectively. Therefore, theoretically, only the protein obtained from the food equivalent to the necessary amount of nitrogen loss can meet the protein requirement of the human body.

Nitrogen balance: Nitrogen balance reflects the relationship between nitrogen intake and output of the body. In fact, catabolism and anabolism are under the dynamic condition with a relative equilibrium state, which can be expressed by the nitrogen balance. The relationship is as follows:

$$B = I-(U + F + S)$$

B: nitrogen balance; I: nitrogen intake; U: urine nitrogen; F: fecal nitrogen; S: loss of nitrogen in the skin.

The intake and discharge of nitrogen is roughly equal in normal adults and B is equal to or close to zero. To avoid negative balance, the intake of nitrogen should be provided more than 5% to meet the zero nitrogen balance in healthy individual; when the intake of nitrogen is more than the discharge, B is a positive number, which is positive nitrogen balance, such as the situation of children during growth and development, women during pregnancy, convalescence of patients; if the discharge is greater than the intake of nitrogen, B will be a negative number, which is called the negative nitrogen balance, such as aging, short−term hunger or some wasting diseases. In these cases, the protein supply should be increased to overcome the negative nitrogen balance.

6.2.1.5 Nutritional evaluation of food protein

Various foods contain different types and amounts of protein, which have different digestibility and the rates of absorption and utilization. To assess the nutritional value of dietary protein, we generally consider these three aspects: quantity, digestibility, and utilization.

(1) Protein content

Protein content is the basis of the nutritional value of food protein. No matter how easy it is digested, if the quantity is not sufficient, it can not meet the physiological need of human body. The protein content in food is generally measured by Kjeldahl method. The content of nitrogen in food is first measured, and then it multiplies by the conversion factor to get the protein quantity. For the same type of food, the conversion factor is usually the same. The nitrogen content of the general food protein is 16%. Hence, the conversion factor for calculating the protein by nitrogen is 6.25, the reciprocal of 16%.

(2) Protein digestibility

Protein digestibility refers to the degree of protein digestion by the digestive enzyme. The higher the digestibility, the greater the likelihood of absorption and utilization by the body, so as the higher the nutritional value. Generally, the digestibility of animal protein is higher than that of plant protein. For the plant protein, its digestibility could be appropriately increased after the processing and cooking by breaking down, softening or even removing the cellulose. For example, the digestibility of protein is only 60% for the whole grain soybeans. However, when they are processed into tofu, protein digestibility could be increased up to 90%. Some plant foods, such as soy, contain anti-trypsin factors, which can reduce the protein digestibility, but could be destroyed by heating. True digestibility and apparent digestibility are generally used to reflect protein digestibility according to whether considering the endogenous fecal nitrogen or not.

1) True digestibility. Both the intake of food nitrogen, excreted fecal nitrogen and fecal metabolic nitrogen (generally 0.9-1.2 g in adults) must be tested to determine protein digestibility, which is calculated as follows:

True digestibility of protein (%) $= I-(F-F_k)/I\times100$

I stands for nitrogen intake, F stands for fecal nitrogen, F_k stands for fecal metabolic nitrogen.

2) Apparent digestibility Fecal metabolism of nitrogen is cumbersome and difficult to determine accurately, so it is not considered in practical work to metabolize nitrogen in feces, especially when the content of dietary fiber is very low. Hence, the measured results is lower than the true digestibility and much safer, which is called apparent digestibility and can be calculated as follows:

Apparent digestibility (%) $= (I-F)/I\times100\%$

I represents nitrogen intake, F represents fecal nitrogen.

(3) Protein utilization

There are many parameters to measure the utilization rate of protein and each of them reflects the degree of utilization of protein from different aspects.

1) Biological Value (BV) reflects the extent to which the protein is utilized by the body after digestion and absorption with the maximum value of 100. The higher the value is, the higher degree of utilization of food protein by the body.

2) Net Protein Utilization (NPU) is the ratio of nitrogen storage to nitrogen intakes in the body and indicates the extent to which the protein is actually utilized.

3) Protein Efficacy Ratio (PER) is a measure of weight gain based on the weight gain of an average of 1 g of protein per animal during the experimental period. This method is quite useful in evaluating enteral and parenteral nutrition prescriptions.

4) Amino Acid Score (AAS), also known as protein chemical score, is a widely used method for evaluating the nutritional value of food proteins. It is not only suitable for the evaluation of single food protein but also for the evaluation of mixed food proteins. The basic steps of this method are to compare the essential amino acid composition of the tested food protein with the recommended ideal protein or reference protein amino acid pattern and calculate the amino acid score.

6.2.1.6 Protein malnutrition and nutritional status evaluation

(1) Protein-energy malnutrition

When energy intake is inadequate, protein intake must be increased because the ingested amino acids are diverted into pathways of glucose synthesis and oxidation. In extreme energy deprivation, protein-energy malnutrition (PEM) may ensue. PEM is a nutritional deficiency caused by inadequate food supply or disease, and it is clinically manifested as Marasmus and Kwashiorkor. Children with Marasmus are deficiency in calorie intake and manifested as progressive weight loss, subcutaneous fat reduction, edema and organ dysfunction. Those with Kwashiorkor are lack of protein in the diet prominently and the total energy might be enough, which is mainly manifested as malnutrition edema. Severe edema may be complicated by bronchial pneumonia, pulmonary edema, sepsis, gastrointestinal infections and electrolyte disorders, often the cause of death. Majority of patients lack protein and energy at the same time, Marasmus and Kwashiorkor. A large percentage of children that suffer from PEM also have other co−morbid conditions. The most common co−morbidities are diarrhea (72.2% of a sample of 66 subjects) and malaria (43.3%). However, a variety of other conditions have been observed in PEM, including sepsis, severe anaemia, bronchopneumonia, HIV, tuberculosis, scabies, chronic suppurative otitis media, rickets, and keratomalacia. These co−morbidities worsen the malnourished children and may prolong hospital stay and increase the likelihood of death.

(2) Excessive protein intake

The right amount of protein intake is essential for human health. Our muscle contractions, access to oxygen, as well as the main components of enzymes and hormones, are inseparable from the protein. However, long−term intake of excessive protein might not benefit our health and even cause disease. Excessive protein intake always accompanied with excessive intake of sulfur−containing amino acids, which will speed up the loss of calcium in the skeleton and consequently cause osteoporosis. Acidic metabolites of proteins increase the burden on the liver and kidneys, causing hypertrophy and fatigue in the liver and kidneys. Large amounts of protein can cause dehydration, decalcification, and gout. In addition, excessive protein intake is also not good for the metabolism of water and inorganic salt and may cause urinary tract stones and constipation. Excessive protein in the body can be converted into fat and sugar, which is one of the causal factors of dyslipidemia and hyperglycemia. The last but not the least, the recommended daily intake of dietary fiber is 25−35 grams. If the protein intake is too much, the fiberrich plant food such as cereals, beans, vegetables and fruits will be at low level, constipation will be the common consequence.

6.2.1.7　Reference intake and food source of protein

Theoretically, 30 grams of protein per day is enough to meet the nitrogen balance. However, the human protein needs are known to be influenced by several factors (e.g., digestion and absorption of protein, energy intake, nutritional and physiological state of the individual). Hence, the recommended protein requirement for adults is 0.8 g/kg body weight per day. For children and adolescents, the recommended allowances decline from 2 g/kg body weight per day during the first year of life to 0.8 g/kg body weight at 18 years of age. It is recommended that protein should not exceed 2 g/kg body weight per day. Generally, protein intake should constitute 10%−12% of the total caloric intake for adults and 12%−15% for children and adolescents.

The food source of protein can be divided into plant protein and animal protein. Because the essential amino acid types, content and proportion are similar to the human body, animal protein has higher nutritional value than plant protein. But plant food contains less saturated fatty acids and cholesterol than animal food. Therefore, appropriate collocation and complementation of the two kinds of dietary protein is essential for human health.

6.2.2　Lipids

Lipids include a wide variety of chemical substances such as neutral fat, fatty acids and their derivatives, phospholipids, glycolipids, sterols, carotenes, and fat−soluble vitamins. Fat (e.g., triglycerides) constitutes about 90% of dietary lipids and provides energy in a highly concentrated form. Phospholipids, glycolipids and sterols are important components of cell membrane, tissues and organs, especially nervous tissue. Fat−soluble vitamins are also crucial for human health.

6.2.2.1　Fats and their functions

The lipids in food are mainly composed of triglycerides, which are formed by three fatty acid chains and one glycerol back bone. Due to the different chain length, saturation and spatial conformation of fatty acids, fats show different characteristics and functions. In general, fats derived from animal foods have long and highly saturated carbon chain as well as a high melting point. Hence, they are solid at room temperature and called as fat. In contrast, fats in plant foods have a high degree of unsaturation and low melting point. They are liquid at room temperature and known as the oil. Triglycerides in human body, mainly distributed in the abdominal cavity, subcutaneous and muscle fibers, have the same or different physiological functions of triglycerides in food.

(1) Biological functions of triglycerides in human body

1) To provide energy. As the largest energy repository, fat is the body's main energy supply material, which provides more energy than the other two energy producing nutrients (carbohydrates and protein). Complete oxidation per gram of fat releases about 9 kcal of heat, which is more than twice the amount of carbohydrate and protein.

2) To maintain normal body temperature. Fat not only provides energy directly, subcutaneous adipose tissue also has thermal insulation effect to maintain body temperature.

3) To Support and protect human organs. Fat often distributes around the internal organs, like a cushion, to prevent and buffer the mechanical friction. For example, fats around heart, kidneys and other organs play protective and anti-shock roles. A large number of abdominal omentum fat play a role in lubrication of the gastrointestinal motility.

4) To form the body composition. Cell membrane contains a lot of fatty acids, which are important for maintaining normal structure and the function of cells.

5) To secret endocrine factor. Adipose tissue is not only an important energy storage device, but also the largest endocrine organ. It can secrete a large number of bioactive substances involved in maintaining body energy metabolism and endocrine homeostasis, such as leptin, adiponectin, tumor necrosis factor α (TNFα), interleukin-6 (IL-6), estrogen, insulin-like growth factor (IGF-1) and so on.

(2) Biological functions of triglycerides in foods

1) To increase satiety. The more fat in the food, the longer time will be for stomach empty.

2) To improve the sensory traits of food. As an important raw material for food processing, fat can improve the color, fragrance, taste and shape of food, and achieve aesthetic appearance and stimulate appetite.

3) To provide the essential fatty acids. Fats also provide the essential fatty acids such as linoleic acid, linolenic acid, arachidonic acid and other unsaturated fatty acids, which are necessary for metabolism and growth.

4) To promote the absorption of fat-soluble vitamins. Fat contains fat-soluble vitamins, such as vitamin A, vitamin D, vitamin E, vitamin K. Fat promotes the dissolution and absorption of fat-soluble substances and fat-soluble vitamins.

6.2.2.2   Classification and functions of fatty acids

Fatty acids are chains of covalently linked carbon atoms, bearing hydrogen atoms, which terminate in a carboxylic group that is responsible for their properties as acids. The naturally occurring fatty acids are, for the most part, unbranched and acyclic, but complex structures with branched or cyclic chains do occasionally occur, particularly in lower biological forms. They have the basic formula $CH_3[CH_2]_n COOH$ where n can be any number 2 to 22 and is usually the even number. The nomination of fatty acids is based on the number of carbons and the number of unsaturated double bonds. For example, palmitic acid, which has 16 carbons and no unsaturated double bond, can be regarded as C 16 : 0; Oleic acid, which has 18 carbons and one unsaturated double bond, is regarded as C 18 : 1.

There are over 40 fatty acids found in nature. Fatty acids of varying chain length occur naturally. They may be saturated (no double bonds) , monounsaturated (one double bond) , and polyunsaturated (two or more double bonds). The relative proportions and intake levels of these acids are of vital importance in determining their significance in nutrition and health. The classification of fatty acids can be done according to their chain length (i. e. , the number of carbon atoms they contain) , saturation , and spatial conformation.

Chain length. Those containing 2 − 4 carbons are called short−chain fatty acids (SCFA) , while those with 6 − 10 and 12 − 24 carbon atoms are called medium − chain (MCFA) and long − chain fatty acids (LCFA) , respectively. The most common fatty acids in food are 18−carbon fatty acids and they have important nutritional values.

Saturation. Fatty acids can also be classified according to the number of double bonds between the carbon atoms (i. e. , the degree of saturation) : saturated , with no double bonds ; monounsaturated , with one double bond ; and polyunsaturated fatty acids (PUFA) , with two or more double bonds. Fatty acids with 2 , 3 , 4 , 5 , and 6 double bonds are called dienoic , trienoic , tetraenoic , pentaenoic , and hexaenoic , respectively. The chemical and physical properties of fat are influenced by the fatty acids they contain. Saturated fatty acids up to 10 carbon atoms are liquid and those containing more than 10 carbon atoms are solid at room temperature. The most commonly consumed are myristic (C 14) , palmitic (C 16) , and stearic (C 18) acids. The first two tend to increase plasma cholesterol , especially for palmitic acid. The SFA is mainly found in animal food , but plant origin coconut oil consists of almost 86% SFA (mostly of the medium−chain length) and palm oil has about 56% of SFA. As with SFA there is no requirement for monounsaturated fatty acids (MUFA) in the human diet. Oleic acid is the most commonly occurring MUFA and is most concentrated in olive oil , but animal fats also contain substantial amounts of these fatty acids. MUFA have no effect on plasma cholesterol. PUFAs are also liquid at room temperature. More about PUFAs are discussed in essential fatty acids and other PUFAs.

Spatial structures. Fatty acids that contain double bonds can exist in either of two geometric isomeric forms ; this is known as *cis* and *trans* isomerism. Because the public fear that saturated fats (usually animal fat) are associated with coronary heart disease (CHD) , margarines and hydrogenated fat are being used in increasing amounts because of their high level of PUFA. The content of *trans* fatty acids generally increases with the extent to which the vegetable oil is hydrogenated. Although hydrogenation offers advantages to the product (e. g. , controlled consistency and improved stability) , questions have been raised about the nutritional and biological effects of the high amount of *trans* fatty acids in the diet , since , at least in rats , the *trans* fatty acids cannot fulfill the role of essential fatty acids. Their biological functions are different from their cis isomers. There is evidence that they can interfere with the biosynthesis of arachidonic acid from linoleic acid (discussed below) through competition for D 6 desaturase and also affect the desaturation of stearic and palmitic acid to their respective monounsaturated acids. They also can be incorporated into the phospholipid fractions of cells. Both metabolic and epidemiological studies have shown that the consumption of *trans* fatty acids increased plasma low−density lipoprotein (LDL) level and decreased HDL level , resulting in the increase of the risk of CHD. Food manufacturers in many countries have reduced or removed *trans* fatty acids from retail margarines and other retail fats.

(1) Essential fatty acids and other PUFAs

1) Essential fatty acids. The essential fatty acids (EFA) are those that cannot be biosynthesized in adequate amounts by human and which are required for growth , maintenance , and proper functioning of many physiological processes. These fatty acids have two or more double bonds situated within the terminal seven carbon atoms (counting from the methyl) and cannot be made de novo ; therefore , these must be supplied in the diet. Linoleic acid (C 18 : 2 , n−6 all cis) and alpha−linolenic acid (C 18 : 3 , n−3 , 6 , 9 all cis) are

two essential fatty acids for human beings. Linoleic acid can be converted by mammals to arachidonic acid ($C\ 20:4, n-6, 9, 12, 15$ all cis).

The biological functions of EFA include stimulation of growth, maintenance of skin and hair growth, regulation of cholesterol metabolism, and maintenance of cell membrane integrity. EFA and other PUFA derived from them play a major and vital role in the properties of most biomembranes. Some specific functions of EFA are given below.

EFA is an important component of phospholipids: phospholipids are the main structural components of cell membranes, so the essential fatty acids are directly related to the structure and function of cell membranes.

Linoleic acid is a precursor of prostaglandin synthesis: the latter has variety of physiological functions, such as vasodilation and contraction, nerve stimulation and so on. Linoleic acid is converted to γ-linolenic acid in our body. γ-linolenic acid is further converted to arachidonic acid. γ-linolenic acid is also converted to eicosatrienoic acid, which is further converted to prostaglandins.

EFA takes part in cholesterol metabolism: About 70% of the cholesterol in the body is esterified with EFA to form esters that are transported and metabolized.

Therefore, the lack of EFA can cause growth retardation, reproductive disorders, skin damage and kidney, liver, neurological and visual diseases. The excessive intake of PUFA is also harmful, since it can increase the oxides, peroxides, etc. , and produce a variety of chronic hazards.

2) Other PUFAs. Mammalian tissues contain four series of PUFA. The four families can be recognized by the location of the first double bond from the terminal methyl group. Two types can be synthesized by animals, namely, those fatty acids in which all double bonds lie between the seventh carbon from the terminal methyl group and the carboxyl group. Such fatty acids may be made by alternate desaturation and chain elongation commencing with palmitoleic ($n-7$) acid and oleic ($n-9$) acid. The other two types of PUFA are necessarily derived from dietary linoleic ($n-6$) and linolenic ($n-3$) acids. These four precursors are alternately desaturated (two hydrogen atoms are removed to create a new double bond) and elongated by the addition of two carbon atoms (by the enzyme system called elongase). Because of competition, retroconversion, and so on, each family has characteristic end products that accumulate in tissue lipids while the intermediates are usually found in much smaller, often trace amounts. Thus, for oleate and palmitoleate, the major PUFA are the trienes $C\ 20:3$ ($n-7$) and $C\ 20:3$ ($n-9$), respectively. For linoleate, the major PUFA are arachidonic acid with four double bonds (tetraene) and some dihomogammalinolenic acid (DHGL). For linolenate, eicosapentaenoic acid (EPA) and docosahexaenoic acid (DHA) are the main end products. The PUFA are necessary components of most biomembranes. Their major function in this role appears to be the regulation of the physical properties of membrane lipids leading to proper transport abilities and osmotic characteristics.

Although other polyunsaturated acids can be converted from EFA in the body, the most efficient way to obtain LCPUFA directly from food is due to competitive inhibition in this process. Because of the lack of desaturases in mammals, $n-3$ and $n-6$ fatty acids can not transform into each other.

Specific role of $n-6$ fatty acids Linoleic acid and arachidonic acid are important fatty acids in $n-6$ PUFA, which come entirely from plants and mainly vegetable oils. $n-6$ PUFA can regulate blood lipids and participate in phospholipid formation, of which arachidonic acid is an important eicosanoid precursor. The lack of arachidonic acid can cause skin irritation and slow wound healing. In addition, $n-6$ can also promote growth and development of human body.

Specific role of $n-3$ fatty acids Linolenic acid is the mother of $n-3$ series FA. Its carbon chain can be extended to longer chain PUFA, such as DHA and EPA. Vegetable oils (containing linolenic acid) and fish oils (mainly EPA, DHA) are the main sources of $n-3$ FA. $n-3$ fatty acids are important components of structural lipids in many tissues, particularly in the brain and retina. Biological structures involved in fast movement or signal transmission appear to have a requirement for the highly unsaturated fatty acid, DHA. The retinal rod outer-segment disk membrane in which rhodopsin rests, the major phospholipid contains 40%-60% of the total fatty acid as DHA. In the cerebral cortex of humans, DHA accounts for approximately one-third of the fatty acid content of phospholipids. The highly unsaturated fatty acids EPA and DHA are particularly concentrated where there is a requirement for rapid activity at the cellular level, such as in the brain and its synaptic junctions, and in the retina where only the long-chain PUFA derived from EFA are found. $n-3$ series FAs have some biological activity in CHD, hypertension, arthritis, other inflammation and tumor prevention and treatment.

(2) Lipoid and functions

Lipids include phospholipids and sterols. The former mainly contain phosphoglyceride and sphingolipid, which are rich in brain, nerve tissue and liver; the latter mainly contain cholesterol and phytosterols. Organ meat, egg yolk and other foods are rich in cholesterol, while phytosterols come mainly from vegetable oils, seeds, nuts and other foods.

Phospholipids are a group of lipoids containing phosphoric acid. There are two major types of phospholipids: one is glycerophospholipid which is composed of glycerol and phospholipid; the other is sphingomyelin which is composed of sphingosine and phospholipid. Phospholipids have both hydrophilic and hydrophobic properties. The hydrophilic head of phospholipidsa (a phosphoric acid linked to the substituent groups) in the cell membrane is located on the surface of the membrane and the hydrophobic tail (the fatty acid chain) is on the inner side of the membrane. Phospholipids are important amphiphilic substances that are important components of biological membrane, emulsifiers and surfactants. In addition, phospholipids can improve cardiovascular function and nervous system function.

Sterols are a class of lipid compounds that contain multiple cyclic structures and vary widely depending on their exocyclic groups, which are widely distributed in animal and plant foods and mainly contain cholesterol and phytosterols. Cholesterol is an important and indispensable material for animal tissues. It not only participates in the formation of cell membranes, but also is the raw material for the synthesis of bile acids, vitamin D and steroid hormones. Cholesterol can be converted into bile acids, steroids, 7-dehydrocholesterol, and 7-dehydrocholesterol will be converted to vitamin D_3 by ultraviolet light. The human body could de novo synthesize endogenous cholesterol. Hence, there is almost no cholesterol deficiency under normal circumstances. On the contrary, long-term and excessive intake of animal foods may lead to elevated plasma cholesterol, which may increase the risk of hyperlipidemia, atherosclerosis, CHD. Dietary phytosterols are known to have the function of lowering plasma cholesterol. Some studies indicated that consuming phytosterol-enriched margarine benefits mild to moderately hypercholesterolemic adults by improving their lipid and lipoprotein levels.

6.2.2.3 Lipids digestion and absorption

The human body absorbs about 50-100 g triglycerides, 4-8 g phospholipids and 300-450 mg cholesterol from the intestine every day. Only a small amount of lipid digestion and absorption occurs in the mouth and stomach. The forceful contraction of the stomach breaks up lipids into fine droplets, which are exposed to bile salts in the duodenum, where they are emulsified into much smaller fat globule with relatively larger surface areas. The emulsified fat is ready for digestion by pancreatic lipase and intestine lipase. Normally, lipid absorption occurs in the upper part of the small intestine. Monoacylglycerol and LCFAs are re-esterified to triglyceride in the smooth endoplasmic reticulum of small intestine cells, and then form chylomicron with phospholipid, cholesterol and a specific protein, finally enter into the blood circulation through the lymphatic system. Chylomicrons, a type of lipoprotein with the largest particle size and the lowest density, are the main transport forms of food fats and are eventually absorbed by the small intestine to meet the body's nefeds for fat and energy. Easily, those with less than $10-12$ carbon atoms pass directly from the mucosal cells into portal blood. SCFA in the stool are primarily acetate, propionate, and butyrate whose chain lengths are 2, 3 and 4, carbons respectively. For example, butyrate, a primary nutrient for colonic epithelial cells, is a representative of SCFA and could be absorbed rapidly and stimulate sodium chloride and fluid absorption in large intestine. The digestion and absorption of phospholipids are similar to triglycerides. Cholesterol can be directly absorbed. However, those cholesterol combined with other lipids need to be hydrolyzed by enzyme first and the free cholesterol then be absorbed.

6.2.2.4 Nutritional assessment

The nutritional value of dietary fat can be evaluated from five aspects.

(1) Fat digestibility. The more unsaturated fatty acids and short-chain fatty acids of fat, the lower the melting point, the more easily to be digested. Generally, plant fat has much higher digestibility than animal fat.

(2) Essential fatty acid content. Because of a higher amount of linoleic acid and alpha-linolenic acid, plant oil is better than animal fat in general.

(3) The proportion of various fatty acids. Except for the quantity, a certain proportion of SFA, MUFA and PUFA are also crucial for human body although further studies are needed to determine the ratio.

(4) Fat-soluble vitamins content. Lipids with high fat-soluble vitamins have high nutritional value. For example, the germ oil of cereal seeds contains a large amount of vitamin E. Some fishes are rich in vitamin A and vitamin D.

(5) Other important fatty acid content. DHA, EPA, arachidonic acid and so on.

6.2.2.5 Reference intake and food source of lipids

Dietary fats and oils are ubiquitous in the food supply and found naturally in both animal foods and plant seeds. They are also presented in prepared and manufactured foods. Fat provides a highly concentrated form of energy (9 kcal/g). In addition to being an important energy source, dietary fat serves as a carrier for fat-soluble vitamins and certain fatty acids that are essential nutrients. Fatty acids are needed to form cell structures and to act as precursors of prostaglandins. These needs can be met by a diet containing $20-25$ g of fat. There are over 40 fatty acids found in nature. Animal fat contains more saturated fatty acids and monounsaturated fatty acids and less polyunsaturated fatty acids. Among the unsaturated fatty acids, oleic acid is the most widely distributed fatty acid in nature. In most fats, it forms 30% or more of the total fatty acids. The polyunsaturated fatty acids are of special interest. Cooking oils (mostly plant derived) supply nearly all of the PUFA consumed in China, of which 80% - 90% is linoleic acid. The most prevalent $n-6$ fatty acid is linoleic acid. It is presented in almost all vegetable oils, such as corn oil, soybean oil, safflower oil, and sunflower oil. Arachidonic acid is found in foods of animal origin. Varieties of fish rich in $n-3$ fatty acids include salmon, mackerel, sardines, scallops, oysters, and red caviar. Most scholars suggest that the ratio of $n-3$ and $n-6$ series of fatty acids should be 1 : (4-6).

In general, people will not lack EFAs, as long as they take a certain amount of vegetable oil. Too much fat intake can lead to an increase in the incidence of obesity, cardiovascular disease, hypertension and some cancers. Therefore, an important measure to prevent the onset of these diseases is to limit and reduce dietary fat intake. The Chinese Dietary Guideline for recommended fat intake is 20% - 30% of total calories and that unsaturated fatty acids should be the primary source of dietary fat and saturated fatty acids should be limited to<10% of calories. SFA can be replaced by MUFA or PUFA depending on the dietary strategy employed, but in either case which will likely result in health benefits. Trans fatty acids appear to provide no specific health benefits beyond providing energy. Therefore, it is recommended that trans fatty acid consumption should be as low as possible while consuming a nutritionally adequate diet. Rather than focusing on total fat, current recommendations and guidelines focus on specific fatty acids due to their individual effect associated with the prevention of disease and health promotion.

6.2.3　Carbohydrates

Carbohydrates are important for the body as the sources of energy. They can be found in a wide range of plant and animal food sources. Roughly half of dietary carbohydrate is in the form of polysaccharides such as starches and dextrins, derived largely from cereal grains and vegetables. The remaining half is supplied as simple sugars, the most abundant being sucrose, followed by lactose, maltose, glucose, and fructose.

6.2.3.1　Classification of carbohydrates

Carbohydrates are polyhydroxy aldehydes or ketones, or substances that produce these compounds when being hydrolyzed. They are constructed from carbon, oxygen, and hydrogen atoms that occur in a proportion that approximates that of a "hydrate of carbon", CH_2O, accounting for the term carbohydrate. According to the structural features and physiological functions, carbohydrates are composed of two major classes: simple carbohydrates and complex carbohydrates. Simple carbohydrates include monosaccharides and disaccharides. Complex carbohydrates include oligosaccharides containing 3 – 10 saccharide units and polysaccharides containing more than 10 units (Figure 6–1).

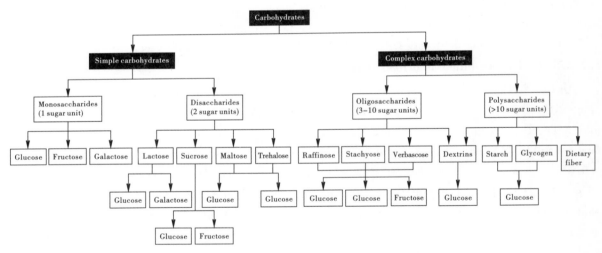

Figure 6–1　Classification of carbohydrates

Source: Beerman/McGuire, Nutritional Sciences, 1/e. Cengage Learning.

(1) Simple carbohydrates

Monosaccharides are structurally the simplest form of carbohydrate and cannot be reduced in size to smaller carbohydrate units by hydrolysis. According to the number of functional carbon atoms, monosaccharides are consequently termed dioses, trioses, pentoses, hexoses and heptoses. In addition to hydroxyl groups, these compounds possess a functional carbonyl group, which can be either an aldehyde or a ketone. The most abundant monosaccharide in nature—and certainly the most important nutritionally—is the six–

carbon sugar, including glucose and fructose. In the case of fasting of human body, the only free monosaccharide is glucose with the plasma concentration of approximately 5 mmol/L. Fructose is a colorless crystal with the same molecular formula as glucose, but a different structure. Just like glucose, fructose is also easily absorbed by animal and human. Fructose is the sweetest sugar with 1. 2 – 1. 5 times the sweetness of sucrose.

Disaccharides consist of two monosaccharide units joined by acetalbond, also called glycosidic bond. Disaccharides are major energy–supplying nutrients in the diet. The most common disaccharides in the diet are sucrose, maltose, and lactose. Within this group, sucrose, consisting of one glucose and one fructose residue, is nutritionally the most significant, furnishing approximately one–third of total dietary carbohydrate in an average western diet. Sucrose is fermentable and can produce substances that dissolve tooth enamel and minerals. It is acted on by certain bacteria and yeast found in the tartar, forming a highly viscous, insoluble sugar on the tooth, producing acid for the teeth and causing dental decay. Maltose is formed primarily from the partial hydrolysis of starch and therefore is found in malt beverages such as beer and malt liquors. It consists of two glucose units linked through the glycosidic bond. Lactose is found naturally only in milk and milk products. It is composed of galactose linked by a glycosidic bond to glucose.

Reducing sugars are the products of monosaccharides reduction and widely found in plant. Because of no need of insulin for their metabolism, reducing sugars are often recommended for use in diabetic patients' diet. In the food industry, they are also important sweeteners and currently often used reducing sugars are mannitol, xylitol, maltitol, etc.

(2) Oligosaccharides

Oligosaccharides consist of short chains of monosaccharide units that are also joined by covalent bonds. Oligosaccharides are polymers composed of three or more, but less than 10 monosaccharide molecules with glycosidic bonds. The functional oligosaccharides known at present include trehalose, xylooligosaccharides, isomaltooligosaccharides and soya oligosaccharides, etc. Some oligosaccharides presented in fruits and vegetables could not or could only be partially absorbed, but can be used by the colon probiotics to produce SCFAs. Some oligosaccharides known as the "atulent sugars" are found naturally in legumes and grains, whereas other oligosaccharides called dextrins are often added to food and beverage products to improve their texture, appearance, and nutritional value.

(3) Polysaccharides

Polysaccharides are long chains of monosaccharideunits that may number from several to hundreds or even thousands. Important polysaccharides include starch, glycogen, and dietary fiber. Polysaccharides are generally insoluble in water and non–reducing. Under the action of enzymes or acids, it can be hydrolyzed into fragments with different numbers of monosaccharide residues and finally become monosaccharides.

Starch is the most common digestible polysaccharide in plants. According to its structure, it can be divided into amylose and amylopectin. The amylose molecule is a linear, unbranched chain, in which the glucose residues are linked solely through 1–4 glycosidic bonds. Amylose chains adopt a helical conformation in water and are responsible for the blue colour produced when starch reacts with iodine. Amylopectin, on the other hand, is a branched–chain polymer, with branch points occurring through (1–6) bonds. Both amylose and amylopectin occur in cereal grains, potatoes, legumes, and other vegetables. Amylose contributes about 15% –20%, and amylopectin 80% –85%, of the total starch content of these foods. The former is easy to make food aging; the latter is easy to gelatinize food. The secondary hydrolyzate of starch is dextrin.

Glycogen, also known as animal starch, is localized primarily in liver (hepatic glycogen) and skeletal muscle (muscle glycogen). It is converted into lactic acid after an animal has been killed. Its structure is very similar to that of amylopectin, but more highly branched. When dictated by the body's energy demands, glucose residues are sequentially removed enzymatically from the non-reducing ends of the glycogen chains and enter energy-releasing pathways of metabolism, and the process is called glycogenolysis. The high degree of branching in glycogen and amylopectin offers a distinct metabolic advantage because it presents a large number of non-reducing ends from which glucose residues can be cleaved.

Dietary fibers include cellulose, hemicellulose, pectins, lignin, gums, b-glucans, fructans, and resistant starches. Functional fiber consists of isolated, extracted, or manufactured nondigestible carbohydrates that have shown benefits to human health. All dietary fibers are functional fibers with the exceptions of hemicellulose, fructans, and lignin. Whole-grain cereals and grain products provide cellulose, hemicellulose, lignin, some gums, b-glucans, some galactooligosaccharides and some fructans. Fruits and vegetables provide almost equal quantities (about 30%) of cellulose and pectin as well as some hemicellulose. Fiber could improve the bowel movement and also plays key roles in the prevention and management of several diseases. The varied health benefits of fiber are related to the fact that fiber is not a single entity or even a group of chemically related compounds, but instead consists of multiple different components with distinctive characteristics.

Cellulose is the major component of cell walls in plants. Being a large, linear, neutrally charged molecule, cellulose is water insoluble, though it can be modified chemically (e. g. , carboxymethyl cellulose, methylcellulose, and hydroxypropyl methylcellulose) for use as a food additive and this modified form may be more water soluble and a little more fermentable by colonic bacteria than naturally occurring cellulose. Because cellulose is not digestible by mammalian digestive enzymes, it is defined as a dietary fiber and is not considered as an energy source. However, colonic bacteria can digest it, resulting in several digestion products including short-chain fatty acids that provide energy to the body and play important roles in the gastrointestinal tract. Examples of some cellulose-rich foods include whole grains, bran, legumes, peas, nuts, root vegetables, vegetables of the cabbage family, seeds, and apples.

Glycemic index (GI) Different carbohydrate-rich foods produce different blood glucose responses despite equivalent quantities of carbohydrate. The GI is a ranking of carbohydrate-containing foods based on their immediate effects in the individual's blood glucose levels. It is expressed as a ratio of the blood glucose level of a certain food to the blood glucose level of a standard food (usually glucose), which refers to how much a person responds to a given blood glucose response. A high GI means that the dietary carbohydrate elevates blood glucose faster and to a higher level than a carbohydrate of lower GI. Simple carbohydrates from commonly used foods tend to raise blood glucose more than complex carbohydrates. Clearly, the glycemic response to 50 g of glucose is much greater than the response to a variety of foods providing 50 g of starch. Although glucose, maltose, and sucrose produce large increase in blood glucose, fructose does not.

6.2.3.2   Digestion, absorption and function of carbohydrates

(1) Digestion

Polysaccharides and disaccharides are the most abundant carbohydrates in the food supply, though some free glucose and fructose are presented in honey, certain fruits and vegetables, "invert" sugar used in confections, and high-fructose corn syrup. Monosaccharides are the form of absorptive carbohydrates for human beings, therefore, the poly-, tri-, and disaccharides must be hydrolyzed before absorption. The hydrolytic enzymes involved are collectively called glycosidases or, alternatively, carbohydrases.

Oral saliva contains alpha-amylase, which can partially hydrolyze starch, but due to the short residence time in the mouth, this hydrolysis is limited. The amylase in the stomach continues to maintain its effect until stomach acid invades the bolus, at which point the amylase is inactivated by the decrease in pH and there is no digestive enzyme for starch in the gastric juice. After the bolus enters the gut, α-amylase is secreted by the pancreas to continue the hydrolysis of undigested and partially digestible starch, resulting in oligosaccharides of smaller molecular mass, as well as maltose and glucose. Followed by the hydrolytic enzymes on the brush border of small intestinal mucosa, such as α-dextrin enzyme, maltase, lactase and sucrase, the final product is monosaccharides.

(2) Absorption

After carbohydrate digestion, glucose and galactose are absorbed into the enterocyte by the same mechanisms involving both active transport and facilitated transport. The relative contribution of active transport versus facilitated transport depends on the amount of carbohydrate consumed; facilitated transport participates to a greater extent following a large carbohydrate meal. The active transport mechanism for glucose and galactose absorption into enterocytes requires energy from ATP and the involvement of a specific transporter protein, designated sodium-glucose transporters.

Some glucose (and galactose) can be absorbed into the enterocyte independent of SGLT1 and thus without the energy expenditure. When glucose concentration in the intestinal mucosa is high, such as after the ingestion of a large carbohydrate-containing meal, glucose is transported into the enterocyte by GLUT2 in the brush border. Glucose is absorbed into the blood and transported to the liver, and then directly used in the corresponding metabolism or deliveried to other organs. Monosaccharides absorbed by the body have three fates: the first is direct access to blood flow; the second is the temporary storage of glycogen in the liver and muscle; the third is converted into fat.

Some people can not digest lactose due to the lack of lactase. After intake of milk products, the non-digested lactose enters large intestine and metabolized by the gut bacteria, which produces large amount of acid, gas, leading to gastrointestinal discomfort, flatulence, cramps and diarrhea, etc. This symptom is called lactose intolerance.

(3) Functions

1) Carbohydrate function

• To supply energy: Carbohydrate is the most important energy producing food. One gram of sugar in the body can produce the energy of 16.7 kJ (4 kcal), in the daily diet about 50% -60% of the energy requirement comes from this source for Chinese. When carbohydrate is severely restricted in the diet, fats are metabolized to provide energy. The accumulation of these incompletely oxidized products leads to ketosis. Therefore, a carbohydrate-free diet leads to ketosis and in an excessive breakdown of tissue proteins, thus causing the loss of cations (especially sodium) and resulting in dehydration. Carbohydrate is also the only source of energy for the brain and red blood cells. Red blood cells depend entirely on glycolysis and the brain uses glucose, but can be partially adapted to use ketone bodies. In an adult, the brain and the red blood cells use about 180 g/d glucose.

• To constitute the human body: Sugar can form important substances with lipids, proteins, glycolipids, glycoproteins, and ribose.

• To save protein: When sugar is sufficient, the body firstly uses sugar to provide the energy to avoid the body uses protein as a fuel to ensure that the protein used to form the body tissue and regulate physiological functions, this role of carbohydrate called Save Protein Effect.

• Anti-ketogenic effect: Fat in the oxidation process must have the participation of sugar in order to completely generate carbon dioxide and water. When there is a lack of sugar, the fat metabolism is not complete and produces ketone body, which builds up to a certain level in the blood causing acidosis. Adequate supply of sugar could prevent ketone body over producing when fat mobilization is under way in energy production.

- To help the role of the liver detoxification and liver protection.
- Special physiological effects of dietary fiber.

2) Physiological functions of dietary fiber

- To enhance intestinal function: Dietary fiber is conducive for the excretion of feces. Most cellulose has the characteristics of promoting intestinal peristalsis.
- Weight control and weight loss: Dietary fiber, especially soluble dietary fiber, can slow down the speed of food entering the intestine from the stomach, and has strong water absorption to increase the gastric volume and produce fullness, so as to achieve the functions of weight control and weight loss.
- To reduce blood sugar and blood cholesterol: Soluble dietary fiber can reduce the intestinal absorption of sugar, so that blood sugar will not rise too fast after meal, and reduce the release of insulin. Insulin is able to promote the synthesis of cholesterol. Dietary fiber can adsorb bile acids, fats and other substances, reducing the body's absorption of these substances to achieve hypolipidemic effect.
- To decrease the incidence of colon cancer: Some stimulants or toxic substances in the food stay in the colon for a long time and are toxic to the colon, which would induce colon cancer.

6.2.3.3 Reference intake and food source of carbohydrates

The main source of carbohydrates in the beginning of this century was the polysaccharide starch derived from cereal; this provided a little over 56% of the total carbohydrates. In recent years, the calories contributed by carbohydrates have dropped to about 48%, and the use of starch as a percent of carbohydrates decreased to 50%. The consumption of sugars increased from 31.7% to 50% of the total carbohydrates. The decreased intake of starch and the increased sugar consumption have been incriminated in the cause of several chronic diseases such as coronary heart disease, hyperlipidemia, obesity, diabetes mellitus, and dental caries.

The main source of carbohydrates in our diet is the plant food. Of the animal products, only milk, oysters, and liver contain significant amounts of carbohydrates. In developing countries, where plant foods are predominant, carbohydrates provide much of the energy, sometimes as high as 90%. It is estimated that in developed countries, carbohydrates provide, on the average, about 50% of calories. For a good health, at least 55% of calories should be derived from carbohydrates.

6.3 Micronutrients

6.3.1 Minerals

The elements contained in the human body, except carbon, oxygen, hydrogen and nitrogen which are mainly existed in organic compounds, are collectively called minerals (also called inorganic salts). Among those minerals, the 25 kinds of elements are necessary for human nutrition, of which the amount of seven elements such as calcium, magnesium, potassium, sodium, phosphorus, sulfur and chlorine are relatively high in the body, accounting for about 60% −80% of the total minerals, are called macrominerals. The content of other 14 elements such as iron, copper, iodine, zinc, manganese, molybdenum, cobalt, chromium, tin, vanadium, silicon, nickel, fluorine, and selenium in the body is extremely lower(<0.005%), known as microminerals.

6.3.1.1 Macrominerals

(1) Calcium

1) Source: The best food sources of calcium are milk, dairy products, especially cheese and yogurt, and selected seafoods, such as salmon, seaweed and sardines. Milk and yogurt, depending on the type, could provide about 100 mg calcium/100 g, and cheese generally provide 700–800 mg calcium/100 g. Meats, grains and nuts are relatively poor sources of calcium. Vegetables such as spinach, rhubarb and swiss chard also are poor source, because they contain large amounts of oxalic acid, which binds calcium and prevents the absorption of calcium.

2) Functions: About 99% of the total body calcium is found in bones and teeth. About 60%–66% of the bone weight largely consist of calcium and phosphorus. Calcium functions in the mineralization of bone, which includes cortical bone and trabecular bone. During the mineralization, calcium, phosphorus, magnesium and other minerals enter bone marrow from the blood and then attach to bone proteins and matrix. The skeletal bone maintains a dynamic balance with the components and blood by the process of osteogenesis and osteolysis, which is called remodeling.

The rest 1% of body calcium is found both intracellularly (0.6%) within organelles such as the mitochondria, endoplasmic reticulum, nucleus and vesicles, and extracellularly (0.1%) in the blood, lymph and body fluids. Of the calcium in the blood plasma, about 50% is ionized (Ca^{2+}). The Ca^{2+} is active, which means that the numerous regulatory functions of calcium are performed by less than 0.5% of the total body calcium. The physiological functions of Ca^{2+} are blood clotting, nerve conduction, muscle contraction, enzyme regulation and membrane permeability.

3) Deficiency: Inadequate calcium intake, poor calcium absorption, excessive calcium losses, or/and some combination of these factors contribute to the calcium deficiency in human body. Poor calcium intake affects mostly the bone and muscle. Low levels of free Ca^{2+} in blood may result in tetany (muscle pain, muscle spasms, and paresthesia are the common signs). For adults, osteoporosis usually occurs when deficient in calcium, which increases bone fragility and fracture risk. And long-term of calcium deficiency is associated with development of hypertension, colon cancer and obesity.

4) Toxicity: Intake of calcium in amount up to 2,500 mg/day appears to be safe for most people. A tolerable upper intake level (UL) of 2,500 mg calcium has been recommended for more than 1 year old. In China, the amount of adequate intake (AI) for adult male is 800 mg/d. The excessive calcium intake may increase the risk of developing calcium-containing kidney stones. And the large intake of calcium resulted in hypercalcemia and deposition of calcium in soft tissue, along with systemic alkalosis. Except this, the high amount intake of calcium interferes with the absorption of iron, zinc, magnesium and phosphorus.

(2) Phosphorus

1) Source: Phosphorus is widely distributed and rich in plant foods and animal foods. Animal products are superior source of available phosphorus (in organic form) compared with most plant foods (inorganic form). More than 80% of the phosphorus in plant foods is found as phytate, which limit its bioavailability up to 50%.

2) Functions: Phosphorus has many functions in our body, which includes bone mineralization, energy transfer and storage, nucleic acid formation, cell membrane structure, and acid-base balance. In adult, there is a total of 600 g phosphorus in the body, of which 85.7% is concentrated in bone and teeth. In bone, phosphorus is in amorphous calcium phosphate forms and crystalline forms (hydroxyapatite). And phosphate is an important component of nucleic DNA and RNA, phosphoprotein, phospholipids, cyclic adenosine monophophate (cAMP), cyclic guanylic acid (cGMP), and some enzymes. Phosphorus is of vital impor-

tance in intermediary metabolism of the energy vector in form of high–energy phosphate bonds (adenosine triphosphate, ATP), creatine phosphate (phosphocreatine), and uridine triphosphate (UTP).

3) Deficiency: Phosphorus deficiency is rare. It is typically confined to people who are receiving large amounts of antacids. And people who are malnourished and being fed enterally through a tube or parenterally without being given additional phosphorus have been known to exhibit phosphate deficiency syndrome.

4) Toxicity: Toxicity from phosphorus is rare, too. Excessive intake of phosphorus may lead to hyperphosphatemia. A tolerable of 4 g/day phosphorus has been recommended for people aged from 9–70 years, and 3 g/day for people more than 70 years old. The 3.5 g and 4 g of ULs are recommended to pregnant and lactating women, respectively.

(3) Magnesium

1) Source: Magnesium is widespread in foods, but varies greatly in content. Chlorophyll in the green leafy vegetables contains rich magnesium, since chlorophyll is a chelate of the magnesium porphyrin. Foods, such as coarse cereals and nuts are also rich in magnesium; while meats, starchy foods and milk are in medium content. In addition to foods, drinking water can also provide a small amount of magnesium. However, due to the impact of water quality, magnesium content varies widely (higher in hard water while lower in soft water). So it is difficult to estimate the intake of magnesium in drinking water.

2) Functions: For adults, there is 25 g of magnesium in the body, of which 60%–65% is concentrated in bone and teeth, where 27% is distributed intracellular. Magnesium in surface layer of bone (30%) acts as an exchangeable magnesium pool for maintaining serum level. And magnesium in the crystal lattice (70%) is probably deposited at bone formation. Within cells, magnesium is bound to phospholipids as part of cell membrane to help the membrane stabilization. Up to about 90% of intracellular magnesium (8– 10 mm) is important for over 300 different enzyme reactions either as a structural cofactor (Mg–ATP or Mg–ADP) or an allosteric activator of the enzyme activity.

3) Deficiency: Deficiency of magnesium is usually associated with inadequate intake, absorption disorders, excessive loss or a variety of diseases. Poor magnesium status may be related to cardiovascular diseases, renal disease, diabetes mellitus, toxemia of pregnancy, hypertension or postsurgical complications.

4) Toxicity: Under normal circumstances, the magnesium metabolism is regulated by gut, kidney and parathyroid, so the significant increasing of magnesium in serum concentration does not occur. Excessive intake of magnesium salts (3–5 g $MgSO_4$) may have a cathartic effect, leading to diarrhea and possible dehydration. Acute magnesium toxicity from excessive intravenous administration results in nausea, depression and paralysis. A tolerable upper intake level of 350 mg/day magnesium from nonfood sources had been recommended for people above 9 years old (women in pregnancy and lactation are included).

(4) Potassium

1) Source: Potassium is widespread in diets and is especially abundant in unprocessed foods, which provide potassium along with anions like phosphate and citrate. Foods rich in potassium are mainly fruits and vegetables. There contains 100–200 mg potassium/100 g cereals, 600–800 mg/100 g beans, 200– 500 mg/100 g fruits and vegetables, 150–300 mg/100 g meats.

2) Functions: Potassium is the major intracellular cation, and in contrast to sodium, about 95%–98% of the body's potassium is found within cells.

Potassium is the basis material to maintain the resting potential of cell membrane. Resting potential mainly depends on the permeability of membrane for potassium and potassium concentration inside and outside the membrane. It is an important factor affecting the excitability of neuromuscular tissue. Potassium is involved in a variety of metabolic processes, and closely related to the synthesis of glycogen and protein.

Some intracellular sugar metabolism related enzymes, such as the active phosphorylase and sulfhydryl-containing enzymes rely on high concentration of potassium. Potassium could maintain intracellular fluid osmotic pressure and acid-base balance, and also affect the extracellular fluid osmotic pressure and acid-base balance.

3) Deficiency: The normal diet is rich in potassium, and the body will not be in potassium deficiency. Patients who have been fasted for a longer period after surgery, cannot eat normally. If they are not given intravenous nutrition with enough potassium, it can lead to different levels of potassium deficiency or hypokalemia. Except reduced potassium intake, excessive potassium excretion can also lead to potassium deficiency, which includes children by the gastrointestinal tract loss, adult kidney loss, and skin sweating loss of potassium. When the body is in potassium deficiency, it can cause weakness, fatigue, dizziness; and severe potassium deficiency can cause paralysis of respiratory muscle. In addition, low potassium will slow down the gastrointestinal motility, leading to intestinal paralysis, increased anorexia, nausea, vomiting, bloating and other symptoms.

4) Toxicity: When serum potassium concentration is higher than 5.5 mmol/L, toxic reaction may occur, which called hyperkalemia.

(5) Sodium

1) Source: Sodium is widespread in many foods, usually the content in animal foods is higher than that in plant foods. The major source of sodium in diets is added salt (sodium chloride) and the processed foods (canned meats, soups, pickled foods, snacks, ham, etc.). And the naturally occurring sources of sodium such as milk, eggs and most vegetables furnish only about 10% of consumed sodium.

2) Functions: Within the body, sodium plays an important role in maintenance of fluid balance, nerve transmission/impulse conduction, and muscle contraction. Sodium is the major cation in the extracellular fluid, accounting for about 90% of the total cation. The osmotic pressure constituted by sodium ions and corresponding anions could maintain a constant fluid balance. Sodium exchanges with H^+ in renal tubular reabsorption by removing the body acid metabolites (such as CO_2) and maintains the fluid acid-base balance. Active movement of sodium and potassium ions (Na^+, K^+-ATPase pump) can proactively excrete sodium ions from the cells to maintain the balance of fluid osmotic pressure between intracellular and extracellular. Sodium is important in ATP generation and utilization, muscle movement, cardiovascular function, and energy metabolism. In addition, glucose metabolism and the use of oxygen also need the sodium participation.

3) Deficiency: Dietary deficiencies of sodium seldom occur because of abundant mineral across a broad spectrum of foods. While with excessive sweating involving a loss of more than about 3% of total body weight, sodium deficiency could happen. And the symptoms include muscle cramps, nausea, vomiting, dizziness, shock and coma.

4) Toxicity: Excessive of sodium intake causes the increase of urinary Na^+/K^+ ratio, which is an important factor in the occurrence of hypertension. Studies have shown that urinary Na^+/K^+ is positively correlated with hypertension, while urinary potassium and blood pressure were negatively correlated. Normally, excessive sodium intake does not accumulate in the body. Poisoning or even death will occur, if mistakenly added salt as sugar to infant food. Acute poisoning may cause edema, high blood pressure, elevated plasma cholesterol, low fat clearance, epithelial damage of gastric mucosa.

(6) Chloride

1) Source: Nearly all the chloride consumed in diets is associated with sodium in salt (sodium chloride). Salt, which is about 60% chloride, is rich in lots of foods, especially in processed foods. And chloride

is also found in eggs, fresh meats and seafood.

2) Functions: Chloride is the most abundant anion in the extracellular fluid, with approximately 88% of chloride in extracellular and 12% intracellular. The total amount of chloride in body is about 82 – 100 g (1. 17 g/kg, 0. 15% of the body weight).

Chloride ion and sodium ion are the main ions that maintain osmotic pressure in extracellular fluid, which account for about 80% of the total ions and regulate the volume and osmotic pressure of extracellular fluid. Chloride could maintain the body fluid acid–base balance, and participate in the transportation of carbon dioxide. Excessive chlorine ion can be used to correct metabolic alkalosis caused by disease or diuretics. Chloride also participates in gastric acid formation in gastric fluid, activates saliva amylase to decompose starch and promote food digestion, stimulates liver function to promote the excretion of metabolic waste in liver, and contributes in stabilizing nerve cell membrane potential.

3) Deficiency: Dietary deficiency of chloride does not occur under normal conditions. A large amount of loss of chlorine, such as sweating, diarrhea, vomiting, kidney function changes, or using diuretics, can cause chlorine deficiency. The lack of chlorine is often associated with the lack of sodium, which causes poor muscle contractions, impaired digestion, and affects growth and development.

4) Toxicity: The harmful effects of excessive chlorine consumption on the health are rare, only in severe dehydration, continuous consumption of high sodium chloride (salt) or excessive ammonium chloride; clinically, ureteral – intestinal anastomosis, renal failure, excessive solute overload, diabetes insipidus and enhanced intestinal absorption of chlorine can be combined with excessive chlorine to cause hyperchloremia.

6. 3. 1. 2 Microminerals

Although the content of microminerals is low in the human body, it is closely related to the survival and health of human beings and plays a crucial role in life cycle. Excessive, inadequate, unbalanced or deficient consumption of microminerals can lead to a different degree of physical abnormality or disease. In 1990, the expert committee of international organizations (FAO/IAEA/WHO) redefined the definition of microminerals and divided them into three categories according to their biological role: ① Eight kinds of essential microminerals in human body, including iodine, zinc, selenium, copper, molybdenum, chromium, cobalt and iron. ② Probably essential microminerals in human body, including manganese, silicon, boron, vanadium and nickel. ③ Potentially toxic, but at low doses, they may be essential for the human body, including fluorine, lead, cadmium, mercury, arsenic, aluminum and tin.

(1) Iron

There is 4 ~ 5 g of iron totally in the body (~ 38 mg/kg body weight for female, ~ 50 mg/kg body weight for male). More than 65% of body iron is found in hemoglobin, 10% is found as myoglobin, 1% – 5% is found as part of enzymes (cytochrome, cytochrome oxidase, peroxidase, catalase, etc.), and the remaining is found in the blood or in storage.

1) Source: Iron is widely available in various kinds of food, but the distribution is very uneven and the absorption rate is very different. The iron content and absorption rate of animal food are higher, so the good source of iron in the diet is mainly animal liver, whole blood of animal, animal and poultry meat, fish. In vegetables, the amount of iron and absorption are not high.

2) Functions: The iron in the body can be divided into functional iron and non–functional storage iron according to the contribution. The functional iron accounts for 70% of the total iron in the body. Functional iron is involved in important physiological processes such as hemoglobin, myoglobin, neuroglobin and DNA synthesis, and cell energy metabolism.

Functional iron participates in the synthesis of haemoglobin, myoglobin, neuroglobin, etc. , which mainly acts as transport and storage of oxygen.

Functional iron participates in energy metabolism, which contributes the activity of catalase, peroxidase, monoamine oxidase and other iron dependent enzymes, and affects the energy metabolism cells.

Functional iron is also the active center of many enzymes. It shows that when iron deficiency occurs, the bactericidal ability of neutrophils is decreased and lymphocyte function is impaired, and the immune function could be improved by supplementing of iron.

3) Deficiency: Iron deficiency implies that the iron content is lower than normal in the body. The degree of iron deficiency is generally divided into three periods. Iron reduction (ID) for the most early iron deficiency, also known as the early stage. Because there is only a decrease in the storage of iron at this period, the iron in the bone marrow cells is decreased, and the serum ferritin is lower than normal. And bone marrow iron granule, serum iron, transferritin saturation, hemoglobin and erythrocyte are all in normal. The second degree is iron deficiency erythropoiesis (IDE) or iron deficiency without anemia. It is characterized by decreasing the loss of iron, loss of myeloid blastocysts, or prototropine/hemoglobin > 4.5, reduced serum iron and transferrin saturation. The third degree is iron deficiency anemia (IDA), in addition to the above abnormal indices, hemoglobin and hematocrit are decreased, and it shows varying degree of hypochromic anemia.

4) Toxicity: Accidental iron overload has been observed in young children following excessive ingestion of iron pills. Other people susceptible to iron overload have a genetic disorder known as hemochromatosis. Excessive iron storage in the body could induce liver damage (liver fibrosis, cirrhosis, hepatoma), catalyze the generation of free radicals, promote the lipid peroxidation (atherosclerosis), damage DNA and induce tumor.

(2) Iodine

1) Source: The iodine needed for human comes mainly from food, which is about 80% –90% of the total daily intake, followed by drinking water and iodized salt. The amount of iodine in food depends on the geochemical status of the area. Seafood is rich in iodine, such as kelp, seaweed, sea cucumber, and lobster. There is very little iodine in soil and air in the hinterland which is far away from the ocean or in the areas easily affected by the sea breeze, and the iodine content in these areas is not high. The iodine content of animal foods is higher than that of plant foods, and the iodine content in eggs and milk is relatively high (40–90 μg/kg), followed by meat, and the iodine content of freshwater fish is lower than that of meat. Iodine is the lowest micro mineral in fruits and vegetables.

2) Functions: Iodine is mainly involved in the synthesis of thyroxine, and its physiological function is expressed by the role of thyroxine. Thyroxine regulates and promotes metabolism and is closely related to growth and development, such as participating in energy metabolism, promoting the growth and development of physique, contributing to the development of nervous system, and related to the action of pituitary hormone.

3) Deficiency: The release of thyroid hormone is related to iodide deficiency. Iodine deficiency prevails in many areas in the world and is associated most often with dietary insufficiency of iodine. Iodine deficiency is the main cause of goiter. Simple goiter is associated most often with inadequate dietary iodine and it's characterized by enlargement of the thyroid gland.

4) Toxicity: The excessive intake of iodine can cause significantly increased incidence of hypothyroidism, autoimmune thyroid disease and papillary thyroid cancer. The harmful effect of excessive intake of iodine on human health is high iodized goiter, which have an impact on mental development. The low observed adverse effect level (LOAEL) occurs at iodine intake of –1,700 μg/d. Some signs of acute iodine toxicity include burning of the mouth, throat and stomach, nausea, vomiting, diarrhea and fever. High iodine

intake may cause problems with the thyroid gland, including both hyper—and hypothyroidism and inflammation of the thyroid.

(3) Zinc

1) Source: Both animal and plant foods contain zinc, but the amount of zinc in foods and the uptake rate is different. In general, shellfish, red meat and organ meat are excellent sources of zinc. Dried fruit, cereal germ and wheat bran are also rich in zinc. Cheese, shrimp, oatmeal, peanut butter, peanuts, corn, etc. are good sources, while animal fat, vegetable oil, fruit, vegetables, white bread and common beverages are poor sources. Fine grain processing can result in a lot of zinc loss. When wheat is processed into fine flour, about 80% zinc is removed; canned soy products is about 60% zinc less than fresh soybeans.

2) Functions: Zinc has many divergent functions. As a component of metalloenzymes, zinc provides structural integrity to the enzyme by binding directly to the amino acid residue, participates in the reaction at the catalytic site, such as oxidoreductase, hydrolase, lyase, isomerase, transferase, and ligase. And zinc is a regulating factor for gene expression, cell replication, membrane and cytoskeletal stabilization, structural role in hormone, and involved in host defenses.

3) Deficiency: The body could cause a variety of symptoms due to lack of zinc. Signs and symptoms are growth retardation (an early response of zinc deficiency in children caused by inadequate cell division needed for growth), skeletal abnormalities from impaired development of epiphyseal cartilage, defective collagen synthesis or cross—linking, poor wound healing, dermatitis (especially around body orifices), delayed sexual maturation in children, hypogeusia (blunting of sense of taste), alopecia (hair loss), impaired immune function, and impaired protein synthesis.

4) Toxicity: Excessive intake of zinc can cause toxicity. Zinc poisoning occurs when adults consume more than 2 g of zinc. One of the main symptoms is that zinc has a direct effect on the gastrointestinal tract, causing upper abdominal pain, nausea and vomiting. Chronic effects can occur as long—term zinc supplementation (100 mg/d), including anemia, decreased immune function, decreased high density lipoprotein cholesterol(HDL), lactate dehydrogenase inactivation, inhibited Na^+, K^+—ATPase, reduced low density lipoprotein and ferulic acid ferroxidase activity. Long—term use of 25 mg/d zinc is accompanied with copper deficiency.

(4) Copper

1) Source: Copper is widely existing in all kinds of foods, including oysters, shellfish, and nut products, (0.3–2 mg/100 g), followed by liver, kidney, germ portions of cereals, beans and other foods (0.1–0.3 mg/100 g). The copper content of plant foods is affected by soil, and processing methods. The lowest copper content is milk and vegetables (not more than 0.1 mg/100 g). Usually 2 mg of copper could be obtained from the daily intake diet in adults, which can basically meet the needs of the human body.

2) Functions: Copper is the original oxidant and antioxidant. The biochemical function of copper in the body is mainly catalytic. Many copper—containing metalloenzymes, as oxidases, are involved in the body's redox process. In particular, oxygen molecules are reduced into H_2O. Many copper – containing metalloenzymes have been identified in the human body and are important to the physiological function, which includes the composition of copper—containing enzymes and copper—binding proteins, participation in iron metabolism and erythropoiesis, promoting the formation of connective tissue, playing an important role in the pathogenesis of some hereditary and sporadic neurological disorders in the central nervous system, promoting the formation of normal melanin, maintaining the normal structure of hair, and protecting the body cells from superoxide anion damage.

3) Deficiency: Various clinical manifestations are associated with copper deficiency, including hypo-

chromic anemia, leucopenia, hypopigmentation or depigmentation of skin and hair, impaired immune function, bone abnormalities, and dysfunction of cardiovascular and pulmonary.

4) Toxicity: Copper is relatively non-toxic to most mammals. Acute copper poisoning in humans is mainly due to the ingestion of copper salt or the consumption of food in contact with copper containers or tubes. Symptoms of acute copper poisoning include: oral metallic taste, salivation, upper abdominal pain, nausea, vomiting and so on. Ingestion of more than 100 g of copper sulfate can cause hemolytic anemia, liver and kidney failure, shock, coma and even death.

Chronic poisoning caused by oral ingestion has not been reported, such as long-term consumption of large quantities of oysters, mushrooms, nuts and other foods containing higher copper, daily intake of copper more than 10 times the normal amount.

6.3.2   Vitamins

6.3.2.1   The water-soluble vitamins

(1) Vitamin C (Ascorbic acid)

Vitamin C, known as ascorbic acid or L-ascorbic acid, is a vitamin found in food and dietary supplement.

1) Source: Vitamin C is the most widely taken nutritional supplement and is available in a variety of forms, including tablets, drink mixes, and in capsules. The richest natural sources are fresh fruits and vegetables. The amount in foods of plant origin depends on the precise variety of the plant, soil condition, and the climate where it grew, the length of time since it was picked, storage conditions, and the method of preparation. Animal-sourced foods do not provide much vitamin C. It is easily to be destroyed by the heat of cooking(Figure 6-2).

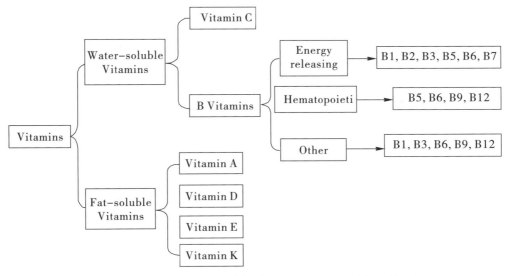

Figure 6-2   The water-soluble vitamins and fat-soluble vitamins

2) Functions: The biological role of vitamin C is to act as a reducing agent, donating electrons to various enzymatic and non-enzymatic reactions, including collagen synthesis, tyrosine synthesis and catabolism, and neurotransmitter synthesis. The one-and two-electron oxidized forms of vitamin C, semi-dehydroascorbic acid and dehydroascorbic acid, respectively, can be reduced in the body by glutathione and NADPH-dependent enzymatic mechanisms.

3) Deficiency: Deficient vitamin C intake results in the deficiency condition known as scurvy, since without this vitamin, collagen made by the body is too unstable to perform its function. Scurvy leads to the formation of brown spots on the skin, spongy gums, and bleeding from all mucous membranes.

4) Toxicity: Despite the less toxicity of vitamin C, overdose can still produce some side effects. It was reported that in adults, vitamin C intake (more than 2 g/d) can cause osmotic diarrhea. When daily intake of vitamin C is no more than 1g, generally there had no hyperuricemia, when daily intake exceeds 1 g, the uric acid output increased greatly. When consumed in 2-8 g/d, nausea, abdominal cramps, excessive iron absorption, red blood cell damage, urinary tract stones and other side effects will happen. Excessive intake of vitamin C during pregnancy can affect embryonic development. Overdose in infancy is prone to bone disease.

(2) B vitamins

B Vitamins includes vitamin B_1, vitamin B_2, vitamin B_6, vitamin B_{12}, niacin, pantothenic acid, folic acid and so on, which are the indispensable nutrients promoting metabolism in the body, and converting the sugar, fat, protein into heat (Table 6-1).

Table 6-1   The description and list of B vitamins

B vitamins	Name	Description
B_1	Thiamin	Conenzymes in the catabolism of sugars and amino acids
B_2	Riboflavin	A precursor of cofactors called FAD and FMN, needed for flavoprotein enzyme reactions, including activation of other vitamins
B_3	Niacin	A precursor of coenzyme called NAD and NADP
B_5	Pantothenic acid	A precursor of coenzyme A, needed to metabolize many molecules
B_6	pyridoxamine	A coenzyme in many enzymatic reactions
B_7	Biotin	A coenzyme for carboxylase needed for fatty acid metabolism and in gluconeogenesis
B_9	Folate	A precursor needed to make, repair and methylate DNA; a cofactor in various reactions; especially important in aiding rapid cell division and growth, such as in infancy and pregnancy
B_{12}	Cobalamins	A coenzyme involved in the metablolism of every cell of the human body (especially affecting DNA synthesis and regulation), fatty acid metabolism, and amino acid metabolism

1) Sources: B vitamins, water-soluble vitamins, are essential to maintain the body's normal metabolism and metabolic activity. The human body cannot synthetize them and must get from food, B vitamins are widely found in rice bran, bran, yeast, animal liver, coarse grains and vegetables. They are sensitive to light, water, and heat, and easily oxidized.

2) Functions: The functions of B vitamins are listed in Table 6-2.

Table 6-2   The functions of B vitamins

B vitamins	Function
B_1 (Thiamin)	It plays a central role in energy generation from carbohydrate, and involves in RNA and DNA production, nerve function. The active form is a coenzyme called thiamine pyrophosphate (TPP), which participates in the conversion of pyruvate to acetyl-coenzyme A
B_2 (Riboflavin)	It is involved in the release of energy in the electron transport chain, the citric acid cycle, and the catabolism of fatty acids

Continue to Table 6-2

B vitamins	Function
B_3 (Niacin)	There are 2 co-enzyme forms of niacin, nicotinamide adenine dinucleotide (NAD) and nicotinamide adenine dinucleotide phosphate (NADP). Both play the important role in energy transfer reaction in metabolism of glucose, fat and alcohol. NAD carries hydrogen and their electrons during metabolic reactions, including pathway from the citric acid cycle to the electron transport chain. NADP is a co-enzyme in lipid and nucleic acid metabolism
B_5 (Pantothenic acid)	It is involved in the oxidation of fatty acids and carbohydrates
B_6 (pyridoxamine)	Its active form pyridoxal 5'-phosphate (PLP) serves as a cofactor in many enzyme reactions mainly in amino acid metabolism including biosynthesis of neurotransmitters
B_7 (Biotin)	It plays a key role in the metabolism of lipids, proteins and carbohydrates and is a critical co-enzyme of four carboxylases (acetyl CoA carboxylase, pyruvate CoA carboxylase, methylcrontony CoA carboxylase and propionyl CoA carboxylase)
B_9 (Folate)	It acts as a co-enzyme in the form of tetrahydrofolate (THF), and THF is involved in pyrimidine nucleotide synthesis for normal cell division, especially during pregnancy and infancy. Folate also aids in erythropoiesis for the production of red blood cells
B_{12} (Cobalamins)	It is involved in the cellular metabolism of carbohydrates, protein and lipids. And it is essential in the production of blood cells in bone marrow, and for nerve sheaths and proteins

3) Deficiency: Deficiency of B_1 causes beriberi. Symptoms of this disease include weight loss, emotional disturbances, impaired sensory perception, weakness and pain in limbs, increased pulse rate and heart failure, and edema. Chronic B_1 deficiency can also cause Korsakoff 's syndrome, an irreversible dementia characterized by amnesia and compensatory confabulation.

Deficiency of B_2 causes ariboflavinosis. Symptoms may include cheilosis, high sensitivity to sunlight, glossitis, seborrheic dermatitis, pharyngitis, hyperemia, and edema of the pharyngeal and oral mucosa.

Deficiency of B_3 accompanies with a deficiency of tryptophan which causes pellagra. Symptoms include aggression, dermatitis, insomnia, weakness, mental confusions and diarrhea.

Deficiency of B_5 can result in acne and paresthesia.

Deficiency of B_6 causes seborrhoeic dermatitis-like eruptions, pink eye, neurological symptoms.

Deficiency of B_7 does not typically cause symptoms in adults, but may lead to impaired growth and neurological disorder in infants. Multiple carboxylase deficiency, an inborn error of metabolism, can lead to biotin deficiency even when dietary intake is normal.

Deficiency of B_9 results in a macrocytic anemia and elevated levels of homocysteine. Deficiency in pregnant women can lead to birth defects.

Deficiency of B_{12} results in a macrocytic anemia, elevated methylmalonic acid and homocysteine, peripheral neuropathy, memory loss and other cognitive deficits. It is most likely to occur among elderly people.

4) Toxicity: Because B vitamins are eliminated in the urine, taking large doses of certain B vitamins usually only produces transient side-effects. General side effects of overdose may include restlessness, nausea and insomnia. These side-effects are almost always caused by dietary supplements, but not food stuffs.

6.3.2.2　The Fat-soluble vitamins

(1) Vitamin A and carotenoids

1) Source: Vitamin A can be found in two principal forms in naturally foods, retinol (preformed vitamin

A) and carotenoids. Retinal, absorbed when eating animal food sources, is a yellow, fat-soluble substance. Since the pure alcohol form is unstable, the vitamin is found in tissues in a form of retinyl esters. It is also commercially produced and administered as esters such as retinyl acetate or palmitate. Carotenoids are syethesiezed by a wide of plants and thus are found naturally in many fruits and vegetables. The most abundant carotenoid is beta-carotene which has the greatest amount or provitamin A activity. In general, yellow, orange, and red fruits and vegetables such as carrots, watermelon, tomatoes, and pumpkins provide large amount of carotenoides.

2) Functions: Vitamin A is a group of unsaturated nutritional organic compounds that includes retinol, retinal, retinoic acid, and several provitamin A carotenoids (most notably beta-carotene). Vitamin A has multiple functions, it is important for growth and development, for the maintenance of the immune system and good vision. Vitamin A is needed by the eyes in the form of retinal, which combines with protein opsin to form rhodopsin, the light-absorbing molecule necessary for both dark-light (scotopic vision) and color vision. Vitamin A also functions in a very different role as retinoic acid (an irreversibly oxidized form of retinol), which is an important hormone-like growth factor for epithelial cell and other cells. Except for that, Vitamin A plays roles in a variety of functions throughout the body, such as gene transcription, embryonic development and reproduction, bone metabolism, haematopoiesis, skin and cellular health, teeth and mucous membrane.

3) Deficiency: Vitamin A deficiency is one of the four major nutritional deficiencies recognized by WHO, which is caused by inadequate intake, impairment of absorption and utilization, increased demand, metabolic disorders, and the effects of other nutrients. The signs and symptoms of deficiency include xerophthalmia, anorexia, retarded growth, increased susceptibility to infections, obstruction and enlargement of hair follicles, and keratinization of epithelial cells of the skin with accompanying failure of normal differentiation. People with chronic nephritis, acute protein deficiency, intestinal parasites, or acute infections may also become vitamin A deficiency.

4) Toxicity: Vitamin A excessive disease is due to a large intake of vitamin A, causing acute vitamin A poisoning, manifested as a temporary increase in intracranial pressure within 24 hours, which including nausea, vomiting, drowsiness, bulging anterior fontanel and other symptoms. After stoping feeding, the symptoms will gradually disappear. The long-term intake of larger amounts of vitamin A or cod liver oil, there will be excessive vitamin A, which shows the loss of appetite, itchy skin, hair loss, irritability, bone and joint pain and other symptoms. It needs to stop the application of vitamin A, until the symptoms ease.

Carotene hyperlipidemia is a yellow dye that is caused by an excess of carotene in the blood. Carotene is a kind of fat pigment which can make the skin yellow. If eating too much carotene-rich carrots, oranges, pumpkin, red palm oil, papaya, blood carotene content will be significantly increased. The only sign of carotenealmia in the blood are yellow or orange-yellow skin without consciousness symptoms occuring in patients with hyperlipidemia, hypothyroidism, diabetes or other congenital defects that cause the conversion of carotenoids to vitamin A, or liver disease, but the sclera is not yellow.

(2) Vitamin D

1) Source: There are two sources of vitamin D, one depending on food (exogenous), and the other from human skin (endogenous) exposed to sunlight (ultraviolet light). Usually in natural foods, the vitamin D content is low. And vegetable foods contain vitamin D_2 and animal foods contain vitamin D_3. Animal foods, such as high fat fish and fish eggs, animal liver, egg yolk, cream and cheese content more vitamin D_3, while lean meat, milk, nuts contain trace, vegetables, cereals and their products and fruits contain little or no vitamin D. The human epidermis and dermis contain 7-dehydrocholesterol, which forms pre-vitamin D_3 upon

exposure to sunlight or ultraviolet light, which can be converted to vitamin D_3. The production of vitamin D_3 is related to season, latitude, UV intensity, age, the area of exposed skin and the exposed time.

2) Functions: The main function of vitamin D is to increase plasma calcium and phosphorus levels to the degree of super-saturation to meet the needs of bone mineralization by promoting intestinal absorption of calcium and phosphorus; promoting growth and bone calcification, and improving tooth health; increasing the absorption of phosphorus through the intestinal wall, and the re-absorption of phosphorus through the renal tubules; preventing the loss of amino acids through the kidneys. The main active form of vitamin D is calcitriol $\{1,25-[OH]_2D_3\}$. Vitamin D is also purported to have a role in regulating blood pressure and preventing autoimmune disorders.

3) Deficiency: Vitamin D deficiency can cause rickets in children and osteoporosis in adults. Rickets occurs in infants and young children, mainly shows as neuropsychiatric symptoms and bone changes. Neuropsychiatric symptoms are hyperhidrosis, night scared, and irritability. The skeletal changes in infants varies with age, growth rate and the degree of vitamin D deficiency, with skull softening, beading of ribs. Osteomalacia occurs in adults, mostly in pregnant women and the frail elderly. The most common symptoms are bone pain, muscle weakness and tenderness. In addition, people living in the polar regions of the earth and some perennial indoor workers cannot synthesize enough vitamin D. Some diseases also affect the absorption of vitamin D, such as Crohn's disease. If their exogenous vitamin D supply is not enough, it will easily lead to vitamin D deficiency.

4) Toxicity: Although excessive exposure to sunlight may be the primary risk factor in developing skin cancer, it poses no risk of toxicity through overproduction of endogenous cholecalciferol. Exogenous dietary ingestion of large amounts of vitamin D is one of the most likely of all vitamin excesses to cause overt toxic reactions. Long-term intake of excessive vitamin D (5,000 IU/d), will cause hypercalcemia and hypercalciuria. The typical symptoms will occur alternately, which includes loss of appetite, excessive thirst, nausea, vomiting, irritability, frail, diarrhea, in severe cases, heart and artery calcification, and death can occur due to renal calcification.

(3) Vitamin E

There are two kinds of vitamin E, which include tocopherol ($\alpha-, \beta-, \gamma-, \delta-$) and tocotrienol ($\alpha-, \beta-, \gamma-, \delta-$) with a total of eight compounds, and α-tocopherol is the most widely distributed in nature, the most abundant and most active.

1) Source: Vitamin E (also called tocopherol) is mainly found in plant foods, especially in vegetable oils. Oils, high in α-tocopherol, include canola, olive, sunflower, safflower, corn, cottonseed and soybean. The bran and germ of cereals are especially rich in tocotrienols. Wheat germ oil and wheat bran represent significant sources of tocopherol. Cabbage, spinach, and asparagus also contain a certain amount of vitamin E. In animal foods, vitamin E is found concentrated in fatty tissues, such as milk, eggs, butter, etc. Tocopherols can be oxidized and destructed with lengthy exposure to air.

2) Functions: Vitamin E can prevent the oxidation of unsaturated fatty acids contained in the phospholipids of the cell membranes, so the principal function of vitamin E is the maintenance of membrane integrity, including possible physical stability in cells. And tocotrienols appears to affect cholesterol metabolism and suppresses the tumor growth and cell proliferation. Vitamin E also has the role of protecting the nervous system, skeletal muscle, and retina from oxidative damage.

3) Deficiency: Vitamin E deficiency is often accompanied by enhanced lipid peroxidation, which lead to decreased energy production of mitochondria, DNA oxidation and mutation, and function changes of plasma membrane. Especially when the cell membrane is exposed to oxidative stress, the cell damage and necrosis

occur quickly, and release the by-products of lipid peroxidation which can attract the accumulation of inflammatory cells and phagocytes.

(4) Vitamin K

Vitamin K is essential for the synthesis of prothrombin and other coagulation factors in the liver. Plant-derived vitamin K is vitamin K_1(phylloquinone). Vitamin K_2 refers to a family of homologues of 2-methyl-1,4-naphthoquinone, which called menaquinone-n [the suffix ($-n$) denotes the number of isoprene units on the side chain, from menaquinone-1 to menaquinone-13]. Menadione is synthesized in the intestine by bacteria and can supply some of the vitamin K needed by humanbody.

1) Source: Dietary vitamin K is provided mostly as vitamin K_1 in plant foods and as a mixture of K_2 in animal products. Bacteria, especially a variety of facultative and obigate anaerobic bacteria in the gastrointestinal tract, can provide a source of K_2 for host. Vitamin K is widely distributed in animal and plant foods, such as citrus fruit (less than 0.1 μg/100 g), milk (1 μg/100 g), spinach, cabbage and turnip green leafy (400 μg/100 g), liver(13 μg/100 g), and cheese (2.8 μg/100 g). Since the human body has a low dietary requirement for vitamin K, most food is basically enough to meet the needs. But breast milk is an exception, with low levels of vitamin K, and cannot even meet the requirement of infants within 6 months.

2) Functions: There are four vitamin K-dependent blood-clotting proteins, called factors II (prothrombin), VII (accelerating factor precursor), IX (the serum factor, plasma thromboplastin component), and X (stuartfactor). Four classic blood-clotting factors (II, VII, IX, X) prevent bleeding and are involved in a series of continuous proteolytic activation that ultimately converts soluble fibrinogen to insoluble fibrin and then inter blocks with platelets to form blood clot. In addition, vitamin K is needed for carboxylation in vitamin K-dependent protein C, S, Z and M to inhibit the coagulation process.

The most characteristic vitamin K-dependent protein in calcified tissue is BGP (bone Gla protein) which is a protein in the rapidly growing bone region. BGP plays a role in regulating the incorporation of calcium phosphate into bone. BGP is the second most abundant protein in bone matrix, accounting for 2% of total bone protein and 10% -20% of non-collagen protein. Because it is the only synthesized by osteoblasts, and can be used as a marker of bone formation.

3) Deficiency: The population groups that appear to be most at risk for a vitamin K deficiency are newborn infants and people with severe gastrointestinal malabsorptive disorders or being treated chronically with antibiotics. Subclinical vitamin K deficiency has been induced in healthy adults fed by a diet providing only about 10 μg phylloquinone per day. Severe vitamin K deficiency is associated with bleeding episodes (hemorrhage) caused by prolonged prothrombin time. Currently, intramuscular injection of 0.5-1.0 mg phylloquinone shortly after birth is recommended for all infants.

4) Toxicity: Vitamin K_1 and K_2 derived from food source are not toxic, and even large doses are not toxic. Menadione, which is a food source, has very low toxicity. Vitamin K precursor, 2-menaquinone (K_3), which is toxic due to its reaction with sulfhydryl groups, can cause hemolytic anemia, hyperbilirubinemia and kernicterus in infants; 2-methylnaphthaquinone should not be used to treat vitamin K deficiency.

6.3.3 Phytochemicals

Phytochemicals refer to a variety of low molecular weight products (secondary plant metabolites) produced by the metabolism of plants, and by degradation or synthesis produce during metabolic processes. These products, in addition to being precursors of vitamins, are all non-nutrients, and broadly, phytochemicals are biologically active molecules that plants maintain their interaction with the environment during their biological evolution. There are many naturally phytochemicals, with about 60,000-100,000 species.

6.3.3.1　Classification

Phytochemicals can be classified according to the respective chemical structure or functional characteristics, as the following categories.

(1) Carotenoids

Carotenoids are plant secondary metabolites that are wide spreading in fruits and vegetables. One of the main functions is to make the plants appear red or yellow. Among the more than 700 natural carotenoids existed in nature, about 40-50 are of benefit to human health. The daily intake of carotenoid is about 6 mg.

(2) Phytosterols

Phytosterols mainly exist in plant seeds and their oil. It could reduce cholesterol level in human body.

(3) Saponins

Saponins, a class of bitter compounds, which can form compounds with proteins and lipids, particularly rich in legumes. It was regarded as harmful compound to health, but the population test failed to confirm it. Now, it is verified that saponins has anti-mutation, anti-cancer, anti-oxidation and immunomodulatory effects.

(4) Glucosinolates

Glucosinolates present in all cruciferous plants, their degradation products have the typical taste of mustard, horseradish and broccoli. Its active compounds are mainly isothiocyanate, thiocyanate, etc., with anti-cancer, inhibition of tumor cell proliferation, anti-inflammatory and other biological role.

(5) Polyphenols

Polyphenols are phenolic derivatives, including phenolic acids and flavonoids. Flavonoids are mainly found in the outer layer of fruits and vegetables, showing anti-oxidation, anti-tumor, cardiovascular protection and other effects.

(6) Protease inhibitors

Protease inhibitors exist in all plants, especially beans, cereals and other seeds which mainly inhibit tumor and anti-oxidation.

(7) Phytoestrogens

Phytoestrogens exist in plants, mainly including isoflavones and lignin, which belongs to both polyphenols and phytoestrogens, with estrogen and anti-estrogen effect.

(8) Sulfides

Sulfides are organic sulfur compounds in garlic and other bulbous plants, with anti-mutation, anti-cancer, and anti-aging effect. The main active substance in garlic is dipropyl disulfide or allicin. The basic material in garlic is allicin. The cabbage also contains sulphide, but lacking of alliinase inhibits the formation of bioactive sulphide metabolites.

(9) Phytic acid

Phytic acid also known as phytate, is naturally found in cereals and beans, a phosphorus-rich organic compounds. In addition, the anti-cancer, anti-oxidant, regulate immune function, anti-platelet and other biological activities have been confirmed.

(10) Others

Such as lectins, glucose diamine, phthalide, chlorophyll and tocotrienols.

6.3.3.2　Physiological function

There are varieties of physiological effects in phytochemicals, which mainly occur in the following areas.

(1) Anti-cancer effect

The occurrence of cancer is a multi-stage process, phytochemicals can inhibit tumor in almost every stage. For example, some phenolic acids can be covalently bound to activated carcinogens and mask the binding sites for DNA and carcinogens; the presence of isoflavin and phytoestrogens in soybean can inhibit the growth and metastasis of angiogenesis and tumor cells under experimental conditions. In addition, glucosinolates, polyphenols, monoterpenes and, sulfides in phytochemicals show the corresponding anti-cancer effects by inhibiting phase I metabolic enzymes and inducing phase II metabolic enzymes.

(2) Antioxidant effect

It has now been found that phytochemicals such as carotenoids, polyphenols, phytoestrogens, protease inhibitors and sulfides also have significant anti-oxidant effects. Certain carotenoids, such as lycopene, have a more potent protective effect on singlet oxygen and oxygen radicals. Polyphenols are the most antioxidant substance in phytochemicals.

(3) Immunomodulatory effects

A number of experimental studies and intervention studies have shown that carotenoids can regulate the body's immune system function. In vitro, it was found that flavonoids have immunomodulatory effect. Saponins and sulfide can enhance the immune function of the body.

(4) Anti-microbial effect

Some plants have long been used to anti-infection. In recent years, due to the toxic side-effects of chemically synthesized drugs, the antimicrobial effect of plant extracts has become a hot research spot. Earlier studies have demonstrated that sulfide in bulbous plants has an antimicrobial effect. Allicin in sulphide, the metabolite isothiocyanate in glucosinolates, also have an antimicrobial activity.

(5) Cholesterol-lowering effect

Animal experiments and clinical studies have found that saponins, phytosterols sulfides, and tocotrienols have the role in cholesterol lowering effect. The serum cholesterol is related to the cholesterol and fat in the diet. The mechanism by which phytochemicals lower cholesterol may be related to the inhibition of bile acid absorption, the promotion of bile acid excretion, and the reduction of cholesterol absorption in the intestinal tract. In addition, phytochemicals such as tocotrienols and sulfides can inhibit key enzymes of cholesterol metabolism in liver, such as hydroxymethyl glutaratemonoacyl CoA reductase (HMG-CoA reductase).

In addition to the above effects, phytochemicals also have the effects of regulating blood pressure, blood sugar and blood coagulation and inhibiting inflammation.

Cheng Yue, Han Bei, Luo Xiaoqin, Yu Yan

Chapter 7

Nutrition in the Life Cycle

Good nutrition during the first 1,000 days of life, before birth—through the time spent in mother's womb—and in the two years of life, helps improve the child's health and social outcomes. Child's development plays an active role in the process from infancy to adolescence and adulthood. Human's development is largely shaped by genetic factors, much evidence reminds us that the environment has profound influence on one's development. Nutrition is no doubt a significant factor.

7.1 Nutrition during pregnancy and lactation

During pregnancy and lactation, nutrition is needed not only to meet the maternal needs, but also to meet the growth and development of the fetus and infant. If a woman is healthy and well-nourished before pregnancy, the risks associated with childbearing for the mother and her baby can be greatly reduced. Proper nutrition during pregnancy and lactation is of great importance to maternal health and development of the offspring.

7.1.1 Pregnancy

7.1.1.1 Physiology of pregnancy

Physiological changes happen to every organ and system during pregnancy. These changes are partially mediated by the placental hormones.

(1) Cardiovascular system

During pregnancy, cardiac output increases compared to non-pregnant status. The increase starts from the first trimester and reaches the peak between 20th and 24th week of gestation. Systemic vascular resistance decreases, leading to a decline of arterial blood pressure.

(2) Gastrointestinal system

Most of pregnancies are accompanied by nausea and vomiting at early stage of pregnancy. Nausea and vomiting can happen any time throughout the day despite the term "morning sickness". These symptoms are the results of the elevated estrogen, progesterone and human chorionic gonadotropin (hCG). In most cases, nausea and vomiting are mild and resolved by 14–16 weeks' gestation. There's a severe form of morning sickness called hyperemesis gravidarum, which means women lose more than 5% of their pregnancy weight due to nausea and vomiting and get ketosis. Ptyalism or acid regurgilation happens during pregnancy resulting from multiple changes such as prolonged gastric emptying time and gastroesophageal sphincter relaxation.

（3）Hematological system

During pregnancy, the maternal plasma volume can be increased by 50%, but the red blood cell volume can only increase 20% to 30%. These facts lead to a decreased hematocrit or 'dilutional anemia'.

7.1.1.2 Nutrients requirement of pregnancy

Nutritional requirements increase during pregnancy. The average Chinese adult woman requires 1,800 kilocalories (kcal) a day. The caloric requirement increased by 300 kcal/d during the second trimester and by 450 kcal/d during the third trimester. Due to differences in region, ethnicity, climate, life style and labor intensity, the maternal need for energy will be different. Therefore, the general recommendation should be adjusted according to the magnitude of weight gain during pregnancy.

In addition to the increased energy requirement, nutritional requirements for protein, calcium, iron, iodine, folic acid, and other vitamins and minerals are also increased. Pregnant women should cousume adequate amounts of protein to meet the needs for maternal health and fetal growth. 400–800 g protein is estimated for a mature fetus plus the growth of placental and other tissue of the pregnant woman. A total of 900 g protein is required for normal pregnancy. The protein requirement increased from 55 g/d to 70 g/d during the second trimester and 85 g/d during the third trimester.

Lipids usually account for 5%–15% of fetal weight. Lipids are vital for fetal nervous system development. Brain cells need a certain amount of essential fatty acids in the process of proliferation and growth. Pregnant women should take a moderate amount of fat, including saturated fatty acids, $n-3$ and $n-6$ polyunsaturated fatty acids, which ensure the needs of the fetus and herself. The Chinese nutrition society recommends that the ratio of energy supplied by fat should vary from 20% to 30% of tatal energy.

The fetus takes a large amount of calcium from the mother for growth and development. If the pregnant woman has insufficient calcium intake mildly or temporally, her serum calcium concentration will decrease, which will trigger the parathyroid hormone synthesis, accelerating the dissolution of calcium salts from the maternal bone and teeth in order to maintain normal serum calcium concentration and to meet the needs of the fetus for calcium. In addition, the mother also needs to store calcium for lactation. The requirement for calcium increases during pregnancy. Pregnant women are encouraged to take foods enriched in calcium. Due to food taboos or habits, in areas where pregnant woman's dietary calcium intake is low or women who are under risk of developing hypertensive disorder, supplementation of pregnant women with 1.5–2.0 grams of elemental calcium per day is advised.

The demand for iron is emphasized during pregnancy considering following situations: Additional iron for pregnant women due to dilutional anemia; storage of a certain amount of iron for pregnant women to compensate for iron loss caused by bleeding during delivery; storage of a certain amount of iron in fetus liver to provide the needs for infant up to 6 months of age.

Adequate intake of zinc in pregnant women is beneficial to the development of the fetus and to the prevention of birth defects. Requirement for zinc by fetus reaches the peak at the later stage of the third trimester. Iodine deficiency in pregnant women can lead to deficient production of thyroid hormone at birth and have an adverse effect on physical and intellectual development during infancy and childhood.

Inadequate folic acid intake has been found to be a risk factor to neural tube defects. Peri-conceptional 400 μg DEF folic acid supplementation per day in prevention of neural tube defects has been supported by many studies.

7.1.1.3 Malnutrition during pregnancy

Malnutrition presents significant threats to pregnant women and their fetuses. Although malnutrition is associated with many factors, such as household food security, maternal and child care, health services and environment, inadequate dietary intake are one of the major causes of malnutrition.

（1）Malnutrition in pregnant women

1）Anemia

Anemia is a condition in which the number of red blood cells or their oxygen-carrying capacity is insufficient to meet physiologic needs. During pregnancy, dilutional anemia occurs. The increased demand on hematopoiesis both by mother and the fetus aggravates the risk of developing iron deficiency anemia, especially for mother in her third trimester. If a woman's haemoglobin concentration during the first, second or third trimester of gestation is lower than 110 g/L, generally, she is considered to be anaemic. Globally, it's estimated that 41.8% of pregnant women are diagnosed as anemia and half of them are assumed to be due to iron deficiency. Iron deficiency anemia occurring in pregnancy is associated with low birth weight and may increase maternal and perinatal mortality.

2）Osteomalacia

Vitamin D deficiency during pregnancy may affect calcium absorption which leads to the decrease of serum calcium concentration. In order to meet the needs of fetal growth and development, calcium in the maternal bone will be dissolved. The dissolution of calcium from maternal bone may cause spine and pelvis osteomalacia.

（2）Malnutrition on fetus

1）Low birth weight

Newborn babies vary in birth weight and size. Low birth weight (LBW) is defined if an infant's birth weight is less than 2,500 g, regardless of gestational age. LBW is closely associated with fetal and perinatal mortality and morbidity. Neonatal deaths account for 46% of all deaths among children under 5 years old around the world, although most neonatal deaths happen in developing countries. Low birth weight has long-term effect on children's physical growth and cognitive development, and increase the risk of chronic diseases in later life. A variety of maternal complications can cause low birth, such as maternal malnutrition, premature birth, and maternal sickness.

2）IUGR

Fetuses whose estimated fetal weight (EFW) less than 10th percentile is defined as small for gestation age (SGA). SGA infants are usually found with higher rates of mortality and morbidity upon their gestational age. Intrauterine growth retardation (IUGR) is one of the factors associated with SGA. Anemia, severe malnutrition, hypertension, chronic renal disease are all maternal risk factors for IUGR.

3）Congenital malformation

Congenital malformation can be caused by environmental or genetic factors. At least 10% of all congenital malformations are known to be caused by environmental factors. Insufficient or excessive intake of certain nutrients during pregnancy, especially during the first trimester is associated with occurrence of a variety of birth defects.

7.1.1.4 Recommendations for pregnant women

（1）Principle of healthy diet during pregnancy

During pregnancy, the diet intake should be adjusted according to the physiological changes and the development of fetal growth, on the basis of balanced diet for non-pregnant women. Diet during the first trimester can be kept roughly the same as non-pregnant woman's balanced diet. Since the second trimester, to meet the nutritional requirement for growth and brain development of fetus, pregnant women are advised to eat a greater amount and variety of foods, such as milk, fish, meat, vegetables, nuts, seeds, cereals and beans to ensure the energy and protein intake. Eating fish 2-3 times per week is the recommended intake for omega-3 fatty acids which are important factors in baby's brain development both before and after birth. The daily recommended dose of iron is 20 mg in the first trimmest, 24 mg in the second trimester and 29 mg in the third trimester according to The Chinese Nutrition Society. Pregnant women are advised to eat iron-rich foods, including lean meat, poultry, fish, beans and bean products.

Gestational weight gain is an indicator that can directly reflect pregnant woman's nutritional status, hence, it's closely associated with many birth outcomes including offspring's birth weight. The recommended weight gain during pregnancy depends on pregnant woman's health and her body mass index before she was pregnant. According to Institute of Medicine (US), if the woman has a normal weight before pregnancy, she should gain 11.5 kg to 16 kg during pregnancy. If the woman is underweight before pregnancy, she should gain more weight than a woman who has a normal weight before pregnancy. If the woman is overweight or obese before pregnancy, she should gain less weight(Table 7-1).

Table 7-1　Weight gain recommendations for pregnancyby institute of medicine

Pre-pregnancy weight	Body Mass Index *	Recommended range of total weight (kg)	Recommended rates of weight gain in the second and third trimesters (kg) [mean range(kg/wk)]
Underweight	Less than 18.5	12.5-18	0.51 (0.44-0.58)
Normal Weight	18.5-24.9	11.5-16	0.42 (0.35-0.50)
Overweight	25.0-29.9	7-11.5	0.28 (0.23-0.33)
Obese (includes all classes)	30 and greater	5-9	0.22 (0.17-0.27)

* Body mass index is calculated as weight in kilograms divided by height in meters squared or as weight in pounds multiplied by 703 divided by height in inches.

Calculations assume a 0.5-2 kg weight gain in the first trimester.

Source: [Institute of Medicine (US) and National Research Council (US) Committee to Reexamine IOM Pregnancy Weight Guidelines; Rasmussen KM, Yaktine AL, editors. Weight Gain During Pregnancy: Reexamining the Guidelines. Washington (DC): National Academies Press (US); 2009. Available from: https://www.ncbi.nlm.nih.gov/books/NBK32813/doi:10.17226/12584].

(2) Supplementation

Neural tube defects (NTDs) are estimated to affect more than 300,000 newborns worldwide each year. These birth defects, which include anencephaly and spina bifida, usually occur in the early weeks of pregnancy and most of the time before a woman is aware of her pregnancy. In order to help prevent NTDs, pregnant women and women who may become pregnant should take folic acid supplementation 400 μg RE per day or daily vitamin supplement that contains folic acid. During pregnancy, women need to consume extra iron, about double the amount that a nonpregnant woman needs, to ensure they have sufficient iron stores to prevent iron deficiency. Iron supplements will be used by pregnant women to prevent and correct iron deficiency and anemia during gestation if she cannot consume enough iron from diet or diagnosed as IDA.

7.1.2 Lactation

7.1.2.1 Physiology of lactation

The mechanism of lactation includes hormonal triggering and oxytocic ejection. During pregnancy, estrogen promotes the development of ducts and progesterone promotes the development of lobular–alveolar. Lactogenesis is inhibited by a direct inhibitory action of steroids on the breast during pregnancy despite the high levels of prolactin. After delivery and clearance of placental steroids, prolactin is involved in breast milk production. Prolactin release is triggered by nipple stimulation. The strength and duration of the suckling process have great effect on the amount of prolactin released. Milk ejection helps the removal of milk from the mammary gland. Oxytocic mechanism can be triggered by factors such as auditory stimuli or other stimuli associated with breast–feeding.

7.1.2.2 The benefits of breastfeeding on mothers

Breastfeeding triggers the release of oxytocin that promotes uterus contraction. This helps the uterus return to its normal size quickly. Breastfeeding is helpful upon the purpose of losing weight gained during pregnancy. Breastfeeding, especially exclusive or predominant breastfeeding can help to prolong the periods of lactational amenorrhoea and play an important role in birth spacing. The risk of breast cancer, ovarian cancer and diabetes can be reduced by breastfeeding.

7.1.2.3 Principle of healthy diet during lactation

The nutritional status of mother has great impact on breast milk. To make breast milk for baby, about 450–500 extra calories a day are needed. If mother's weight is in the normal range, she needs about 2,300 total calories per day. During lactation, healthy diet which contains a variety of dietary foods is still recommended. Quality and quantity of dietary protein is closely related to the quality of breast milk. Women during lactation are encouraged to have protein through the following food groups, which are thought to be the good sources of protein. They are beef, pork, fish, poultry and eggs, dairy products beans, peas and nuts. The amount of drinking water is closely related to the amount of milk secretion. So, drinking plenty of fluids and paying attention to additional oil and sodium intake are highly recommended.

7.2 Nutrition during infancy, in childhood and adolescence

Infant and childhood nutrition is one of the critical components of childhood care. Better nutrition can stimulate intellectual development and is also associated with improved infant and child health, and stronger immune systems. There are some long–term health outcomes of good nutrition during childhood, such as lower risk of non–communicable diseases and longevity.

7.2.1 Infancy and childhood

Child from birth to 1 year old is defined as infant. It's the first phase of rapid growth of human life. Increase of body weight is the first presentation of infant development. Baby's body weight doubles at around 5–6 months after delivery and it can be triple at the age of 1 year old. Body length usually signifies the growth of skeleton. Body length usually doubles during the first year. From birth to age 1, children should be weighed every month and from age 1 to age 2, at least every three months. If a child does not appear to be growing, the child should be treated by a trained health worker. The growth of head circumference is rapid in the first two years. It's an easily gained parameter and can be a sign of abnormal brain development. Gastrointestinal function of infant is not fully developed and there are many limitations regarding digestion, absorption and utilization of food. Breast milk contains protein, fat, vitamin A and vitamin C, iron, and lactose. It also contains fatty acids essential for the infant's growing brain, eyes, and blood vessels. Nutrients are more easily absorbed from breast milk than from other milk. During the first year, infant's immune system has not fully developed, however breastfeeding can protect against illness since breastmilk contains antibodies transferred from the mother's immunite system. Infancy is a key period of rapid development of cognition, behavior and perception. The brain develops most rapidly before birth and during the first two years of life. It canhelp the brain to develop if we make infants use their eyes and ears, touch and explore things because children can see and hear things at birth. Breast milk also helps young children free from illness so that they are strong enough to explore and learn something.

7.2.1.1   Breastfeeding and food complementation

Breastmilk alone is the best food and drink for an infant for the first six months of life. Exclusive breastfeeding means only breastmilk and no other liquids or solids can be taken by the infants, not even water (the child can take medicine and vitamins, if needed). If children continue to be breastfed up to two years and beyond, the health and development of children would be greatly improved. If a woman can't breastfeed her infant, the baby can be fed expressed breastmilk or, if necessary, a quality breastmilk substitute from an ordinary clean cup. Infant's sleep pattern is not well established until 6 months old and it varies among individuals greatly. It is recommended that mothers feed as much as the baby wants. Normally, the baby should be breastfed at least eight times daily, day and night. Almost every mother can breastfeed successfully. Under some special circumstances that mother cannot produce breastmilk, infant formula can be substituted with bottle feeding. Feeding the baby with just infant formula (breastmilk substitutes) in the first six months is necessary.

Breastmilk should be continually fed to children older than 6 months up to two years and beyond. To meet infants' growth and development needs, other nutritious foods should be given to infants. Infants may lose weight and have fluctuated weight during this critical period if additional food hasn't been complemented with the breast milk. Good complementary foods should first be nutrient-rich, energy-rich, and locally available. Foods should be prepared safely and hygienically. They should be prepared in a consistency that is nutritionally rich and adapted to a child's requirements and eating abilities. It is important to start with soft, mushy foods and move gradually to more solid foods. Greater the variety of healthy foods is a key component to the balanced nutrition of the child's diet. Introducing foods to a child who has been exclusively breastfed may be difficult at first. It should start by giving 2–3 tablespoons of well mashed food, 2–3 meals each day and gradually encourage—but do not force—the child to eat more.

7.2.1.2   Children's nutrient needs and diet principle

Children of 6–8 months old should be breastfed frequently and receive other foods have the two to three times a day. Infants can eat pureed or mashed foods, thick soups and porridges, and gradually increased consistency (thickness) food. Animal foods such as meat, eggs and fish can be given, but they should be mashed, minced or cut into very small pieces. One should start with one kind of complementary food and add a new type of food until infants get used to the previous food.

Most infants by 8 months of age can also eat 'finger foods' (snacks that children can eat by themselves). By 12 months, most children can have table food. Children age 9–24 months should receive other food three to four times a day in addition to breastfeeding. Food from animals, such as meat, fish and eggs, should be included. If the child is no longer breastfed, 300 mL of milk plus one or two extra meals should be added each day.

Sometimes, it may be difficult to meet all the child's nutrient requirements without enough food from animal sources. So, it may be necessary to give the child fortified foods or spreads or multiple vitamin and mineral supplements, such as powders, syrups or dissolvable tablets. For example, iron fortified rice powder is recommended as complementary food after 6 months old to increase the iron intake and prevent infant anemia.

The diet of children of 2-5 years old follows the principles of healthy diet that can provide balanced nutrients intake. The food variety should be adequate and similar to adult's diet. The frequency of foods should be set up as a routine gradually with certain amount of foods to help in developing a good habit. Snacks, preferably raw fruits and vegetable should be given between meals. Avoiding commercial snacks and sugared beverages. Meals with great look and taste can improve children's appetite. Proper cooking methods should be considered in order to promote food intake and nutrients absorption. During cooking, salt reduction should be carried out to develop a healthy appetite for children.

Children of 6-9 years old is similar to that of 2-5 years on the base of balanced diet. Children at this age are active in exercise and learning, which need much energy expenditure. Energy and other nutrients should come from a variety of foods with regular meals and healthy snacks. Quality and quantity of breakfast has much effect on learning, so does milk and other dairy products which are also good sources of protein and calcium.

7.2.1.3　Childhood obesity prevention

Children need a well-balanced diet which includes adequate protein and energy as well as vitamins and minerals to ensure good health and development. Overweight or obesity is caused by multiple factors, such as over nutrition and lack of physical activity. Childhood obesity is associated with increased risk of diabetes and cardiovascular disease and other diseases in adulthood. Sometimes children eat large quantities of foods that are high in energy but not rich in other necessary nutrients, such as sugary drinks or fried, starchy foods. In such cases, improving the quality of the child's diet is crucial along with increasing his or her level of physical activity.

7.2.2　Adolescence

Adolescents are often thought of as a group young people whose age is between 10 and 19. Adolescence is a period consising of the physical changes of puberty as well as cognitive, social, and psychological changes. There are some serious diseases in adulthood originated in adolescence. For example, tobacco use, poor eating and exercise habits, sexually transmitted infections including HIV, leading to illness or premature death later in life.

Promoting healthy behaviors during adolescence, and taking steps to better protect young people from health risks are critical for the prevention of health problems in adulthood.

In developing countries, there are many boys and girls who enter adolescence in a malnutrition state, leaving them more vulnerable to physical and psychological diseases. At the other end of the spectrum, there is a large amount of adolescents with overweight and obesity around the world. Developing adolescence's healthy eating and exercise habits are foundations for good health in adulthood and later life.

Sufficient protein and carbohydrate are essential to provide energy and nutrients needs for adolescents. Whole grains can provide energy for development and physical activity. Dietary fiber and vitamin B can be found in whole grains. In addition, adolescents should take animal foods, such as fish, meat, poultry, and eggs in order to meet the needs for protein. Green vegetables and dairy products along with adequate physical activity play a key role for bone health. Besides the dietary guides for healthy diet, regularly consuming foods high in saturated fats, trans-fatty acids, free sugars, or salt, should be avoided. Engaging in physical activity is important for all but especially children and adolescents. About 60 minutes of moderate to vigorous physical activity daily are recommended to improve the physical development and to prevent the overweight and obesity. Female adolescence tends to lose iron due to the menstrual period and are under threat of iron deficiency anemia so they need extra iron, preferably from foods, including lean meat, poultry and beans.

7.3 Nutrition in the adult years and aging

7.3.1 Adulthood

Healthy diet helps prevent malnutrition (both under-nutrition and over-nutrition) and diet-related non-communicable diseases. The exact make-up of a diversified, balanced and healthy diet will vary depending on each adult's needs (e. g., gender, lifestyle, degree of physical activity), cultural context, locally available foods and dietary customs. But basic principles of what constitute a healthy diet remain the same.

A healthy diet for adults contains the following.

A variety of foods should be considered. Fruits, vegetables, legumes (e. g., lentils, beans), nuts and whole grains (e. g., unprocessed maize, millet, oats, wheat, brown rice).

Fresh vegetables and fruits should be consumed every day. At least 400 g (5 portions) of fruits and vegetables, not including potatoes, sweet potatoes and other starchy roots, are recommended per day.

Identify the existence of free sugar and limit the intake of free sugar to less than 10% of total energy intake, which is equivalent to 50 g for a person of healthy body weight who consumes approximately 2,000 calories per day. Ideally, if one person takes free sugar that is less than 5% of total energy intake, it has additional health benefits. Free sugars are those monosaccharides (such as glucose or fructose) and disaccharides (such as sucrose or table sugar) added to foods or drinks by the manufacturer, cook or consumer, and can also be found in sugars naturally present in honey, syrups, fruit juices and fruit juice concentrates.

Limit the intake of fat at 20% –30% of total energy intake from fats is recommended. Unsaturated fats, usually found in fish, avocado, nuts, sunflower, canola and olive oils, are preferable to saturated fats, usually found in fatty meat, butter, palm and coconut oil, cream, cheese and lard. Industrial trans fats, most of time found in processed food, fast food, snack food, fried food, frozen pizza, pies, cookies and spreads, are not part of a healthy diet and should be avoided. Decreasing the salt intake to less than 5 g of salt per day and use iodized salt are suggested.

Besides principle of healthy diet listed above, additional advice on diet during adulthood can play a positive role to bone health, especially for females. Skeleton supports the body and protects internal organs from injury. There is a continuing process of bone renewal in adults. The renewal process of bone includes bone resorption (break down of small amounts of bone) and bone formation (replaced by new bone). There is a shift of minerals like calcium phosphate and calcium carbonate, fluorides and chlorides from other parts of the body to the bone and back again, under the regulation of hormones, specialized bone cells and the stresses and strains of weight-bearing activities. The bone hardness is primarily decided by the amount of mineral in bone, with the contribution of substances like the structural protein collagen. Osteoporosis is diagnosed when the loss of bone density and strength leads to an unacceptably high tendency for bones to fracture. Many factors are associated with the increased risk of developing osteoporosis, such as sex, age, race and menopausal status, family history of osteoporosis, lean body mass, smoking, excessive alcohol intake, a lifestyle with little physical activity and inadequate calcium intake or poor vitamin D nutrition. Although the problem of osteoporosis is shared by both elderly man and elderly women, in most western countries the risk of the condition is about twice as high in women at the age of 60. Adulthood is the period that is essential for reduction of risk to osteoporosis through daily healthy diet.

The reference nutrient intake of calcium for non-pregnant women is 800 mg/d. Dairy products, such as fresh milk is good source of calcium. Also, 300 mL fresh milk per day is recommended. Other than dairy products, bean products are also good source of calcium. The reference nutrient intake of vitamin D is 400 IU/d. Vitamin D is not rich in most foods. The good source of Vitamin D is marine fish liver oils. The other source of Vitamin D from diet is foods fortified with vitamin D, such as some fruit juices. Adequate amounts of vitamin D can be produced with enough sunlight exposure.

7.3.2 Ageing

Life expectancy is extending around the world. Populations are rapidly ageing. The meaning of the longer life is not only for older people and their families, but also for societies as a whole. The elderly can take advantage of the additional years to make valuable contributions to family and community and pursue new activities such as a long-neglected hobby. The biggest problems for older people are heart disease, stroke and chronic lung disease in low-and middle-income countries. Disability is also threatening the health of the elderly. Sensory impairments and chronic obstructive pulmonary disease are particularly severe in low- and middle-income countries.

Ageing is a result of accumulation of a wide variety of molecular and cellular damage over time. The elderly's physical and mental capacity decrease gradually and risk of death increases. Disease is inevitable to most ageing population. The absence of disease is not a sign of good health, but the combination of a person's physical and mental capacities is a better predictor of the elderly's health.

Nutrition plays an important role in terms of keeping good physical and mental capacities. Loss of muscle mass and strength, reduced flexibility, and problems with balance can all impair mobility. Ageing is a process of physiological change including lowered basal metabolic rate (BMR), disorder of lipid metabolism, impaired digestive system, enhanced oxidative damage, and decreased immunologic function. The principle of balanced diet should be followed by ageing people.

Energy input should be adjusted to meet the decreased energy expenditure by the standard of keeping the healthy body weight, for example BMI is between 18.5-23.9. Protein rich foods such as lean meat, eggs or bean products are recommended but with limited amount due to the need to control the serum lipid concentration. If inadequate intake of protein happened with inactivity, lean body mass (mainly muscle) loss can great harm to balance and flexibility. Whole grains are good sources of carbohydrates, (including dietary fiber and polysaccharide) and vitamin B. Fresh fruits and vegetables can provide nutrients against oxidative damage.

With the improved nutrition, multimodal exercise, especially strength resistance training should be introduced to ageing people to improve their physical capacity and mental capacity. Low vitamin D level is possibly associated with the lack of exposure to sunlight due to insufficient outdoor activity. Foods with vitamin D fortified or supplementation should be consumed if the ageing people have difficulty to access outdoor activity.

Cheng Yue

Chapter 8

Community Nutrition

8.1 Dietary reference intakes

8.1.1 Introduction of dietary reference intakes

The recommended dietary allowances (RDAs) were established by the Food and Nutrition Board (FNB) of the Institute of Medicine (IOM) in 1941 as American standards for nutrient requirements. Revised approximately every 10 years, the RDAS have kept pace with current research and population needs. The first editions of the RDAs were developed at a time when the U. S. population was recovering from a major economic depression and World War Ⅱ, so nutrient deficiencies were a concern.

As the science of nutrition advances, it is becoming abundantly clear that other components of food besides essential nutrients affect health. It is also becoming apparent that levels of nutrient intake associated with deficiency disease prevention may be too low to help prevent cancer, heart disease, and osteoporosis. Excessively high intakes of nutrients from fortified foods and supplements are other problems that were not considered when previous editions of the RDAs were prepared.

The recommended daily levels of intake not only meet the nutrient needs of almost all healthy people (97%–98%) but also promote health and help reduce the risk of chronic disease.

In 1993 the FNB developed a framework for the development of nutrient recommendations, called dietary reference intakes (DRIs). DRIs encompass four types of nutrient recommendations for healthy individuals—adequate intake (AI), estimated average intake (EAR), recommended nutrient intake (RNI), and tolerable upper intake level (UL).

8.1.2 DRIs components

The DRI model expands the previous RDA, which focused on establishing AIs of nutrients for healthy populations to prevent deficiency diseases. To respond to scientific advances in diet and health throughout the life cycle, the DRI model now including seven reference points (Figure 8–1).

(1) The EAR is the average requirement of a nutrient for healthy individuals a functional or clinical assessment has been conducted, and measures of adequacy have been made at a specified level of dietary

intake. An EAR is the amount of a nutrient with which about one half of individuals would have their needs met and one half would not. The EAR should be used for assessing the nutrient adequacy of populations, not individuals.

(2) RNI corresponds to the traditional RDA, the daily dietary intake level of a nutrient considered to be sufficient to the majority of individuals (97% –98%) of a certain gender, age and physiological status group.

RNI is based on EAR, if the standard deviation (SD) of the EAR is available and the requirement for the nutrient is symmetrically distributed, the RNI is set at two SDs above the EAR (RDA = EAR + 2SD). Long-term intake of RNI can meet the body's need for this nutrient and maintain healthy and adequate reserves in the organization.

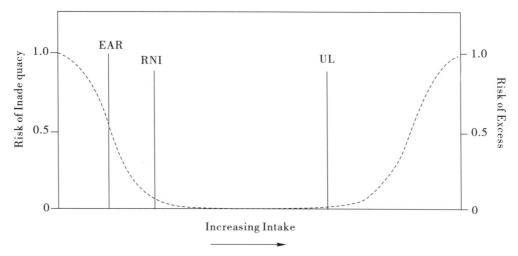

Figure 8-1　Terms and abbreviations used in DRIs and a graphic representation of their meaning

(3) The AI is a nutrient recommendation based on observed or experimentally determined approximation of nutrient intake by a group (or groups) of healthy people when sufficient scientific evidence is not available to calculate an RNI or an EAR.

(4) Tolerable upper intake levels (ULs) have been established (for nutrients for which adequate data are available) to reduce the risk of adverse or toxic effects from increased consumption of nutrients in concentrated form–either alone or combined with others (not in food) –or from enrichment and fortification. The UL is the highest level of daily nutrient intake that is unlikely to have any adverse health effects on almost all individuals in the general population.

In China, except the four indexes, we had other 3 reference indexes for different nutrients.

(5) Acceptable macronutrient distribution ranges (AMDR) are ranges of intakes of macronutrients associated with reduced risk of chronic disease. The AMDRs for fat, carbohydrate, and protein are based on energy intake by age group.

(6) Proposed intake for preventing non–communicable chronic diseases (PI–NCD) is the daily intake of essential nutrients, aiming at the primary prevention of non–communicable diseases (NCDs). NCDs, including cancer, cardiovascular disease and stroke, diabetes mellitus, and chronic obstructive pulmonary disease (COPD), have become the primary causes of death in both developed and developing countries.

(7) Specific proposed level (SPL) is used to evaluate and assign the intake value for bioactive substances. In 2010, China Nutrition Society, initiated the incorporation of a SPL for non–nutrients and a proposed intake that is based on reducing the risk of non–communicable chronic disease and improving optimal

health. Their stated rationale as to why they consider the SPL a DRI value is that both traditional medicine and modern nutrition research have deepened the understanding of plant compounds; and because consumers are widely consuming these bioactive substances in China.

8.2 Nutrition survey and nutrition assessment

8.2.1 Introduction

Nutrition and health surveys at the national level provide information on the dietary status of a population, the nutritional adequacy of the food supply, the economics of food consumption, and the effects of food assistance and regulatory programs. Public guidelines for food selection are usually based on the survey data. The data are also used in policy setting and program development.

Measures of nutritional status are usually valuable in as much as they may be predictive of health outcomes. The practical requirements for assessment of nutritional adequacy arise from the need to intervene, either by advice or by more aggressive strategies, to improve the nutrition of individuals or populations, and thereby to reduce the risks and the burdens of those diseases that have, or may have a nutritional component. Such diseases may range from the classical single nutrient deficiency diseases such as beriberi or scurvy to multifactorial diseases such as cardiovascular diseases or cancer, where nutrition is thought to play a modulating role as one of many aetiological factors.

The major categories of nutritional assessment strategies include: dietary, anthropometric, biochemical status and functional and clinical status.

Dietary assessment can be performed by weighed or household-measures-intake records, usually for 3 or 7 days. It can be done by diet histories or recalls, usually for the previous 24 hours, or by a food frequency questionnaire to probe the frequency with which specified food items are usually eaten per week for instance.

Anthropometry measures typically include weight and height with body mass index being calculated from these; mid-upper arm circumference, and perhaps others such as skinfold thicknesses.

Biochemical status measures or indices are selected and tailored for each nutrient, and are often the concentration of the nutrient or its derivatives in a body fluid such as serum or plasma. Thus plasma retinol is an index of vitamin A status, 25-hydroxy-vitamin D is an index of vitamin D status and the activation of the flavin-dependent red cell enzyme erythrocyte glutathione reductase is an index of riboflavin (vitamin B_2) status.

Functional indices assess the integrity and efficiency of metabolic processes that are nutrient dependent. Thus plasma homocysteine concentration is influenced by several B vitamins and is a functional index for their adequacy. Dark adaptation is influenced by vitamin A and zinc. Blood clotting is influenced by vitamin K.

Clinical indices comprise clinical signs or symptoms of nutrient deficiency: rickets is a sign of vitamin D deficiency and impaired blood clotting is a symptom of vitamin K deficiency. To some extent, these indices may overlap: for instance, some biochemical indices are based on nutrient concentrations in body fluids which are, in turn, highly dependent on recent dietary intake, where others are based on related biochemical functions and metabolic-pathway adequacy which is more dependent on the tissue status and more closely related to functional adequacy.

8.2.2　Methods of dietary assessment

There are five stages at which food availability and consumption can be measured, including domestic food production, total food available, household food purchases, food available in household and food consumption by individuals. In this chapter, the main focus is on how to measure food consumption among individuals.

There are two main approaches to individual dietary assessment, prospective and retrospective. Prospective methods involve collecting or recording current diet by the subjects, while retrospective methods require subjects to recall their recent or past diet. Both types of assessment have strengths and limitations.

8.2.2.1　Prospective method

(1) Duplicate diet method (nutrient composition analysis). This technique requires subjects to weigh and record their food consumption at the time of eating. At the same time, they put aside an exact duplicate portion of each food consumed which is analyzed chemically for energy and nutrient content. The main advantage of this method is that it is independent of errors associated with the use of food composition tables. It is best suited to metabolic balance studies in free-living population.

(2) Weighed inventory method. The weighed inventory is one of the most widely used techniques. It was first described by Elsie Widdowson in 1936. Subjects keep a record of all food and drink consumed. Each food item is weighed prior to consumption using portable food weighing scales. Items left over are also weighed. In practice, most weighed inventories include a proportion of items recorded in household measures.

(3) Household measures method. The method is similar to the weighed inventory, except that subjects record portion sizes in household measures (cup, bowl, spoonful, etc.) rather than weigh their food. In more recent, sets of food photographs are provided to aid subjects with recording portion size. Records in household measures have the advantage of simplifying the recording process for subjects.

(4) Food checklist method. Respondents are provided each day with a pre-printed list of foods and asked to tick a box each time an item consumed. A space is usually provided to record foods eaten but not listed. Standard portion sizes may be indicated, or portion descriptions entered. The method is simple to use and well-liked by respondents, but the information collected is less detailed than other prospective methods and food consumption and nutrient intakes are less precise as a result.

8.2.2.2　Retrospective method

(1) 24-hour recall method. The 24-hour recall (originally attributed to Wiehl in 1942) involves a trained interviewer asking subjects to recall and describe every item of food and drink consumed over exactly 24 hours. The information is obtained through systematic repetition of open-ended questions. Amounts may be described in household measures or using food photographs. Interviewers must be thoroughly familiar with both the local diet and the food composition tables to be used to estimate nutrient intakes, in order to probe subjects effectively and obtain adequate details for subsequent coding of data. The 'multiple-pass' 24-hour recall is now in widespread use (consisting of several stages including an uninterrupted 'quick list' of items recalled; a detailed interview elaborating the quick list that determines detail and amounts; and a thorough review of the detailed interview). This multiple pass method minimizes the opportunity for items to be forgotten.

(2) Diet history method. The diet history which was originally described by Burke in 1947 is one of the oldest approaches for assessing diet though used less frequently today. It is used to assess 'usual' diet over the recent past. Typically, a trained interviewer begins by carrying out a 24-hour recall which is elaborated

in an interview lasting up to 2 hours. For each meal, subjects are asked to describe the range of foods that would be likely consumed, the frequency of their consumption, and typical amounts. Differences between weekdays and weekends are clarified, and seasonal variations are elaborated.

(3) Food frequency questionnaire. Food frequency questionnaires (FFQ) are pre-printed lists of foods on which subjects are asked to indicate the typical frequency of consumption and to state in household measures the average amount consumed on the days when the food is eaten. The number of foods on the list varies. Optically scannable questionnaires speed up the coding of information.

Brief dietary assessment methods are useful when total diet does not need to be assessed. For example, simplified FFQs that contain far fewer food items than that typically be included may be used in instances where a single nutrient or type of food is being estimated. Although such assessments can be made at a low cost with a low respondent and interviewer burden, they have several limitations including an inability to assess entire diet and provide quantitatively precise information.

8.2.2.3 Prospective methods-advantages and disadvantages

The main advantage of prospective methods is that they provide a direct measure of current diet. Also, they can be carried out for varying lengths of time according to the level of accuracy of the estimate of food consumption or nutrient intake required. In general, for a given food or nutrient, the more days of information collected, the better precision of the estimate. However, there is a balance to be found between achieving precise estimates of intake and maintaining recording enthusiasm of the subjects so as to minimize changes in patterns of usual consumption.

The main disadvantage of prospective methods is that they are labor-intensive for both the respondent and the interviewer. The respondent needs good literacy, language and numeracy skills in order to provide an accurate record. This limits the usefulness of prospective methods in populations where literacy levels are low, unless trained recorders are present, but the presence of an observer may result in a distortion of usual diet. Good subject motivation and a commitment to complete the record accurately and objectively are needed.

8.2.2.4 Retrospective methods-advantages and disadvantages

Retrospective methods require subjects to recall their current or past diet. This may involve remembering the type and amount of all individual items consumed over a specified period of time (e.g., 24-hour recall), or creating a mental construct of 'usual' consumption involving recollection of both the frequency of consumption of specific foods or food groups and the amounts consumed.

The main advantages of the retrospective methods are that they are relatively quick to administer compared with prospective methods. They are also less expensive in terms of equipment and (except for repeat 24-hour recalls, see below) resources considering the time taken for interviewers to meet subjects. A further advantage of retrospective methods is that because there is a lower respondent burden than for prospective methods, the chances of obtaining a more representative sample of all consumers is increased. They can also be used to assess diet in the past, which may be relevant to studies where the underlying causes of chronic diseases such as heart disease or cancer may lie in past rather than current diet.

The main disadvantage of retrospective methods relates to sources of bias. Errors in memory result in the omission of foods from the assessment. This may be a problem for some elderly subjects and for children under the age of about 12. Subjects and interviewers must have good skills relating to the perception and conceptualization of food portion size (the ability to develop an accurate mental construction of the amount of food consumed and to translate that construction into a description or selection of an appropriate food portion photograph which corresponds to the amount actually consumed). Among respondents, this is a problem especially in children under 12 years of age. The presence of an observer (interviewer) may cause subjects to overemphasize what they perceive as the 'healthy' aspects of their diet and to minimize the 'unhealthy aspects' (social desirability and social approval bias). Daily variation in diet is less readily assessed using retrospective methods (unless using repeat 24-hour recalls). Subjects who do not have regular eating habits will have difficulty describing the usual frequency of consumption and, as with most prospective methods, the use of food composition tables will introduce error into the estimates of energy and nutrient intake.

8.2.3 Anthropometry assessment

Anthropometry is the scientific study of variation in the size and shape of the human body. Compared with the dietary biochemical status, and functional and clinical status methods, anthropometry may provide a relatively quick and inexpensive measurement for the assessment of nutritional status. Anthropometric nutritional assessment involves the measurement of aspects of body size. These are then related to references or standards according to the age and sex of the subject, which reflect the body growth of healthy and well-nourished individuals. Differences from the reference values are taken to be outcomes of nutritional experience. The WHO states that anthropometry reflects both health and nutritional status and predicts performance, health and survival. As such, it is a valuable, but currently underused tool for guiding public health policy and clinical decisions.

The reasons why the WHO and other health authorities recommend anthropometry as the primary method of nutritional assessment is the relatively low cost and portability of equipment needed, the relatively low level of training required to use this equipment, and the high accuracy and precision relative to dietary methods.

Although a wide range of anthropometric measurements can be made for ergonomic, anthropological, physiological, medical and sports purposes, a rather more limited list is appropriate to nutritional anthropometry. All of the measurements given in this book are appropriate for the assessment of under-nutrition at all ages. For older children, adolescents and adults, waist and hip circumference, in addition to weight, height, arm circumference and skinfolds, are useful in the assessment of over-nutrition. The following are instructions for the main anthropometric measurement techniques, height, length, weight, arm circumference and skinfolds (triceps skinfold). All measurements should be taken by at least two people, one is primarily responsible for positioning the subject and reading the measurement, and another makes sure the positioning is correct and records the measurement. The recorder must repeat the measurement aloud and receive confirmation before finalizing the record.

(1) Height

The measurement of the maximum distance from the floor to the highest point on the head, when the subject is facing directly ahead, with shoes off, feet together, arms by the sides, and heels, buttocks and upper back in contact with the wall. The equipment requires a stadiometer, portable anthropometer or steel ruler placed against a wall. Experienced technicians achieve a reliability of ± 1.0 mm on repeated height measurements of the same person. Height is greater in the morning as it should be at the same time of day each time, especially if the same person is measured on two or more occasions.

(2) Recumbent length

As infants under 2.0 years old cannot stand erect well enough for a useful measure of height, body length is measure lying down (recumbent). A measuring board is used, normally with a fixed headpiece and an adjustable foot piece. It is placed so that—it is stable on a hard, flat beside the board surface, such as the floor. Place the record form and kneel at the base of the board to the right side of the child so that you can move the foot piece with your right hand. With the help of mother or an assistant, gently lower the child onto the measuring board. With your hands cupped over the child's ears and your arms straight as well as place the child's head against the base of the board. The child should look straight up and lie flat in the centre of the board. With your left hand on the child's shins press them gently but firmly against the board and check the position of the child's. When the child's position is correct, move the foot piece with your right hand until it is firmly against the child's heels and read the measurement to the nearest 0. 1 cm.

(3) Body mass/weight

The person stands (or sits) on the balance with minimal movement and with hands by his/her side, or a young child can be placed in a sling attached to a hanging spring scale. Shoes and excess clothing should be removed so that the subject is dressed in light gown, bathing suit or minimal clothing. The spring scale, or a balance is calibrated for accuracy using weights authenticated by a government department of weights and measures. Weight measurements are generally reliable, with most errors due to mis-calibration or mis-reading of the equipment.

(4) Arm circumference

The person stands with his back to the examiner and the right arm flexed. The examiner locates the acromion of the scapula (tip of the shoulder) and the olecranon of the ulna (tip of the elbow) and measures the distance between these two points. A mark is placed on the triceps muscle at the mid-point between the shoulder and elbow. A flexible tape, made of non-stretchable plastic, is wrapped around the arm at the level of the mark and tightened to just touch the skin in all places, without compression. The circumference is read from the tape measure.

(5) Skinfolds

The measurement of skinfolds can use between three and nine different standard anatomical sites around the body. The right side or the left side of the body only is usually measured for consistency. The tester pinches the skin at the appropriate site to raise a double layer of skin and the underlying adipose tissue, but not the muscle. The skinfold calipers are then applied 1 cm below and at right angles to the pinch, the jaws of the caliper are released and a reading in millimeters (mm) is taken 2 seconds later, as fat tissue is compressible under continuous pressure. The mean of two measurements is calculated. If the two measurements differ by more than 10%, a third one is taken and the median value will be used. The triceps site is the most commonly measured for nutritional assessment.

The most common anthropometric measures of under-nutrition in children are weight and height, either individually or combined, relative to refer for age and weight for height, since they can be used to discriminate between acute and chronic under-nutrition. Weight for height can also be used to assess over-nutrition in children, and the body mass index, (BMI) [weight(kg)/height (m)^2] is now the most widely used measure for this purpose, though it is a less sensitive marker of body fatness than skinfold thicknesses values.

For adults the most commonly used measure of under-nutrition and over-nutrition is the BMI. Adult under-nutrition, which called chronic energy deficiency (CED), is classified by the following BMI cut-offs 17-18. 5, grade I ; 16-17, grade II ; below 16, grade III CED. BMI cut-offs of 25, 30 and 40 are used inter nationally to define mild, moderate and severe obesity respectively, though various nations may have differently defined criteria. The cut-off of 25 is also called overweight. BMI is an appropriate index in the general population especially in the wealthier nations of North America, western Europe, Australia and Japan. However, in these nations, people in better than average physical condition, especially athletes with considerable muscle mass, will have a higher BMI but not excessive fat. In many poorer nations, malnutrition and chronic disease can result in short stature due to relative stunting of the legs. Because the trunk of the body is more massive than the legs, such people will have a normal to high BMI but may have low fat, and may even be undernourished. Because of these limitations of BMI, waist and hip circumferences, and waist–to–hip ratio, are often preferred measures of the central distribution of body fatness.

8.2.4　Biochemical assessment

Biochemical assessment ideally forms part of a coordinated set of nutritional investigations that may also include diet estimates, anthropometry, functional and clinical investigations. These are used to distinguish between physiological deficiency, adequacy and overload of nutrients, and to assist in the diagnosis of nutrition–related factors that are relevant to the causation and treatment of disease states. The design of the biochemical part of the nutritional assessment depends on an available and suitable sample of body fluid or tissue for analysis and feasible biochemical tests to estimate the concentrations or functional adequacy of key nutrients. The results must then be interpreted in the light of established normal ranges. Therefore, it is essential to have access to suitable analytical equipment, suitable laboratory facilities and relevant expertise for sample collection, storage, analysis and interpretation.

Biochemical markers are specific diagnostic analytes that can be measured in accessible human body fluids and tissues such as blood, urine, saliva, hair and nails, used as predictors for the different levels of nutrient intake and of tissue status adequacy that occur in human individuals and populations.

Biochemical markers are potentially useful for the following reasons.

They can often be measured with high specificity and excellent accuracy and objectivity and unlike diet assessments they can be obtained without reliance on the accuracy of information being provided by the individuals being studied. Unlike clinical signs and symptoms of deficiency disease, biochemical markers can be nutrient–specific, rapidly and predictably responsive to the correction of nutrient deficiencies. Some, however, may reflect adequacy or deficiency of multiple nutrients, and should be interpreted accordingly.

In a few cases, dietary nutrient intakes can be predicted more accurately from biochemical indices than from diet assessment, especially urinary sodium, potassium and fluoride, used as markers for intakes of these elements, and urinary nitrogen and iodide, used as markers for protein and iodine intakes, respectively.

8.2.4.1　Protein and essential amino acids

There are no good indices for tissue protein status in the sense of reflecting the adequacy of dietary protein as distinct from metabolic processes. The most commonly used index is serum (or plasma) albumin. This is lowered (in conditions such as kwashiorkor) attributable to low protein intakes or poor protein quality. However, serum albumin may also be lowered by the acute phase reaction, and indeed severely malnourished children commonly also present with infections that affect their acute phase status.

Serum albumin is traditionally measured by a dye–based assay, or by more specific and reliable immunoassay. An alternative, possibly more reliable index of inadequate protein supply is the plasma amino acid profile, since the essential amino acids, notably the branched–chain amino–acids, are lowered when dietary protein is inadequate. Protein intakes can be monitored fairly accurate by nitrogen excretion rates, though protein is not the only dietary contributor to urinary nitrogen.

8.2.4.2　Essential fatty acid status (and fatty acid profiling)

Serum or plasma is frequently used for fatty acid profiling, and hence for monitoring of essential fatty acid (EFA) intakes. However, its interpretation is complicated by variability of lipoprotein profiles and by diurnal variation More promising, but less explored, are new techniques for fatty acids in red cell membranes, fat biopsies (reflecting long–term fat store composition), etc. New research into relationships with alternative, critical sites, such as nerve cell membranes, is needed.

8.2.4.3 Fat-soluble vitamins

(1) Vitamin A and Vitamin E are commonly measured in serum or plasma together with the carotenoid pigments, by high-performance liquid chromatography.

(2) Plasma vitamin E (tocopherol) levels are usually expressed as a ratio to cholesterol or total lipids, since the vitamin E content of plasma is highly dependent on its lipid content, and this ratio is a reasonably reliable indicator of vitamin E status, though it is not ideal in terms of its specificity and sensitivity.

(3) Vitamin D status is usually assessed by the concentration of 25-hydroxyvitamin D in serum or plasma. Levels may vary enormously between the seasons and with variable sunlight exposure.

(4) Vitamin K status is measured crudely by the rate of blood clotting, or more sensitively and specifically by PIVKA (protein induced by vitamin K absence or antagonism) and recently by vitamin K serum or plasma levels or the degree of under-carboxylation of osteocalcin, a bone-related peptide, in plasma. There is a need for more research on vitamin K indices and their functional interpretation.

8.2.4.4 Water-soluble vitamins

(1) Vitamin C status is usually measured by serum or plasma vitamin C concentrations or in older studies by the vitamin C content of buffy coat (i. e. , unfractionated white cells). The latter index is more closely related to body stores and long-term status for vitamin C, but it requires a cumbersome assay, creating heavy demands for fieldwork. Like the plasma index, which is subject to several ambiguities of interpretation. Despite confounding influences of acute phase processes in some studies, plasma vitamin C has been found to correlate relatively well with recent intakes (the most recent 1-2 weeks) of this vitamin, from foods and supplements.

(2) Of the B-vitamins, thiamin (B_1), riboflavin (B_2) and pyridoxine (B_6) levels are commonly assessed by the activation coefficients specific erythrocyte enzymes that require these vitamins as a part of the essential cofactors, such as transketolase for thiamin; glutathione reductase for riboflavin, and certain erythrocy amino acid aminotransferases for the vitamin B_6 coenzymes for vitamin B_6, direct measurement of plasma or red cell pyridoxal phosphate concentration is often preferred. Folate, vitamin B_{12}, biotin and pantothenic acid status are commonly assessed by serum or plasma concentrations. Red cell folate is a better index of long-term folate takes and body-stores than plasma or serum folate, but it is more difficult to measure accurately. Niacin status is usually assessed by its urinary breakdown products: n-methyl nicotinamid (NMN) or pyridones.

8.2.4.5 Mineral nutrients

Macro-essential elements include sodium, potassium, calcium, phosphorus, magnesium and chlorine (Na, K, Ca, P Mg and Cl). Some of these (notably Na, K) can be monitored by 24 h urine collections, or by spot urine samples with creatinine as the denominator; others (e. g. , Mg) are best studied in blood serum or plasma; yet others (e. g. , Ca, P) are best studied in relation to their functional effects—e. g. , on bone related enzymes and bone turnover markers. Micro-essential elements include iron, zinc, copper, selenium, chromium, manganese and iodine (Fe, Zn, Cu, Se, Cr, Mn and I). Zinc can be assessed by plasma zinc levels but this index is strongly (negatively) affected by acute phase effects and by any reduction in plasma protein concentration, notably albumin. Copper can, albeit with caveats, be assessed by the copper-zinc erythrocyte enzyme superoxide dismutase however there are no robust status indices for this element. Se can be assessed by serum, plasma or red cell Se levels, or by the selenium enzyme glutathione peroxidase usually in whole blood or red cells. Chromium and manganese have been assayed in blood fractions but interpretation is difficult. Direct iodine measurements are: usually performed on urine samples however there are also some plasma analytes (e. g. , thyroid-stimulating hormone, thyroglobulin, T_4 and T_3, thyroid hormones and their ratios), which can be used as indirect indicators of iodine status.

8.2.5   Clinical Assessment

Nutrition assessment may be completed within the context of a traditional medical model or a functional integrative medical model. Clinicians must demonstrate critical thinking skills to observe, interpret, analyze, and infer data to detect new nutrition diagnoses or determine that nutrition-related issues have resolved (Charney et al. ,2013). The three sources of information—biochemical data, physical attributes, and functional changes—are viewed in the context of each other, and the trends of data over time are useful to identify patterns consistent with nutrition and medical diagnoses.

(1)Clinical signs and symptoms of human nutritionrelated diseases

The purpose of the clinical examination is to determine the occurrence and progress of nutrition related diseases caused by under-nutrition or over-nutrition according to the symptoms and signs.

Due to a variety of nutrition related diseases, symptoms and signs will be different because of its stage of development, from the point of view, the long-term intake of each nutrient deficiency or excess will cause a corresponding change in the characteristic, but specific to an individual, may also exist many kinds of nutrient intake deficiency or excess, caused by the symptoms and signs are not typical.

Registered dietitian nutritionists (RDNs) evaluate all of the information from the nutrition assessment to determine a nutrition diagnosis. Accurate diagnosis of nutrition problems is guided by critical evaluation of each component of the assessment combined with critical judgment and decision-making skills. The purpose of identifying the presence of a nutrition diagnosis is "to identify and describe a specific nutrition problem that can be improved or resolved through nutrition treatment/ nutrition intervention by a food and nutrition professional". Patients with nutrition diagnoses may be at a higher risk of nutrition-related complications, such as increased morbidity, increased length of hospital stay, and infection with or without complications. Nutrition-related complications can lead to a significant increase in costs associated with hospitalization, lending support to the early diagnosis of nutrition problems followed by prompt intervention.

(2)Common clinical signs with corresponding lack of nutrients such as Table 8-1.

Table 8-1   Common clinical signs and possible deficiency of nutrient relations

Position	Signs	Nutrients that may be lacking
From head to foot	Emaciation or edema, dysplasia.	Energy, protein, zinc
	Anemia	Protein, iron, folic acid, Vitamin B_{12}, B_4, B_2, C
Skin	Dry skin, hair follicle keratosis	Vitamin A
	Haemorrhage point around hair follicle	Vitamin C
	Dermatitis	Nicotinic acid
	Scrotal inflammation, seborrheic dermatitis.	Vitamin B_2
Hair	Scarce and tarnish	Protein, Vitamin A
Eyes	Bitot's spots and night blindness	Vitamin A
Lip	Angular cheilitis	Vitamin B_2
Oral cavity	Gingiva bleeding Gingival loosening	Vitamin C
	Glossitis, Scarlet tongue and Pinkish red tongue	Vitamin B_2 and Nicotinic acid
	Geographic tongue	Vitamin B_2, Nicotinic acid and zinc

8.3　Dietary guidelines

An appropriate diet is adequate and balanced and incorporates the individual's variations such as age and stage of development, taste preferences, and food habits. It also reflects the availability of foods, socioeconomic conditions, storage and preparation facilities, and cooking skills. An adequate and balanced diet meets all the nutritional needs of an individual for maintenance, repair, living processes, growth and development. It includes energy and all nutrients in proper amounts and proportion to each other. The presence or absence of one essential nutrient may affect the availability, absorption, metabolism, or dietary need for others. The recognition of nutrient interrelationships provides further support for the principle of maintaining variety in foods to provide the most complete diet.

Dietitians translate food, nutrition, and health information into food choices and diet patterns for groups and individuals. With increasing knowledge of the relationship of diet to incidence of chronic disease among Americans, the importance of an appropriate diet cannot be overemphasized. In this era of vastly expanding scientific knowledge, food intake messages for health promotion and disease prevention change frequently. Numerous standards serve as guides for planning and evaluating diets and food supplies for individuals and population groups. Many countries have issued guidelines, which are appropriate for the circumstances and needs of their populations. The Food and Agriculture Organization (FAO) and the world health organization (WHO) of the United Nations have established international standards in many areas of food quality and safety, as well as dietary and nutrient recommendations.

8.3.1　Dietary guidelines for chinese

China issued the first Chinese dietary guide in 1989, and made two revisions in 1997 and 2007 to reflect the progress of nutrition science and to contrapose actual dietary and nutrition problems of Chinese populations. In order to match the nutritional status and health needs of the Chinese residents better, the Chinese Nutrition Society started the revision again in 2014, and released the 2016 edition of Chinese dietary guidelines in 2016. Compared with the 2007 version, the number of guidelines is reduced from ten to six, and recipes as well as visual graphics and charts are enhanced to make them easy for people to read, understand, accept, and use. The current guidelines consist of three parts: the dietary guidelines for general population, the dietary guidelines for specific population, and the practice of balanced diet of Chinese residents. The dietary guidelines for the general population form the core of the guidelines. The six guidelines proposed for healthy people over 2 years of age in the general population are as follows.

(1) Eat a variety of foods, with cereals as the staple.

(2) Balance eating and exercise to maintain a healthy body weight.

(3) Consume plenty of vegetables, milk, and soybeans.

(4) Consume an appropriate amount of fish, poultry, eggs and lean meat.

(5) Reduce salt and oil, and limit sugar and alcohol.

(6) Eliminate waste and develop a new ethos of diet civilization.

The Chinese government has produced a new version of the Dietary Guidelines for Chinese Residents in the form of the Chinese Food Pagoda (Figure 8−2). The new 2016 dietary pagoda is a revision of the 2007 Food Pagoda.

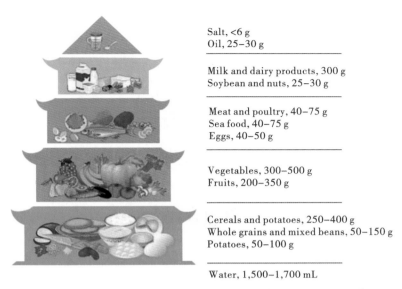

Salt, <6 g
Oil, 25–30 g

Milk and dairy products, 300 g
Soybean and nuts, 25–30 g

Meat and poultry, 40–75 g
Sea food, 40–75 g
Eggs, 40–50 g

Vegetables, 300–500 g
Fruits, 200–350 g

Cereals and potatoes, 250–400 g
Whole grains and mixed beans, 50–150 g
Potatoes, 50–100 g

Water, 1,500–1,700 mL

Figure 8–2   Food guide pagoda for chinese residents (Chinese Nutrition Society,2016)

8.3.2   Dietary guidelines for the other country's people

8.3.2.1   Dietary guidelines for Americans

The U. S. Departments of Agriculture (USDA) and Health and Human Services (DHHS) have a shared responsibility for issuing dietary recommendations, collecting and analyzing food composition data, and formulating regulations for nutrition information on food products. The Dietary Guidelines for Americans was first published in 1980. With the passage of the Nutrition Monitoring Act in 1990, the dietary guidelines are required to be reviewed every 5 years.

In 1969, President Nixon convened the White House Conference on Nutrition and Health (White House,1970). Increased attention was being given to prevention of hunger and disease. The development of dietary guidelines in the United States began with the 1977 report of the U. S. Senate Select Committee on Nutrition and Human Needs called Dietary Goals for the United States (the U. S. Senate Select Committee on Nutrition and Human Needs,1977).

Dietary recommendations have evolved during the past 30 years. Although numerous federal agencies are involved in the issuance of dietary guidance, USDA and DHHS lead the effort. Following the Senate's Dietary Goals report, the Dietary Guidelines for Americans was first published in 1980. The guidelines were revised in 1985(second edition),1990(third edition), and 1995(fourth edition). With the passage of the Nutrition Monitoring Act in 1990, the dietary guidelines are now required to be reviewed every 5 years.

The most recent guidelines were released in 2015 (8th edition). This edition is very interesting in providing key recommendations for selecting healthy food choices. It centers on preventing diet–related chronic diseases that afflicts people (the U. S Department of Agriculture,2015). The guidelines aim to support individuals to improve and maintain overall health and to decrease their risk of chronic disease through adopting healthier eating patterns and making healthy choices in their daily lives. The focus is on disease prevention, not treatment. The US government has characterized five dietary guidelines plus two important key recommendations (a healthy eating pattern and physical activity) in the eighth edition of the Dietary Guidelines for Americans,2015—2020. And the My Plate Food Guidance System, shown in Figure 8–3, replaced the previous My Pyramid diagram.

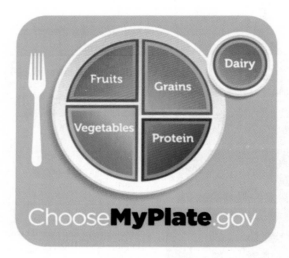

Figure 8-3　My plate showing the five essential food groups

(1) The Dietary Guidelines for Americans (8th edition, 2015—2020)

1) Follow a healthy eating pattern across the lifespan. All food and beverage choices matter. Choose a healthy eating pattern at an appropriate calorie level to help achieve and maintain a healthy body weight, support nutrient adequacy, and reduce the risk of chronic disease.

2) Focus on variety, nutrient density, and amount. To meet nutrient needs within calorie limits, choose a variety of nutrient-dense foods across and within all food groups in recommended amounts.

3) Limit calories from added sugars and saturated fats and reduce sodium intake. Consume an eating pattern low in added sugars, saturated fats, and sodium. Cut back on foods and beverages higher in these components to amounts that fit within healthy eating patterns.

4) Shift to healthier food and beverage choices. Choose nutrient-dense foods and beverages across and within all food groups in place of less healthy choices. Consider cultural and personal preferences to make these shifts easier to accomplish and maintain.

5) Support healthy eating patterns for all. Everyone has a role in helping to create and support healthy eating patterns in multiple settings nationwide, from home to school, work, and communities.

(2) Key recommendations of Dietary Guidelines for Americans (2015—2020)

To consume a healthy eating pattern that accounts for all foods and beverages within an appropriate calorie level.

1) A healthy eating pattern includes

● A variety of vegetables from all of the subgroups dark green, red and orange, legumes (beans and peas), starchy, and other.

● Fruits, especially whole fruits.

● Grains, at least half of which are whole grains.

● Fat-free or low-fat dairy, including milk, yogurt, cheese, and/or fortified soy beverages.

● A variety of protein foods, including seafood, lean meats and poultry, eggs, legumes (beans and peas), and nuts, seeds, and soy products.

● Oils.

2) A healthy eating pattern limits

● Saturated fats and trans fats, added sugars, and sodium.

Key Recommendations that are quantitative are provided for several components of the diet that should be limited. These components are of particular public health concern in the United States, and the specified limits can help individuals achieve healthy eating patterns within calorie limits.

- Consume less than 10% of calories per day from added sugars.

- Consume less than 10% of calories per day from saturated fats.

- Consume less than 2,300 milligrams (mg) per day of sodium.

- If alcohol is consumed, it should be consumed in moderation—up to one drink per day for women and up to two drinks per day for men—and only by adults of legal drinking age.

In tandem with the recommendations above, Americans of all ages—children, adolescents, adults, and older adults—should meet the Physical Activity Guidelines for Americans to help promote health and reduce the risk of chronic disease, Americans should aim to achieve and maintain a healthy body weight. The relationship between diet and physical activity contributes to calorie balance and manage body weight. As such, the Dietary Guidelines includes a Key Recommendation to:

- Meet the Physical Activity Guidelines for Americans.

8.3.2.2　Dietary guidelines for Japanese

The Dietary Guidelines for Japanese, released in 2000, provides the basics of a healthy diet for the people of Japan. In July 2005, the Ministry of Health, Labor and Welfare and the Ministry of Agriculture, Forestry and Fisheries of Japan jointly released a new pictorial guide, The Japanese Food Guide Spinning Top, to help people implement the Dietary Guidelines for Japanese. It guides people as to what kinds and how much food they should eat each day to promote health (Figure 8-4). The food guide comprises five categories of dishes: grain dishes (rice, bread, and noodles), vegetable dishes (vegetables, mushrooms, potatoes, and seaweed), fish and meat dishes (meat, fish, egg, and soybeans), milk (milk and dairy-products), and fruits (fruit and 100% fruit juice). To propose reference values of desirable dietary intake of energy and nutrients for Japanese people to maintain and promote their health, the Minister of Health, Labor and Welfare published the latest edition of Dietary Reference Intakes for Japanese (2015).

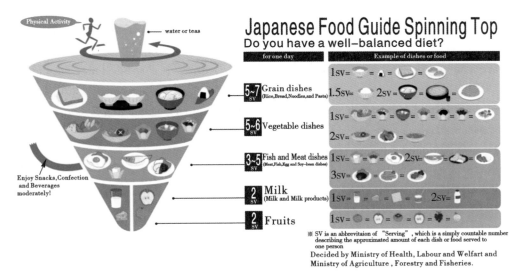

Figure 8-4　Japanese Food Guide Spinning Top, 2015

8.3.2.3　Dietary guidelines for Englishmen

The latest edition dietary guidelines for Englishmen was published by Public Health England (PHE) on 17th March 2016. The Eatwell Guide is a pictorial representation of government healthy eating advice showing the proportions in which different types of foods are needed to have a well−balanced and healthy diet (Figure 8−5). The proportions shown are representative of your food consumption over the period of a day or even a week, not necessarily each meal time.

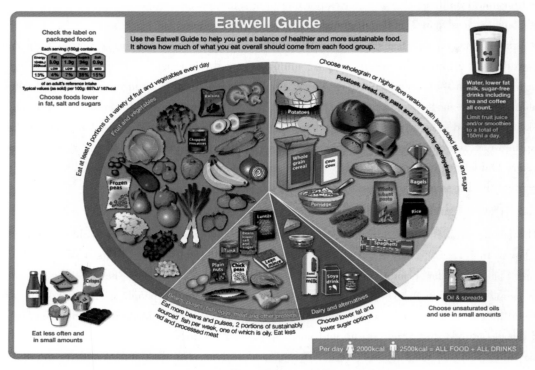

Figure 8−5　The Eatwell Guide of England, 2016

The Eatwell Guide shows the proportions of the main food groups that form a healthy, balanced diet:

(1) Eat at least 5 portions of a variety of fruit and vegetables every day.

(2) Base meals on potatoes, bread, rice, pasta or other starchy carbohydrates; choosing wholegrain versions where possible.

(3) Have some dairy or dairy alternatives (such as soya drinks); choosing lower fat and lower sugar options.

(4) Eat some beans, pulses, fish, eggs, meat and other proteins (including 2 portions of fish every week, one of which should be oily).

(5) Choose unsaturated oils and spreads and eat in small amounts.

(6) Drink 6−8 cups/glasses of fluid a day.

If consuming foods and drinks high in fat, salt or sugar, please have these foods less often and in small amounts.

8.3.2.4　Dietary guidelines for Australian

The Australian Guide for Healthy Eating uses a pie−shaped image with the five food groups represented proportionally in terms of recommended intakes (Figure 8−6). There are five principal recommendations featured in the Australian Dietary Guidelines. Each Guideline is considered to be equally important in terms of public health outcomes:

(1) To achieve and maintain a healthy weight, be physically active and choose amounts of nutritious food and drinks to meet your energy needs.

（2）Enjoy a wide variety of nutritious foods from these five groups every day.

（3）Limit intake of foods containing saturated fat, added salt, added sugars and alcohol.

（4）Encourage, support and promote breastfeeding.

（5）Care for your food; prepare and store it safely.

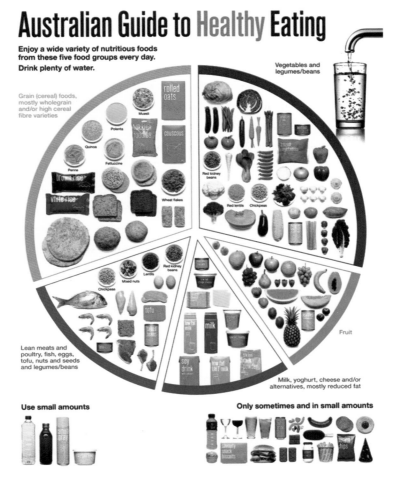

Figure 8-6　Australian Guide to Healthy Eating, 2015

8.4　Policies measures and approaches

8.4.1　Legislation and advocacy

Nutrition and health professionals can be valuable advocates for legislation (local, state, or federal) that supports the nutritional well-being of the population, especially of those who are under served or under represented. They can advocate in the following ways.

（1）Visiting, writing, or calling legislators and their aides to provide important information and establish communication links.

（2）Encouraging community members to provide testimony on their successes or the consequences of having unavailable or insufficiently funded medical nutrition therapy or nutrition services—a step that is especially important when legislation is pending.

(3) Inviting legislators to visit local agencies, schools, or hospitals to showcase the benefits of nutrition services provided by qualified professionals.

(4) Serving on campaign committees, donating time and money, or running for office.

8.4.2 Food fortification and enrichment

Assuring and improving the nutritional adequacy of an ever–changing food supply includes both enrichment and fortification of foods that are widely consumed enrichment is the addition of nutrients to restore the nutritional value lost in processing. An example is enriched flour with addition of iron and certain vitamin B lost in the milling process. Iron enrichment is considered to be a major public health measure to improve the iron status of the U. S. population. Fortification is the addition of nutrients to enhance the food's nutritional value; adding folate to flour and grain products, iodine to salt and calcium to orange juice are examples of fortification being used as a public health measure.

8.4.3 Nutrition education

The Cooperative Extension program is a USDA initiative administered by land grant or state universities. The program provides hands–on training in homes and community settings for community residents. Originally intended for rural settings, Cooperative Extension is still active in such programs as 4H and homemaker training. Since 1969, one component of the program has been the Expanded Food and Nutrition Education Program (EFNEP), which serves low–income families, many in urban settings. Childcare, nutrition education, food preservation, food safety and budgeting are some of the major topics addressed by these programs. EFNEP is also involved in food stamp recipient education.

8.4.4 Food labeling

Helping consumers make choices between similar types of food products that can be incorporated into a healthy diet, the Food and Drug Administration (FDA) established a voluntary system of providing selected nutrient information on food labels. The regulatory framework for nutrition information on food labels was revised and updated by the USDA (which regulates meat and poultry products and eggs) and the FDA (which regulates all the other foods) with enactment of the Nutrition Labeling and Education Act (NLEA) in late 1990. The new labels became mandatory in 1994. According to nutrition labeling regulations, almost all multiple–ingredient foods must be labeled with nutrition information. Labeling of fresh vegetables and fruits and raw meats is voluntary because these foods are often sold individually and without packaging. All labeled foods must provide the information shown on the Nutrition Facts panel in Figure 8–7. Additional information on specific nutrients can be added to the panel on a voluntary basis. However, if the package makes a claim about the food's content of a particular nutrient not on the "mandatory" list, then information about that nutrient must be added to the Nutrition Facts panel. In 2014 changes to the layout of information on the food label were proposed, to help consumers make better informed decisions, placing greater emphasis on calorie content and serving size, as well as replacing nutrients abundant in the food supply (e. g. , vitamin A) with those that are under consumed by certain population groups (e. g. , potassium). The new labels also include a separate line for added sugars, because many health experts recommend decreasing intake of sugars in favor of more nutrient–dense foods, as well as to help decrease overall caloric intake.

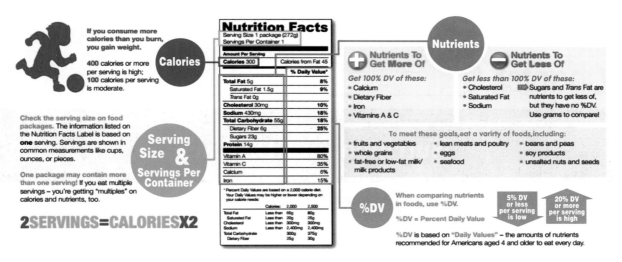

Figure 8-7　Nutrition facts label information

Ma Yuxia

Chapter 9

Nutrition and Diseases

9.1 Nutrition and obesity

Obesity has become one of the major nutrition-related diseases of this century, and has defined as excessive fat accumulation that may have adverse effect on health. Obesity is classified by body mass index (BMI, weight-for-height, kg/m^2), where the body fat composition also should be taken into consideration. Obesity is at high risk factor for many health problems, such as the majority of new cases of type 2 diabetes mellitus, other metabolic complications, cardiovascular, respiratory, digestion, reproductive system diseases, bone and joint disease, cancer, and mental and psychological problems.

9.1.1 Causes, types and diagnosis of obesity

Although obesity could be preventable by changes of lifestyles, diet, physical activities, and psychological assistance, there still exist some powerful causes that can drive it to develop in a more serious direction and challenge the preventing progress. The incidence and development of obesity are single or multifactorial, generally the following factors are regarded as the important causes.

Environmental factors: With the development of the social economy, people's living quality continue to improve, and the daily calorie-intake gets highly increased, while the physical activities are constantly reduced, so the excess energy could not be consumed in a short time. The excess energy will be transformed into fat and stored in the body, which causes obesity. Beyond these traditional environmental risk factors, many non-traditional factors, such as the short sleep duration and less calcium in diet have shown as higher risk for both children and adults clearly. Mental stress has been demonstrated to cause an increased energy intake.

Genetic factors: A small percentage of obesity is caused entirely by genetic factors. However, it is undeniable that chromosomal aberrations and mutations can cause pathological changes in individuals that ultimately affect the amount and distribution of body fat. Genome sequencing has identified that many genes related to body fat mass and distribution. For example, the fat mass and obesity-associated (FTO) gene is the gene that changes the amount of body fat. Currently, only 15 genes have been found to change body fat distribution, and studies have found that these genes play a stronger role in women than men. Epigenetic changes have also played a significant role in the obesity in pregnant women, and obesity during pregnancy can also affect the fetus, changing its susceptibility to obesity and metabolic diseases.

There are two types of obesity: the simple obesity and the secondary obesity. In most cases, The obesity we mentioned refers to the simple obesity and also the most common type. As for this type, obese size is the main clinical manifestations with no obvious nerve or endocrine system morphology and function changes, but which usually is accompanied with fat and glucose metabolism disorders. Secondary obesity is a symptom derived from a certain metabolic or endocrinal disease and is rarely seen clinically, accounting for only about 5% of obese patients.

There are three methods used to diagnose obesity.

Body weight and standard body weight. Body weight refers to the total weight of body. Standard body weight refers to analyze the data statistically collected from the survey of a cohort in different countries or regions with different age, height and other demographic characteristics to come to the standard weight values of all ages.

The method can be found in the following table. The formula for adult standard body weight is (Table 9-1):

standard adult body weight (kg) = [height(cm) - 100] ×0.9

The evaluation criteria for the degree of obesity can use this formula:

Degree of obesity = actual body weight (kg)/standard body weight (kg) × 100%

Table 9-1 Adult standard body weight

Values	Degree of obesity
90% -110%	Normal
110% -120%	Overweight
120% or more	Obesity
120% -130%	Mild obesity
130% -150%	Moderate obesity
150% -200%	Severe obesity

It should be pointed out that the above method is simple and suitable for self-assessment. However, it is far from accurate and reliable methods and need to combine with other methods such as body mass index, waist circumference and waist-to-hip ratio.

BMI, waist circumference and waist-to-hip ratio Evaluation criteria for the degree of obesity using BMI can be found in Table 9-2.

Table 9-2 The classification of adult overweight and obesity according to BMI

WHO	Asia	China	Degree of obesity
18.5-24.9	18.5-22.9	18.5-23.9	Normal
25-29.9	23-24.9	24-27.9	Overweight
≥30	≥25	≥28	Obesity
	25-29.9		Mild obesity
	30-34.9		Moderate obesity
	≥35		Severe obesity

Also, BMI has its limitation and need to combine with other methods such as waist circumference and waist-to-hip ratio (WHR). WHO also suggested that persons with the waist circumference of more than 102 cm for male or 88 cm for female can be diagnosed as upper body obesity; so does the waist-to-hip ratio of more than 0.9 for male or 0.8 for female. BMI is recognized as one of the best indicators of obesity assessment and widely used worldwide. But it is not suitable for all, such as the growing infants and children, muscular athlete or pregnant women, patients suffering from edema and ascites.

Besides the methods mentioned above, physical measurements and chemical measurements for obesity are also used.

9.1.2　Health risks of obesity

9.1.2.1　Health risks of obesity to children

As for childhood obesity, it is related to higher blood pressure and LDL-C, combined with an increased risk of steatohepatitis, T2DM and psychosocial problems. Even in moderately obese children, the health risks are mainly associated with the ongoing obesity into later life, or the concomitant risk of some serious diseases, such as diabetes, cardiovascular disease and cancer.

In fact, the impact of childhood obesity on their growth and development is more serious. Although their energy intake usually exceeds the recommended standards, they still have the signs of calcium and zinc deficiency. Also, childhood obesity can impact children's mental and psychological behavior.

Population surveys have found that the secondary sexual development of female obese children was significantly earlier than that in the control children. The behavior quotient of obesity children was significantly lower than that in the control group. Obese boys tend to be depressed and emotionally instable, while obese girls tend to be self-abased and incompatible. Obese children's reaction speed, readings and brain capacity index were lower than that in the control group.

9.1.2.2　Health risks of obesity to adults

Population studies have found a convincing relationship between obesity and mortality, mainly because of the increased risk of chronic diseases due to obesity, such as T2DM and cancer. If people have a high genetic susceptibility to insulin resistance, these individuals with normal body weight can still develop T2DM. T2DM has serious health impact and maybe the most serious health effects for obesity.

For the health risk of obesity to the cardiovascular disease, it seems to be associated with metabolic syndrome, which links obesity with almost all significant health complications. If other factors added, such as the physical activities, genetic disposition, and body-fat distribution, the more serious health complication can be found with obesity. This link may be contributed by the hormones and the substrates may be secreted by the adipose tissue.

Meanwhile, in an obese person, it has greater risk to develop hypertension than that in the non-obese people. Though there are many other factors contribute to the hypertension, obesity is the main and obvious co-morbidity of that.

Obesity also can greatly increase the risk of cancer developing. Many solid tumors and hematological malignancy are related to obesity and the mechanism is very complex but different. This is generally associated with endocrine chaos in obese individuals, so obese patients are more likely to suffer from endocrine-related tumors, such as prostate and colorectal cancer for male, breast cancer and endometrial cancer for female. The latest studies have found that there are some relationship between obesity-causing tumors and the host intestinal flora.

9.1.3   Relationship between nutrition and obesity

9.1.3.1   Energy metabolism and obesity

The vast majority of obesity is simple obesity which is caused by imbalanced diet, unreasonable lifestyle or other preventable factors. Obesity is a manifestation of energy imbalance. Energy intake comes from daily food, and energy consumption is due to the work or physical/mental activities. So, if the energy intake is more than the energy consumption, the excessive energy will be stored in human body as the fat tissue leading to obesity. Therefore, it's important to be on reasonable diet to maintain proper body weight to prevent obesity.

Carbohydrates: Levels of plasma insulin play a dominant role in the process of carbohydrate metabolism. Obese people have higher plasma insulin than normal people. They have 4-fold plasma insulin levels, however the higher plasma insulin can not work effectively as that in the normal and form the insulin resistance. In other words, obese people must secrete more than normal amount insulin to meet the body's requirements for glucose metabolism.

Lipids: The body fat metabolism is related to the characteristics of fat cells. Adipose tissue consists of white fats and brown fats. Current studies have suggested that the incidence of obesity may be related to the dysfunction of brown fat. Brown fat dysfunction can cause thermal energy imbalance, so that the consumption of the energy taken from the food reduces and is stored in the body as fat. The nutritionists also have demonstrated that in some cases that eat less and have adequate physical activities still come to obesity. The mechanism underlain may be the dysfunction of the brown adipose tissues, that is to say, it can not consume the energy normally.

9.1.3.2   Diet and obesity

If the obesity is induced by traditional risk factors, it is good news for the patients with obesity to overcome. And it is also easier to develop effective strategies to counteract the increasing prevalence of this simple obesity and its co-morbidities.

Actually, it should be paid great attention to the content of dietary fiber in the diet. Dietary fiber with high expansibility and water-holding capacity can make a variety of nutrients absorbed slowly to prevent obesity. Dietary fiber also can adsorb bile acids and cholesterol to lower plasma cholesterol, which can prevent obesity as well. On the other hand, most foods rich in dietary fiber contain only a small amount of fat and the namely low energy density, which can control the intake of dietary energy. At the same time, dietary fiber can delay the absorption of carbohydrates and reduce the digestibility of other foods, so it can also play a role in weight control. Therefore, dietary fiber is an important nutrient to prevent obesity.

9.1.3.3   Strategies of body weight management

Identification of healthy body weight is a usual indicator for health status. Recently, health professionals and scientists have become aware of the risk of many diseases, such as hypertension, stroke, heart disease, diabetes, osteoarthritis, infertility and some cancers (breast, colon and kidney), increasing with excess body fat. Due to the fact that body fat is hard to evaluate, body weight is a good proximate indicator in general population. Changes of body weight usually stand for imbalanced energy intake. On the contrary to excessive body weight, a low body weight may imply the malnutrition or an eating disorder and may pose risks to other diseases(including sarcopenia and osteoporosis, etc.). To what extent the body weight is too much or too less for a given height, so far there isn't a final agreement reached yet.

Body mass index (BMI) is commonly used index. Body fat in both men and women is widely accepted as indicator classifying overweight and obesity. According to WHO's definition, overweight is a person whose BMI equals to or more than 25 and obesity is when a person's BMI equals to or more than 30. Despite the fact that the BMI is a valuable tool for assessing body weight for height, this method still has limitations. BMI cannot determine the body composition precisely. BMI cannot estimate the proportion of fat body mass corresponding to lean body mass. There's a possibility of overestimating the overweight among athletes and underestimating the overweight among aged population. There are many methods for measuring body composition, such as neutron activation analysis, total body potassium, total body electrical conductivity and bioelectrical impedance analysis. BMI is just a practical indicator during weight management for convenient measurement and easy calculation.

Prevalence of overweight and obesity: The prevalence of obesity nearly tripled between 1975 and 2016 all over the world. Once obesity is common in high income countries, now it's also prevalent in low and middle-income countries. In 2016, more than 1.9 billion adults were overweight and 650 million were obese. Childhood obesity is one the of most serious public health challenges of the 21st century. Overweight children are more likely to become obese when growing. They are also more likely to develop diabetes and heart diseases than non-overweight children resulting in a higher chance of premature death and disability.

Strategies of overweight and obesity prevention: In most cases, overweight and obesity is the result of energy imbalance caused by excessive calorie consumed and inadequate physical activity. Consumption of energy dense foods contributes much to the excessive calories intake. Decreasing levels of exercise may also lead to weight gain. Generally, principle of overweight and obesity prevention includes healthy diet and regular physical activity.

Methods of weight management: Finding out how many calories should be taken each day for the individual's level of activity and staying within the limits of the ideal. To lose weight, it is perfect to only lose body fat and keep lean body mass as much as possible. Not only should more calories be used up than taken in, but also composition of macronutrients in diet should be carefully calculated. To successfully lose weight and maintain a healthy figure, most people need to subtract about 500 calories per day from their diet to lose about 1 pound per week.

Regular physical activity has many proven benefits, such as helping to control weight and blood pressure, as well as decrease the risk of heart diseases and stroke. All healthy adults (ages 18-64) should get at least 2 hours and 30 minutes (150 minutes) of moderate-intensity aerobic physical activity (e.g., brisk walking) every week or 1 hour and 15 minutes (75 minutes) of vigorous intensity aerobic physical activity (e.g., jogging, running) every week. Additionally, individuals need 2 or more days a week for muscle-strengthening activity.

The amount of physical activity any individual needs for weight loss varies, but it is recommended to have both regular physical activity and follow a healthy eating plan. Keeping a food diary may help you control your daily intake. Whether the quantity or the quality of food you consumed do good or harm, body weight management is still essential. Building a habit, such as taking diet diary, in managing your diet and maintaining a healthy life is a good choice.

9.1.4 Strategies for obesity prevention and body weight control

Prevention of obesity is more effective and meaningful than treatment. Health education should be strengthened, for example, through media such as television, newspapers, radio and internet, to educate the public. The most basic and effective way to prevent obesity is weight loss. The guideline for prevention of obesity can be found in the following paragraphs.

Regular eating, less snacks Various desserts, candies, chocolates and beverages have a very high sugar (sucrose or fructose) and relatively lower other nutrients with high energy density. Fried foods and ice cream are high-sugar and high-fat foods. Alcohol is pure-energy food and all kinds of alcohol have different ratios of ethanol, so long-term drinking can easily lead to obesity.

Less carbohydrates Daily intake of carbohydrates should account for 55% -65% of the total energy. People should also insist on eating high-dietary-fiber foods, but low other monosaccharides and disaccharides.

Adequate protein Daily intake of protein should account for 15% -20% of the total energy. In the case of strict control of energy, excessive protein intake can cause damage to liver and kidney function, so daily intake of protein should not be too high. Adequate milk, eggs and meat can supply proper quantity of protein.

Strict restrictions of fats Studies have shown that daily fat intake of patients with obesity are often above 35% of the total energy, while those with normal weight are often below 30%. So, the daily intake of fat should be 20% -30% of the total energy. And do not use or use less saturated animal fat prior to use vegetable oil rich in essential fatty acids.

Adequate minerals and vitamins Supplement of minerals and vitamins can smoothly lubricate the body machines and make them work more harmoniously.

Reasonable diet Staple foods, meats, poultries, dairy products, vegetables and fruits should be included in three meals of obese patients, as well as low-fat, high-protein foods.

Adequate excise Appropriate exercises can reduce appetite to decrease the food intake. Weekly playing football, walking or swimming and other appropriate regular exercise can effectively prevent the formation of obesity.

9.2   Nutrition and diabetes

As one of the severer chronic disease, diabetes mellitus (DM) is caused either due to pancreatic secretion of insulin at inadequate amount or ineffectively use of insulin by the body. Hyperglycemia is the most remarkable metabolic disorder of DM. The poor glycemic control of DM could influence many systems, especially the nerves and blood vessels and cause some serious complications, such as stroke, coronary heart disease, and renal failure, which inducing disability and pre-mature death.

9.2.1   Prevalence of diabetes mellitus

Based on the newly released report from the WHO, the global incidence of DM in people aged 18 and above has almost doubled in the past a few decades, from 4.7% in 1980 to 8.5% in 2014, while the total number of diabetic individuals has increased from 108 million in 1980 to 422 million in 2014, which has more than tripled. In 2015, diabetes directly caused 1.6 million deaths.

The incidence of DM is higher in obese, sedentary, favorite high fat diet individuals. A survey data from 2008 showed that the prevalence of DM doubled in the past ten years. The morbidity of DM in aged 18 and over was 9.7% in 2012, but has risen to 10.9% (close to 100 million cases) in 2013. The morbidity of pre-DM (intolerant glucose and impaired fasting glucose) was 35.7% in 2013. The morbidity increased with aging. The growth rate of morbidity is significant in middle aged people. Body weight is positively associated with the incidence of DM. The visceral obesity had even higher incidence of DM. Lifestyle is closely related to the DM prevalence. Globally, the rapid increase of DM prevalence happens in the middle-and low-income countries. In China, the morbidity is higher in cities (12.3%) than that in rural area (8.4%). The variation of physical activity and dietary patterns between the people living in rural and urban areas might contribute the difference of morbidity for the two population groups. The majority of DM is type 2 diabetes mellitus (T2DM), which counts for more than 90% of total DM. Approximate 80% of DM patients died of cardiovascular diseases. Along with the fast urbanization, lifestyle has been changed markedly. The incidence of DM in urban area significantly increased, and most of the T2DM patients are accompanied with obesity, lipid disorder, and fatty liver, which in turn, increase the coronary heart disease (CHD) risk.

9.2.2　Pathogenesis and types of diabetes mellitus

The basic pathophysiological change of diabetes is hyperglycemia which causes by either insulin deficiency and/or insulin dysfunction. There are four types of diabetes mellitus, that are type I diabetes mellitus, type II diabetes mellitus, gestational diabetes mellitus and other (e.g., secondary to other clinical situations). Type I diabetes mellitus (formerly called as insulin dependent diabetes mellitus) is common in young population under 25 years of age. Due to the damage of pancreatic β-cells, the individual can not produce insulin and then develop diabetes mellitus. The etiology of type I diabetes mellitus is not completely known yet. The autoimmune which caused by virus infection destroys β-cell. This might be one of the causal factors. The patients with type I diabetes mellitus must rely on the injection of insulin for the glucose control. Type II diabetes mellitus (T2DM), formerly known as non-insulin dependent diabetes mellitus, is the majority of diabetes mellitus (over 90% of total diabetes). In T2DM, plasma insulin level might be higher than normal, but the tissue cells respond to it abnormally, which is called as insulin resistant(IR). The most patients do not need or at least do not rely on the insulin therapy. In general, T2DM occurs at middle and aged people. Overweight/obesity, physical inactivity, and smoking are known the risk factors of T2DM. The gestational diabetes mellitus (GDM) is the diabetes mellitus occurring during pregnant period, mostly presented at second trimester of pregnancy and progressed into the third. Its pathology is mainly insulin resistant. The risk factors of GDM include age (the older age, the higher risk), obesity, and over gestational weight gain. GDM has the high risk for the future obesity and T2DM of the offspring. Other specific type of diabetes mellitus depends on the original diseases, such as genetic defect of β-cell function, genetic defect of insulin action, other condition e.g., infection, immune-induced, medicine-induced pancreatic damage. The other condition is called pre-diabetes. The pre-diabetes is the condition of abnormal glucose condition either impaired fasting glucose or impaired glucose tolerance, which is the case of high risk of diabetes mellitus, especially the T2DM.

9.2.3　Diagnosis of diabetes mellitus

The classical symptoms of diabetes are polyuria, polydipsia, and polyphagia. Symptoms may develop rapidly (weeks or months) in T1DM, while in T2DM they usually develop much more slowly and are even subtle or absent. Some patients are diagnosed by screening. Blood glucose test is an important measure for the diagnosis of DM and pre-DM. The DM criteria is listed in Table 9-3.

Table 9-3　Criteria of diabetes diagnosis

Condition	Fasting glucose (mmol/L)	2hour glucose (mmol/L)
Normal	<6.1	<7.8
DM *	≥7.0	≥11.1
Impaired glucose tolerance [§]	<7.0	7.8-11.0
Impaired fasting glucose [#]	6.1-6.9	<7.8

* HbA1c ≥6.5% is also a parameter of DM diagnose.

[§] Impaired glucose tolerance (IGT): Two hours after a 75 g oral glucose load, plasma glucose is in the range between 7.8 mmol/L and 11.0 mmol/L.

[#] Impaired fasting glucose (IFG): It is a special glucose metabolic status between normal and DM. Fasting glucose level is between 6.1 mmol/L and 6.9 mmol/L.

9.2.4　Complications of DM

Clinical complication is the common consequence of poorly managed DM. In numerous cases, the complication is the first reason to see the doctors for the T2DM patients. The diabetic complications include acute and chronic, the later one is more insidious.

Bacterial infection happens if elevated plasma glucose is poorly controlled, e.g. furuncle and carbuncle of skin, pulmonary tuberculosis, and infection of urinary tract, gallbladder, sinus, and periodontal tissue. The skin infection makes the wound difficult to heal.

9.2.4.1　Acute complications

Ketoacidosis is the most common complication in untreated T1DM patients and poorly controlled T2DM patients characterized by hyperglycemia and ketonemia. It is a metabolic state associated with high concentrations of ketone bodies, formed by the breakdown of fatty acids and the deamination of amino acids. Ketoacidosis occurs when the body is producing large quantities of ketone bodies via the metabolism of fatty acids and the body could not effectively process the over-produced substrates. The ketone bodies accumulated in the blood can significantly acidify the blood causing water-electrolyte and acid-base imbalance. Ketoacidosis is an emergency situation. The patients appear as hyperglycemia, dehydration, metabolic acidosis and even coma.

Nonketotic hyperosmolar coma also termed as hyperosmolar hyperglycemic nonketotic coma (HHNKC), is a type of diabetic coma associated with high mortality. It is usually precipitated by an infection, myocardial infarction, stroke or other acute illness and usually happened in elder T2DM patients. A relative insulin deficiency leads to the plasma glucose being higher than 33 mmol/L, which results in plasma osmolarity greater than 350 mOsm. This causes polyuria, which in turn, inducing hemoconcentration through decreasing blood volume and further increasing blood glucose level. Ketosis is absent at this case, because the presence of some insulin inhibits lipolysis, unlike diabetic ketoacidosis. The patients present more serious diabetes symptoms accompanied with apathia, slow response, severe dehydration, drowsiness and even coma. It is a life-threatening situation.

Hypoglycemia happens when patients are under medication at a high dosage medicine and/or along with inappropriate dietary control. The clinical presentations include lower plasma glucose, sweating, weakness, hunger, dizziness, palpitation, pale, hypotension and coma for severe case.

9.2.4.2 Long term complications involved in vessel pathogenesis

Macrovascular complications: Although microvascular complications are the major cause of morbidity of diabetes, macrovascular complications represent the primary cause of mortality with heart attacks and stroke which account for around 80% of all deaths. Atherosclerosis is the most common complication of diabetes. Diabetes patients have 2－4 folds higher risk of CHD, stroke, and peripheral vascular disease than matched nondiabetic people. Lipoprotein abnormalities play a major role in atherosclerosis. Increased plasma LDL-C but decreased HDL-C are common lipid disorders in atherosclerosis development, which are also risk factors of DM.

Microvascular complications: Diabetic retinopathy, nephropathy, neuropathy, and foot disease are the common microvascular complications. Data showed that after 15 years of diabetes, about 2% of patients became blind and about 10% developed severe visual handicap. Diabetes is one of the leading causes of renal failure. Diabetic neuropathy is the most common complication of diabetes. It leads to sensory loss and limb damage. Diabetic foot is the result of both vascular and neurological disease processes. Diabetes is the most common cause of non-traumatic amputation of the lower limb.

9.2.5 Principles of diabetic control and dietary management

DM is a complicated metabolic disorder disease with multiple fatal complications. Its management includes health education, dietary therapy, hypoglycemic medicine, physical activity and self-monitoring.

Health education: The goals of education are to make the patients aware of DM and get to know glucose self-test methods, to be confident for the treatment and be actively involved in the treatment.

Nutritional therapy: Nutritional measures include maintaining desirable body weight, keeping a diet rich in dietary fiber, soy protein, antioxidant, and water-soluble vitamins, but low in fat and cholesterol. General goals are providing balanced and appropriate diet. The objectives of nutritional plan are to have good body weight control, improve metabolic disorder, and reduce pancreatic β-cell load. At the stage of pre-DM, the appropriate dietary plan could effectively prevent it from DM development. Obesity prevention and management by dietary intervention are critical at this period. The total energy requirement should be calculated based on age, physical activity level and body weight. For the obese patients, to lose body weight, the calculated energy based on the body weight should be cut 500-600 kcal/d. Weight loss for the obese individuals could improve insulin sensitivity and lipid disorder, and help to lower plasma glucose.

Dietary therapy is the fundamental measure of diabetes treatment and should be carried out during the entire process of diabetes treatment. The dietary plan should be personalized and persistent. The energy distribution in daily meals should be rational and the energy producing nutrients should be in a suitable proportion. Food diversity is encouraged. Enough vitamins and minerals should be included in daily diet.

Macronutrients: Protein intake for diabetic people should be more than non-diabetes people. It is suggested to have protein accounting for 15% of total energy intake. High biological value protein should be included at a certain amount. Soy protein intake benefits cardiovascular health, weight control, and insulin sensitivity, and is recommended for diabetes patients. Fat intake should not exceed 30% of total energy. Saturated fatty acid (SFA) should not be more than 10% of total energy. Carbohydrates should provide 55% to 65% of total energy. Unrefined carbohydrates with intact natural fiber have distinct advantages over highly refined versions because of their other health benefits, such as lower glycemic index, greater satiety, and cholesterol lowering properties.

Glycaemic index (GI) is a measure of the effects of carbohydrate consumption on blood sugar levels. High GI carbohydrates refer that the carbohydrates break down quickly during digestion and release glucose rapidly into the bloodstream, while the low GI carbohydrates refer that carbohydrates break down more slowly, releasing glucose more gradually into the bloodstream. The GI of a food is defined as the area under the two hour blood glucose response curve (AUC) following the ingestion of a fixed portion of carbohydrate (usually 50 g). The AUC of the test food is divided by the AUC of the standard (either glucose or white bread) and multiplied by 100. Low GI foods are healthy choices for persons with diabetes and dyslipidemia. Low GI foods significantly decrease fasting plasma glucose in DM patients. In general, simple carbohydrates (monosaccharides and disaccharides) have higher GI than the complex ones (starch). Bread has higher GI value than beans. The GI values of some commonly consumed food are listed in Table 9-4.

Dietary fiber has therapeutic value in diabetes and may even reduce the prevalence of diabetes. It is recommended to consume 25-35 g/d or 15-25 g/1,000 kcal of dietary fiber for diabetic patients. This amount is easily to achieve by choosing whole grain cereals, high fiber cereals, plenty of vegetables and fruits and beans.

Table 9-4   GI for common foods in China

Grain	GI	Fruits	GI	Sugar	GI
Soba noodle	59.3	Cherry	22	Fructose	23
Soba steamed bun	66.7	Plum	24	Lactose	46
White rice	80.2	Grapefruit	25	Sucrose	65
Wheat flour steamed bun	88.1	Peach	28	Honey	73
White bread	105.8	Apple	36	Glucose	97
Bean products		Pear	36		
Haricot bean	18.5	Grape	43		
Dry green bean	27.2	Banana	52		
Dry tofu	23.7	Kiwi	52		
Stewed tofu	31.9	Mango	55		
Green bean dried noodles	33.4	Pineapple	66		
Soy flour dried noodles	66.6	Water melon	72		

Vitamins and minerals: Hyperglycemia induces more free radical production which increases plasma oxidized LDL level. Intake of some anti-oxidant vitamins e. g. , β-carotene, vitamin E, and vitamin C may prevent the oxidation process, which in turn, may prevent vessel complications, e. g. , atherosclerosis, diabetic retinopathy, nephropathy, and neuropathy. The family of vitamin B plays an important role in carbohydrate metabolism and is crucial for nerve function. Therefore, the diet of diabetic patient should include enough vitamin B. Minerals commonly mentioned in relationship to diabetes are chromium, zinc, and selenium. Zinc is involved in insulin synthesis and degradation. Zinc deficiency is associated with insulin resistant. Trivalent chromate is the component of glucose tolerant factor. Intake of plenty trivalent chromate may improve glucose tolerance. Selenium is the structural component of glutathione peroxidase and has scavenging capacity of free radicals, which helps to prevent diabetic complications. Seaweed and laver are great sources of dietary selenium.

Alcohol: In diabetes patients, alcohol could induce fasting hypoglycemia by inhibition of gluconeogenesis. Alcohol may also provoke hypertriglyceridemia in DM patients. Persons with poorly controlled diabetes should avoid alcohol consumption.

Physical activity:Routine physical activity benefits all people. Exercise is important for weight control, fitness,better working capacity and body composition improvement. Exercise is even more important for DM patients. Physical exercise has advantages for diabetes people through weight control,improving dyslipidemia,blood pressure control,increasing insulin sensitivity and lowering risk of CHD. Because highly intense exercise might cause some negative consequences for diabetes patients,moderately intense exercise is usually recommended. Aerobic exercise that uses large muscles throughout the whole body is preferred. Walking 6,000-10,000 steps (about three to five kilometers) per day may be one of the best modes of exercise. Moderate jogging,biking and swimming are also good activities.

Pharmacotherapy:For the DM patients, if nutritional therapy and physical activity could not control plasma glucose well,providing hypoglycemic medicine should be taken into account. Oral pills of hypoglycemia are priority for T2DM patients,while insulin is suitable for T1DM and poorly controlled T2DM.

Self-monitoring:Patients should be trained to do self-test of blood and urinary glucose and to have appropriate judgment of their glucose control,which would help them to make a good plan for their diet. It is also necessary to educate how to recognize common complications and time frame to visit doctors.

Dietary design for diabetes mellitus:The goal of dietary therapy for diabetes mellitusis is to supply enough nutrient and energy to the person and at same time to help control the plasma glucose level at relatively stable range.

The first step is to calculate the total energy requirement of the person, which is based on the body weight and physical activity level. If the person is under-weight or overweight,the energy should be adjusted upper or lower, in other words, the energy basically should be given by referring to the ideal body weight. Once the daily energy is defined,the proportion of energy producing macronutrients could be calculated, such as, the protein occupies up to 15% of the total energy, less than 30% of the total energy from fat, and the rest from carbohydrates. To design a dietary menu for a period of time,e. g. a week or longer, it should be kept in mind to make a good variety of food items, and to choose low glycemic index food and make a low glycemic load diet.

Wang Ling

9.3 Nutrition and cardiovascular diseases

9.3.1 How atherosclerosis develops

Currently,cardiovascular diseases,cancer and diabetes are the main chronic diseases that pose a threat to human health. These diseases are closely related to the dietary structure and nutrients intake. Among them,the cardiovascular diseases,with its top-1 incidence,disability rate,and mortality rate have become the leading risk to our health.

Atherosclerosis,as one of the representative cardiovascular diseases, is an inflammatory, multi-stage degenerative complex disease. The pathological changes of atherosclerosis can be classified into four stages: a ruptured thin-cap fibroatheroma (TCFA), thick-cap fibroatheromas, pathological intimal thickening, fibrotic plaque, and fibrocalcific plaque. The components of atherosclerotic plaque consisted of calcium, fibrous tissue,fibrofatty tissue, and necrotic core. Briefly, the pathological process of atherosclerosis begins from the affected endocardial damage, which is its initiation factor, and aggravated by the atherosclerotic plaque formation. The molecular process is that the long–term hyperlipidemia could cause oxidized–low–density lipoprotein and cholesterol increased, which will lead to the functional impairment of the intima of the arteries, and changes of the cell surface properties of endothelial cells and leukocytes. Meanwhile, High–cholesterol enhances the adhesion of monocytes to arterial endothelial cells, which will migrate through the endothelial cells by ways of chemotactic attraction to form phagocytes, foam cells and leading to the formation of lipid stripes, smooth muscle cell migration and proliferation, collagen secretion, until the formation of arterial intima with lipid as the core, wrapped with fiber cap.

The plaque could be divided into two types: stable and instable types. In the stable type, the convex atherosclerotic plaque will narrow the arterial lumen to reduce blood supply to the distal tissue; while in the instable type, the plaque rupture will stimulate platelet aggregation and induce thrombosis leading to tissue ischemia or even necrosis. Coronary atherosclerosis mainly caused by arterial lumen stenosis or obstruction and led to ischemia or hypoxia of the myocardial and its surrounding tissues. Unstable–atherosclerotic–plaque–rupture and secondary complete or incomplete occlusion thrombosis can lead to acute coronary syndromes, which is a critical illness clinically.

Causes of plaque rupture and thrombosis include: ① the damage of endothelial cell and release of thrombotic factors; ②destruction of microvessels at the plaque leading to bleeding or thrombus formation at the plaque; ③weakening or degeneration of the fibrous cap leading to rupture. Instable–plaque rupture is the leading cause of coronary syndrome and death. Therefore, preventing the plaque formation, promoting the regression of plaque and improving the stability of plaque are the main strategies for prevention and treatment of atherosclerosis.

A large number of studies have shown that there are multiple risk factors for the disease. The convincing risk factors for coronary heart disease include smoking, dyslipidemia (elevated total cholesterol, triglycerides and LDL–C, decreased HDL–C), overweight and obesity, hypertension, diabetes, stress, sedentary lifestyle and so on. Changing diet and behavior could help to reduce the risk factors.

High morbidity and mortality are the defining characteristics of atherosclerotic cardiovascular diseases in western and eastern countries. In the eastern developing countries, especially in China, atherosclerotic cardiovascular disease has its evidently upward trend. While improving the dietary nutrition or behavior can reduce this kind of risk.

9.3.2 The relationship of nutrition and atherosclerosis

9.3.2.1 Lipids and atherosclerosis

Atherosclerosis is closely linked to dyslipidemia. Increased plasma total cholesterol, LDL and other lipids, and decreased HDL are the main risk factors for atherosclerosis. Dietary lipids are the main factors that affect cardiovascular diseases.

A large number of epidemiological studies showed that the total dietary fat intake, especially the saturated fatty acid, is positively correlated to cardiovascular disease. The intake of saturated fatty acids can cause atherosclerosis by inhibiting LDL receptor activity and increasing plasma LDL–C levels. Therefore, saturated fatty acids in the diet are considered as the main fatty acids that increase blood cholesterol. Monounsaturated fatty acids (MUFA) such as olive oil and tea oil can reduce blood total cholesterol and LDL, without reduce HDL–C levels. Monounsaturated fatty acids have less unsaturated double bonds and less sensitivity to oxidation, which may be more advantageous in the prevention of cardiovascular disease.

However, polyunsaturated fatty acids, are prone to be oxidized due to the presence of many double bonds. So excessive intake of polyunsaturated fatty acids can lead to an increase of the levels of oxidative stress in bodies, sequentially promote the formation and development of atherosclerosis and increase the risk of cardiovascular diseases. While at the adequate intake levels, n-6 polyunsaturated fatty acids can reduce plasma cholesterol, LDL-C, as well as HDL-C. Linoleic acid can inhibit platelet aggregation and reduce plasma LDL-C to prevent cardiovascular disease. Dietary n-3 polyunsaturated fatty acids, such as alpha-linolenic acid, eicosapentaenoic acid (EPA), and docosahexaenoic acid (DHA), can lower plasma cholesterol levels and triglyceride levels, and increase HDL-C levels. The mechanism is that they could prevent the incorporation of triglycerides into the liver VLDL particles, resulting in a decrease in hepatic secretion of triglycerides to plasma. In addition, n-3 polyunsaturated fatty acids also have the role of preventing cardiac arrhythmia caused by myocardial ischemia and improve the function of the intima of blood vessels.

Trans-fatty acids, produced in the hydrogenation of plant oils, can increase plasma LDL-C levels and decrease the HDL-C levels, which could significantly increase the risk of cardiovascular disease. Studies have shown that the risk of trans-fatty acids to atherosclerosis is even stronger than saturated fatty acids. Phospholipids is a strong emulsifier, which can make the blood lipid particles smaller and easy to permeate the blood vessels for tissue to reduce the concentration of plasma cholesterol, and avoid the deposition of cholesterol in the blood vessels. Therefore phospholipids can be conducive to the prevention and treatment of cardiovascular disease. 30% - 40% of human cholesterol is exogenous, high cholesterol intake in the diet is an important factor leading to elevated serum cholesterol. When large amounts of cholesterol are ingested, the risk of developing atherosclerosis increases. Plants-derived cholesterol-like compounds called phytosterols, which can compete with the endogenic cholesterol to inhibitthe absorption of cholesterol to lower plasma cholesterol levels.

It should be noted that dietary guidelines in many countries recently removed the cholesterol dietary intake limit. However, this does not mean that it is good for the body and safe to consume large amounts of cholesterol.

9.3.2.2   Carbohydrates and atherosclerosis

Carbohydrates are closely related to cardiovascular diseases. Excessive energy intake in the body will be transformed into fat and store subcutaneously, or in other tissues, such as fatty livers.

The type and amount of dietary carbohydrates have a greater impact on blood lipid levels. Excessive intake of fructose and sucrose can easily lead to elevated serum triglyceride levels, which is the cause of excess carbohydrates in the liver to form triglycerides for storage. Sugar intake is more closely related to cardiovascular disease incidence and mortality.

9.3.2.3   Protein and atherosclerosis

The relationship between protein and atherosclerosis remains unclear. Protein intake does not affect blood lipids levels. There must be a sufficient amount of protein, with good-quality protein in daily diet. Individuals should also pay attention to the balance of protein sources, preferably plant-original and animal-original protein each accounted for 50%. Myocardium and vascular tissues contain a lot of protein. If insufficient supply, the function of these two tissues will be affected.

Some amino acids can affect cardiovascular function, such as taurine cannot only reduce the production of oxygen free radicals and increase reduced glutathione to protect the stability of cell membranes, but also decrease the blood cholesterol and liver cholesterol. Lysine and tryptophan can lower serum cholesterol and triglycerides. Arginine helps to regulate vascular tone and to inhibit the platelet aggregation factors for the prevention of vascular damage. Methionine is a precursor of homocysteine, which is a risk factor for atherosclerosis and confirmed by animal studies.

9.3.2.4　Vitamins and atherosclerosis

Vitamin E has been widely accepted for its prevention and treatment function to atherosclerotic cardiovascular disease. Epidemiological studies have shown a negative correlation between vitamin E intake and the risk of cardiovascular disease. At the same time, it was found that vitamin E can not only prevent the occurrence of cardiovascular diseases, but also play an important role in retarding and regulating this disease.

Vitamin C plays an important role in prevention and treatment of atherosclerosis in vivo. The deficiency of vitamin C leads to liver cholesterol accumulation and the elevated blood cholesterol. At the same time the antioxidant effect of vitamin C can reduce LDL oxidation and prevent vascular endothelial and smooth muscle cell oxidative damage. Vitamin C has the effects of increasing HDL–C and inhibiting platelet aggregation, thus helping to prevent and treat atherosclerotic cardiovascular diseases.

B vitamins in the body play the roles as coenzymes, such as vitamin B_{12}, B_6 and folate, to improve the transformation of homocysteine to methionine and cystine, thus the deficiency of B vitamins will lead to high homocysteine, and increase the risk of atherosclerosis. In addition, vitamin B_6 also is involved in the synthesis of acid mucopolysaccharides and the activity of lipoprotein lipase, which are the matrix components that make up the arterial wall. So dyslipidemia and atherosclerosis will happen because of the absence of vitamin B_6.

9.3.2.5　Minerals and atherosclerosis

Minerals and cardiovascular disease are also related closely. The main minerals related to atherosclerosis are copper, zinc, magnesium, calcium, chromium and selenium. Copper and zinc are the components of superoxide dismutase, while zinc also has antioxidant function, which helps to protect the integrity of vascular cells. Chromium is a component of human glucose tolerance factor, and the deficiency of chromium can cause metabolic diseases, resulting in arterial injury. Selenium is the core component of glutathione peroxidase, which can reduce the oxygen free radicals' injury on the blood vessels and myocardial. Magnesium can lower blood cholesterol and regulate blood pressure. Calcium can inhibit platelet aggregation and its deficiency can cause the rise of blood cholesterol and triglycerides.

9.3.3　Nutrition prevention for coronary atherosclerotic heart disease

In general, many factors can affect the development of coronary atherosclerotic heart disease(CHD), and dietary prevention of coronary atherosclerotic heart disease is one of the important positive measures. For coronary atherosclerotic heart disease, the main risk factors are hypercholesterolemia, hypertriglyceridemia, hypertension and diabetes. The strategies in preventing CHD are as follows:

(1)To limit the total calorie intake and maintain the ideal body weight.

(2)To limit fat and cholesterol intake.

(3)To increase plant protein intake and eat less sweet food.

(4)To ensure adequate dietary fiber intake.

(5)To keep adequate supply of vitamins and minerals.

(6)To have light diet and less salt.

(7)To have more protective foods at appropriate quantities.

9.4 Nutrition and hypertension

Hypertension, or high blood pressure is a chronic disease characterized by a continuous increase in arterial blood pressure accompanied by progressive damage to the structure and function of the heart, brain, kidney and blood vessel walls. It has a very silent onset and progress, and eventually leads to the cause of death which are heart failure, kidney failure and stroke. So it is also called "silent killer".

9.4.1 How hypertension develops

Blood pressure is regulated by the vascular elasticity, peripheral vascular resistance, cardiac output, and neuro-humoral receptors. The hypertension develops because of increased systemic vascular resistance. Under the condition of atherosclerosis, vascular degeneration, increased vascular resistance, neuro-humoral dysregulation, increased renin-angiotensin secretion, hypertension will be formed.

9.4.2 Causes, diagnosis and risk factors of hypertension

Generally, hypertension can be divided into primary and secondary types.

The primary hypertension is an independent disease characterized by elevated blood pressure, unknown cause, accounting for more than 95% of hypertension, may be the result of a combination of genetics and poor lifestyle choices. Poor lifestyle includes poor diet (high sodium, etc.), less physical activities, stress, smoke, and overweight/obesity. Secondary hypertension may arise as a complication of another disease, especially with the disease of endocrine system. The patients with secondary hypertension can be recovered after the treatment of the underlying condition.

Etiology of primary hypertension is unknown, generally which could relate to the following causes.

9.4.2.1 Causes

(1) Genetics

It's complex and combined contribution of many genes with mild effects responses to the different environmental stimuli. Previous reports have shown that 30% -50% of the variance of hypertension in familial and twin studies attributed to genetic heritability. These genes are mainly implicated some specific enzymes, channels and receptors involved in sodium handling and the renin-angiotensin-aldosterone system.

(2) Diet

Hypertension is associated with several dietary factors, such as high alcohol intake, high salt intake, low dairy fruit, and vegetable intake. Hypertension is the most closely related to salt intake. The mechanism of salt's effects on hypertension is that the salt (sodium) works on the sympathetic tone and peripheral vascular resistance. Thus, deficient dietary K^+, Ca^{2+} intake, or high dietary Na^+/K^+ ratio will increase the susceptibility to hypertension, and high K^+, Ca^{2+} diet may reduce the incidence of hypertension, which also confirmed by the animal experiments. The latest proofs showed that the gastrointestinal microbiome might be the pivotal bridge between diet and hypertension. The reduction of total fat intake and the proportion of saturated fatty acids as well as the increase of the unsaturated fatty acids ratio will decrease the average blood pressure in these population. The prevalence of high blood pressure in long-term drinkers increases, and is directly proportional to the amount of alcohol consumed, which may be correlated to the promoted corticosteroids.

(3) Occupational and environmental factors

Workers with high intensity, long-term stress, long-term exposure to environmental noise and adverse visual stimuli are prone to hypertension.

(4) Other factors

People with smoking and obesity will have high prevalence of hypertension.

9.4.2.2 Diagnosis

The diagnosis of hypertension discussed here refers to the clinical symptoms, the grades and the stages of the primary hypertension.

The main symptoms of the primary hypertension are dizziness, headache, irritability, heart palpitations, and insomnia. There are also other symptoms for the primary hypertension, such as vertigo, tinnitus, hand numbness, backache, leg weakness and hemorrhinia.

Without treatment, high blood pressure or hypertension is defined as systolic blood pressure of 140 mmHg or above for Chinese population, 130 mmHg or above for American population, and diastolic blood pressure of 90 mmHg or above for Chinese population, 80 mmHg or above for American population (Table 9-5). Two or more careful readings of the blood pressure on more than 2 occasions should be conducted. Meanwhile, before measuring blood pressure, the patient should be in relax, sitting in a chair (feet on floor, back supported) for >5 minutes. Proper technique should be used for blood pressure measurement.

Table 9-5 Categories of BP in adults from China and USA

BP Category	China			USA		
	Systolic BP		Diastolic BP	Systolic BP		Diastolic BP
Ideal	<120	and	<80	<120	and	<80
Pre-hypertension	120-139	or	80-89	120-129	and	<80
Hypertension						
Grade 1	140-159	or	90-99	130-139	or	80-89
Grade 2	160-179	or	100-109	≥140	or	≥90
Grade 3	≥180	or	≥110			
Isolated systolic hypertension	≥140	and	<90			

Combined with clinical symptoms, in China, the clinicians developed the diagnosis of hypertension and created the staging theory of hypertension. Staging of hypertension is based on brain, heart, kidney damage and other vital organs, divided into three levels. ①Stage I hypertension: hypertension is clinically without brain, heart, kidney and other important organ damage performance. ②Stage II hypertension: if one of the following symptoms happens, it can be included in stage II, which includes left ventricular hypertrophy or strain, narrowing of the retinal artery, increased proteinuria, or elevating the serum creatinine. ③Stage III hypertension: if one of the following symptoms happens, it can be included in stage III, which including left ventricular failure, renal failure, strokes, retinal hemorrhage, exudation, with or without papilledema.

Systolic blood pressure is the maximum pressure during a heartbeat, when the heart is sending blood throughout the body.

Diastolic blood pressure is the lowest pressure between heartbeats, when the heart is filling with blood.

9.4.2.3　Nutritional factors and other factors to hypertension

(1) Proteins

The dietary protein comes from two ways, one is from animal foods such as fish, eggs, meat which contains more protein, and the ratio of essential amino acids in such foods is more suitable for the human body; The other one is grains, which contains non-ideal essential amino acids whose utilization is low.

Previous studies have shown that the caloric supply of dietary protein is negatively correlated with mean systolic blood pressure. That means the higher caloric supply of dietary protein, the lower average systolic blood pressure; vice versa. On the other hand, proteins are also involved in the pathological process of hypertension. That's to say, the amino acid composition of dietary protein has effects on the blood pressure. Such as methionine, cystine and methionine are abundant in the fish, eggs and meat, and its metabolite taurine can significantly decrease blood pressure and prolong life expectancy. On the contrary, reduced intake of those amino acids can reduce the body taurine levels and elevate blood pressure.

In addition, tyrosine in meat and poultry foods is the precursor of neurotransmitter catecholamines, so with the lack of tyrosine in the diet, the central sympathetic neurons will reduce the release of catecholamine, which will increase peripheral sympathetic release of catecholamines and elevate the blood pressure.

(2) Lipids

Increasing dietary polyunsaturated fatty acids and reducing dietary saturated fatty acids will help to reduce blood pressure. Cohort studies showed that supplement of fish oil will reduce blood pressure in a dose-dependent manner. $n-3$ polyunsaturated fatty acids can change the metabolism of prostaglandins, improve the function of vascular endothelial cells and inhibit the cell proliferation of vascular smooth muscle, which plays a key role in anti-hypertension.

(3) Minerals

Salt (sodium chloride) intake is positively correlated to the blood pressure levels and the prevalence of hypertension. Cohort studies have shown that dietary sodium intake increased by an average of 2 g/d, systolic and diastolic blood pressure would increase by 2.0 mmHg and 1.2 mmHg respectively. Excessive sodium intake can increase blood volume and then increase blood pressure. In addition, high sodium intake can increase blood pressure by other ways, such as enhancing sympathetic excitability and improving cardiac output and peripheral vascular resistance; inhibiting vascular smooth muscle sodium ion transport; increasing intracellular calcium content and interfering with the synthesis of nitric oxide to increase vasoconstriction and peripheral resistance.

Potassium intake and blood pressure levels are negatively correlated. Potassium intake can be overt anti-high-sodium-induced hypertension. High sodium, low potassium diet is the most important risk factor for the incidence of most patients with hypertension in the developing countries.

Insufficient dietary calcium intake also causes elevated blood pressure. The National Health and Dietary Survey of US found that persons with daily calcium intake less than 300 mg had 23 folds of risk to have high blood pressure than persons with daily calcium intake at 1,200 mg. Supplemental calcium also has the effects against high-sodium-induced hypertension.

Magnesium intake and the incidence of hypertension are negatively correlated. Increasing dietary magnesium intake helps to lower blood pressure. The underlying mechanisms may include that magnesium can reduce vascular tone and contractility, decrease the content of intracellular calcium and improve vasodilation.

In addition to nutrients, there are other risk factors involving the onset and the development of hypertension, such as overweight and obesity, drinking, mental stress and less physical activities.

9.4.3 Nutrition prevention for hypertension

For patients with hypertension, they should pay attention to their lifestyle and make an active treatment to avoid aggravating the status of hypertension. To inhibit the development of hypertension, we should do more in the nutritional prevention as following description.

9.4.3.1 Body weight control

Overweight and obesity are the major causes of hypertension. Abdominal obesity increases the risk of cardiovascular and metabolic diseases. It can reduce the incidence of hypertension by controlling total energy intake and increasing physical activity to reduce body weight.

As for the diet, a balanced diet is suggested, including control high-energy food and the staple intake. While in lifestyle, regular physical exercise can lower blood pressure and improve glucose metabolism. Therefore, at least 30 minutes of moderate-intensity aerobic activity should be performed daily, and more than once a week of aerobic physical activity such as walking, jogging, cycling should also be done. Regularly, moderate-intensity aerobic exercise is an effective way to control weight.

9.4.3.2 A balanced diet

Eat less, increase meals and avoid over-fed. We should choose to eat low-calorie foods (such as vegetables, coarse grains), and eat less than a proper quantity of foods. At the same time, the plant oil should be used as edible oil mainly in the cook. We also need to avoid sugary foods and eat more high-fiber foods.

9.4.3.3 DASH

Dietary approaches to stop hypertension (DASH) is a hypertension-based dietary model developed by the National Institutes of Health and National Heart, Lung and Blood Institute of the USA. DASH is characterized by rich in fruits and vegetables, including whole grains, poultry, fish and nuts, which are rich in potassium, calcium, magnesium as well as low protein, total fat, saturated fatty acids and cholesterol. Studies have found that DASH diet can reduce mild systolic and diastolic blood pressure.

9.4.3.4 Limit sodium intake

Low-sodium diet is very important for individual health, especially for hypertensive patients or individuals with family history. According to the recommendation of WHO about the sodium intake, adult people should take no more than 6 g salt daily.

9.4.3.5 Moderate intake of high-potassium foods

Accompanied low-sodium diet, potassium-rich foods are able to counteract the effects of sodium-induced vasopressor and vascular injury. There are many types of high-potassium foods, including walnuts, peanuts, potatoes, lean meat, fish, beans, mushrooms, black dates, almonds, poultry meat, root vegetables, bananas, dates, peaches, and oranges.

9.4.3.6 Life styles

Quit smoking and control alcohol intake.

Periodically measure blood pressure Out-of-office measurement of BP can be good for confirmation and management of hypertension. Self-monitoring of BP refers to the regular measurement of BP by oneself at home or somewhere outside the clinic setting. Out-of-office measurement and Self-monitoring of BP can be very convenient real-time monitoring of blood pressure changes.

9.5 Nutrition and gout

9.5.1 Definition and clinical manifestation

Gout is a chronic and progressive disease caused by purine metabolism disorder that results from an o-verload of uric acid in the body (either over-produced or less discharged of uric acid). This overload of u-ric acid leads to the formation of tiny crystals of uric acid that deposit in tissues of the body, especially the joints. When crystals form in the joints, they cause recurring attacks of joint inflammation (arthritis). The clinical symptoms of gout include hyperuricemia, recurrent attack of acute inflammatory arthritis, and kidney stones, or urate nephropathy. The crystals found in white blood cells of synovial fluid are the definitive proof of gout. Gout frequently occurs in combination with other medical problems. Metabolic syndrome, a combination of abdominal obesity, hypertension, insulin resistance and abnormal lipid levels occurs in nearly 75% of gout cases.

9.5.2 Prevalence of gout

Gout has been common in Europe and America for a period of time, affecting approximately 1% –4% of the population. The incidences are 3% –6% and 1% –2% for male and female respectively. Since 90's, the incidence of gout has been increased rapidly in Asia, e. g. China, Japan, and Indonesia. The incidence is associated with social-economic development and dietary pattern change. In some countries, the prevalence has reached 10%. In general, there are 2-6 folds more incidence in male than that in female. The graduate increase of gout incidence worldwide is largely due to unhealthy life-style, such as high energy diet and sedentary living pattern.

9.5.2.1 Metabolism of uric acid and gout

In the body, uric acid comes from two major sources, e. g. , endogenous (damaged or dead cells which release nucleic acid to provide the substrates for urate synthesis) and exogenous (from diet). Uric acid is the end product of purines and primarily synthesized in liver, intestines and the vascular endothelium. In the physiological level, uric acid has protective roles for the body, such as antioxidant effect (scavenging reactive oxygen species and peroxynitrite), which in turn, playing the function of endothelial tissue healing in case of oxidative stress, and immune protective effect.

The synthetized uric acid is discharged from body mainly via kidney and intestine. The filtrated uric acid from glomerulus is re-absorbed by kidney tubules and only 8% –12% is discharged from urine. The factors result in either over-producing or less discharging of uric acid could build up plasma uric acid level, which might be crystallized in tissues like joint and kidney, named as gout. The prevalence of hyperuricemia is much higher than that of gout, approximately, around 10% of hyperuricemia might eventually develop to gout.

9.5.2.2 Pathogenesis and diagnosis of gout

Gout is a metabolic disorder caused by hyperuricemia, while hyperuricemia can be induced by genetic and environmental factors. Renal under-excretion of uric acid is the primary cause of hyperuricemia accounting for about 90% of cases, while over production of uric acid accounting for less than 10% of the cases. The occurrence of gout is partly genetic, contributing to about 60% of variability in uric acid level. Dietary causes account for about 12% of gout cases and include a strong association with the consumption of alcohol, fructose–sweetened drinks, meat and seafood. The factors promoting purine synthesis or uric acid production and/or reducing uric acid excretion are all the contributors of hyperuricemia development, of which, about 10% will eventually contribute to gout. Hyperuricemia can also be induced by some chronic diseases, e. g. obesity, hypertension, chronic renal failure, and diabetic acidosis and drug use, such as diuretics and aspirine.

The diagnostic criteria of gout are:

(1) Hyperuricemia, plasma uric acid >420 μmol/L (male); >350 μmol/L (female).

(2) Uric acid crystal is found in synovial fluid under microscope.

(3) Identified chalkstone as uric acid crystal.

(4) Therapeutic effect is positive after colchicine treatment.

9.5.2.3   Nutritional therapy of gout

Dietary pattern of patients with gout should follow the dietary guideline. Energy proportions of carbohydrate, lipids, and protein should be appropriated. The intake of total fat and SFA should be well controlled. Adequate energy is required to prevent ketosis. When accompanied with renal failure, the quantity of protein intake should be limited to minimize renal workload.

(1) Weight control

Obesity is shared by the incidence of lipid disorder, hypertension, hyperuricemia, and gout. Data showed that hyperuricemia is positively associated with body weight, BMI, and WHR. Lower energy intake to reduce body weight is a good way to control gout. However, since acidosis can reduce uric acid excretion, extremely energy restriction should be avoided to prevent ketosis.

(2) Dietary category

Abundant of plant foods, e. g. , vegetables, fruits, potatoes, and seaweed are rich in sodium, potassium, calcium, and magnesium. The basic ions produced from these elements promote uric acid dissolution and excretion through increasing uric pH value.

(3) Plenty of liquid intake

To help the excretion of uric acid, drinking plenty of liquid is strongly recommended, at least two litters per day, even three litters in the case of kidney stone. The types of liquid include water, vegetable juice, fruit juice, tea, and soy bean milk.

(4) Alcohol

Alcohol consumption should be avoided in gout patients. Lactate metabolized from alcohol can reduce uric acid discharge through inhibiting excretion of uric acid in nephridial tubule. Beer is rich in purine, which in turn can increase plasma uric acid.

(5) Dietary behavior

Engorgement or consumption of large amount of meat in one meal can trigger the attack of acute inflammatory arthritis. Broth generally is high in purine, if meat is included in the meal, broth should be discarded.

(6) Diet selection

Inside the body, 20% of purine is exogenous and 80% is endogenous. Dietary restriction may reduce 10 mg/L to 20 mg/L of plasma uric acid. At acute stage of gout, purine intake should be less than 150 mg/d. At remittent stage, meat consumption should be controlled under 120 g/d. All kinds of soup made from animal organs, fish, and other animal sources should be avoided.

Based on the purine contents, foods are sorted as low–, mid–, and high–purine groups. They are listed below as reference for gout patients.

(7) Low-purine group

Containing purine at<50 mg/100 g of food.

1) Grain and potatoes: Rice, rice flour, millet, sticky rice, barley, wheat, buckwheat, flour, macaroni, noodle, bread, steamed bun, oat, sweet potato, potato, taro, and greens.

2) Vegetables: Cabbage, Chinese cabbage, celery, pickpurse, water spinach, kale, crown daisy, Chinese chive, cucumber, bitter melon, whitegourd, pumpkin, sponge cucumber, summer squash, cauliflower, eggplant, bean sprout, green pepper, turnip radish, carrot, onion, tomato, green onion, ginger root, and garlic.

3) Fruits: Orange, tangerine, apple, pear, peach, water melon, cantaloupe, banana, and dried fruits.

4) Eggs and dairy products: Chicken egg, duck egg, cow milk, powder milk, cheese, and evaporated milk.

5) Others: Coagulated pig blood, hogskin, sea cucumber, jelly fish, seaweed, dry date, dry grape, agaric, honey, sunflower seed, water melon seed, almond, chestnut, lotus seed, peanut, walnut, tea, coffee, and chocolate.

(8) Mid-purine group

Containing purine at 50-150 mg/100 g of food.

1) Grain and beans: Rice bran, wheat bran, wheat germ, dry green bean, red bean, pea, tofu, black bean, and soy bean.

2) Meats: Pork, beef, lamb, chicken, goose, ham, and turkey.

3) Fishes: Eel, carp, grass carp, cod, salmon, black pomfret, flounder, lobster, cuttlefish, and crab.

4) Vegetables: fresh mushroom, asparagus, green bean, peas, seaweed, and spinach.

(9) High-purine group

Containing purine at 150-1,000 mg/g of food.

Organ meat, e. g. , liver, kidney, brain, intestine; some fishes, e. g. , belt-fish, sardine, anchovy, chub, herring; shellfish, e. g. , oyster and clam; broth; and yeast.

▶▶ *Summary*

Diabetes mellitus results from insulin inadequate or resistance. It is characterized as metabolic disorders of carbohydrate, lipid, and protein. The typical symptoms are hyperglycemia, polyuria, polydipsia, and polyphagia, plus lose weight. DM often induces complications, e. g. CHD, retinopathy, nephropathy and neuropathy which may shorten life expectation or result in handicap. The comprehensive measure is needed for DM management, e. g. education, dietary therapy, drug therapy, physical activity, and self-monitoring. The general principles of dietary intervention include personalized diet plan, rational dietary pattern, proportional meal distribution, and persisting. The goals of treatment are plasma glucose control, β-cell function recovery.

Gout is a chronic and progressive disease caused by purine metabolism disorder that results from an overload of uric acid in the body. Its clinical manifestations include hyperuricemia and recurrent attack of acute inflammatory arthritis, and kidney stones, or urate nephropathy. Gout frequently occurs in combination with other medical problems, e. g. obesity, hyperlipidemia, diabetes, hypertension, and CHD. Its dietary interventions include energy control, increased basic foods intake and water drinking.

Questions:

(1) Please state the relationship between dietary factors and diabetes, the principle of dietary prevention and treatment for type 2 diabetes.

（2）What are the metabolic characteristics of gout? How do we manage the daily dietary guide for gout patient?

Wang Ling

9.6   Nutrition and cancer

Since the 21st century, cancer has become a major issue that threatens human health and life. Cancer in China has been listed among the top 10 causes of death. In the next 10 years, the incidence and mortality of cancer in China will continue to rise. Behind the "Cancer County" and "Cancer Village", There are decades of fast social-economic development and quick changes of lifestyle. In fact, besides Chinese who are suffering from cancer, some developed countries are also plagued by cancer. Data released by the International Union against Cancer showed that the number of people worldwide died of cancer was more than total people with AIDS, malaria and tuberculosis. Without effective measures, it is estimated that by 2030, there will be 26 million new cases of cancer each year and the number of deaths will reach 17 million. Low-and middle-income countries will become the "hardest hit areas" for cancer.

WHO pointed out that more than one-third or even about half of the cancers are preventable. The prevention measures include tobacco control, developing healthy eating habits, increasing physical activity, reducing occupational hazards and environmental pollution. In the carcinogenesis, nutrition plays an important role.

9.6.1   Nutrition, food and cancer

The reasons for the neoplasia development have not yet been fully understood. They are multifactorial interactions, including genetic, environmental and psychological factors. 80% of cancer is caused by poor lifestyle and environmental factors. Among them, unreasonable diet, smoking and drinking accounted for 35%, 30% and 10%, respectively.

Foods is the most direct, common and largest amount of media that can contact between the human body and the external environment and are also the material basis of the structure, microenvironment and metabolism of the body. Diet and nutrition can affect the initiation, promotion and progress of malignant tumors. There are carcinogenic and anti-cancer factors in food, both of which can affect the onset of cancer.

9.6.2   Energy and cancer

Humans need energy generated from their foods to maintain their normal physiological functions. Insufficient caloric intake will cause weight loss and impair the immunity to weaken the prevention of cancer from some energy-rich foods in long-term. While the energy supply is too much, excess energy will be converted into fat and accumulated in the body, leading the body to be overweight and obese. For those people, they will get a higher risk of cancer than the normal weight. Simultaneously, among them the excess calorie will cause breast cancer in female and colorectal cancer in male. So, the limitation of calorie intake and control of excessive weight gain are beneficial for prevention of such cancers. Studies suggested that dietary fiber rich food may reduce the risk of colon and pancreatic cancer. In contrast, excessive refined starches diet may increase the risk of gastric cancer and colorectal cancer.

9.6.3　Protein and cancer

Both of excessive and insufficient protein intake will promote tumor growth. Epidemiological data showed that the patients with esophageal cancer, gastric cancer before diagnosed had been taking less protein than that in the normal ones. Reports also suggested that those who have milk regularly have less risk of gastric cancer than those who never have milk. However, excessive protein intake will increase the risk of some cancers, such as colon cancer, breast cancer and pancreatic cancer, the underlying mechanisms are still unknown.

9.6.4　Lipids and cancer

The dietary lipids are mainly from the cooking oils, meat and other foods. Previous researches find that the high-fat diet is related to the colorectal cancer and breast cancer. Recent studies suggested that high-fat diet is also related to prostate cancer, testicular cancer and ovarian cancer. Surveys of immigrants from different countries and regions all over the world agree that the incidence and mortality of colon cancer and breast cancer in high-fat-consuming areas are higher. Total lipids intake and animal fat intake are both positively correlated to the morbidity and mortality of cancer. Such as the colorectal cancer has a higher prevalence in Western Europe and North America as well as having a low prevalence in Asia and Africa. Japanese-Americans also have a higher prevalence than Japanese lived in Japan. After World War II, the diet of Japan gradually Europeanized and the incidence of colon cancer gradually increased. There are similar findings epidemiologically in dietary lipids and breast cancer.

However, the relationship between total lipids intake and the risk of cancer has been debating, and there is a number of data showing that the main effect of dietary lipids on some cancer risk depends on the types rather than the total intake. The researches of fatty acids on tumor growth, improvement or inhibition mainly focus on $n-3$ and $n-6$ series fatty acids. EPA and DHA in the $n-3$ fatty acids are all derived from fish oil, and α-linolenic acid is derived from vegetable oil.

Pharmacological experiments showed that α-linolenic acid, EPA, DHA and other $n-3$ polyunsaturated fatty acids not only inhibit platelet aggregation, prevent thrombosis and reduce serum total cholesterol, low density lipoprotein, very low density lipoprotein and elevate serum high density lipoprotein, but also inhibit the production and metastasis of cancer. The scholars suggested that $n-3$ fatty acids have an inhibitory effect on tumor cells, while other fatty acids may improve tumor growth or without any effects.

Conjugated linoleic acid (CLA) is a group of linoleic acid geometric isomers and positional isomers of conjugated diene acid, which is a natural ingredient in foods. Previous data showed that CLA can not only inhibit the growth of breast cancer, skin cancer, colon cancer and gastric cancer, but also inhibit other malignant tumors.

In spite of this, the indirect effect of dietary lipids on cancer risk through obesity must not be neglected. Considering the relationship between lipid-obesity-cancer and controlling the dietary fat intake should be the direct measures to prevent obesity, which is also a positive way to prevent the onset of cancer.

9.6.5　Carbohydrates and cancer

People with high starch intake accompanied by low protein intake have a higher incidence of gastric cancer and esophageal cancer. Dietary fiber plays an important role in the prevention of cancer through its absorption of harmful substances in the intestine to increase the volume of intestinal contents. At the same time, these fibers can dilute the carcinogens in intestinal tract and reduce the risk of colorectal cancer. Polysaccharides in edible fungi and marine organisms have anti-cancer effects, such as mushroom polysaccharides, Ganoderma lucidum polysaccharides via improving human immunity.

9.6.6　Vitamins and cancer

Vitamin A plays an important role in the differentiation of epithelial cells. Vitamin A and retinoids can stop, delay cancer or restore precancerous lesions. Many epidemiological data have shown that the quantity of vitamin A or beta-carotene is negatively correlated to cancer. Animal experiments confirmed that chemical carcinogens on vitamin A—deficient animals tend to induce mucosa, skin and gland tumors; while vitamin A or synthetic retinol or retinoic acid derivatives can inhibit the occurrence of chemical carcinogens-induced tumors.

Epidemiological surveys find that people with high incidence of esophageal cancer and gastric cancer have low vitamin C intake. The data also showed that the prevalence of cancer is inversely proportional to the amount of daily vitamin C intake. And the patients with cancer have lower vitamin C level in blood and urine than that in the normal patients. Vitamin C can block the synthesis of N-nitroso compounds both in vitro and in vivo, thus preventing tumors. It also inhibits the growth of leukemia cells, treats some precancerous lesions, and enhances the function of the connective tissues and immune system.

Vitamin E is a natural lipid-soluble antioxidant that protects the bio-membrane and proteins from oxidative stress. Vitamin E could inhibit the synthesis of N-nitroso compounds and therefore has anti-cancer effects. Animal experiments have confirmed that vitamin E also can suppress some other chemical carcinogens. Foods that are rich in antioxidants such as vitamin C, beta-carotene, vitamin E, and vitamin A have protective effects to cancer, which may due to the joint efforts of these vitamins. Therefore, people should not only understand the relationship between different vitamins and cancer, but also pay attention to the synergy of different vitamins.

9.6.7　Minerals and cancer

Both of excessive or deficient iodine intake can increase the risk of thyroid cancer. There is higher prevalence of thyroid cancer in the area with higher incidence of goiter. Low-iodine diet can also promote the formation of hormone-related breast cancer, endometrial cancer and ovarian cancer. So the diet with adequate iodine-rich food should be increased, such as kelp, sea cucumber, seaweed, jellyfish, etc. In addition, the lack of minerals such as iron, zinc, molybdenum, selenium also contributes to the carcinogenesis of certain types of cancer.

Selenium can be found in cereals, vegetables, seafood and meat. Although selenium is not an independent antioxidant, it acts as a cofactor for glutathione peroxidase, protecting body tissues from oxidative damage. Other protective mechanisms of selenium include the change of carcinogens, the production of cytotoxic selenium metabolites and the inhibition of protein synthesis, stimulate cell apoptosis, and so on.

Milk and dairy products are rich in calcium Long-term drinking of milk can have a significant effect of prevent gastric cancer and colorectal cancer because of adequate calcium in milk. Calcium can reduce the risk of colorectal cancer by binding to potential carcinogens such as secondary bile acids and by reducing mucosal proliferation and increasing cellular differentiation. An interesting finding is that the changing from a dairy-rich diet to a dairy-free diet can significantly increase the cytotoxicity of human fecal fluid, which is considered as a risk biomarker for colon cancer, but has no genotoxicity.

9.6.8　Dietary fibers and cancer

Since the preventive effect of dietary fiber on rectal cancer was firstly proposed in 1971, the relationship between dietary fiber and human health has been paid more and more attention. Some nutritionists regard dietary fiber as the "seventh nutrient" and more and more researches have been conducting worldwide.

Dietary fiber in the body cannot be digested and absorbed, but can promote intestinal peristalsis, which is conducive to excretion and shortening the stay of potential carcinogens in the intestine tract. In addition, the understanding of the relationship between dietary fiber intake and breast cancer, endometrial cancer, prostate cancer and other cancer mainly based on the epidemiological survey data. Dietary fiber intake and the incidence of cancer were negatively correlated. Some scholars speculated that dietary fiber may affect the above pathological process by changing the metabolism of sex hormones.

9.6.9　Nutritional prevention of cancer

Numerous findings showed that most cancers are preventable. Nutrition plays a very important role in cancer prevention. The incidence of cancer has been rising globally. Although doctors are constantly striving to explore effective treatments and methods, the cure rate of cancer is still limited. So effective prevention is an important way to reduce the morbidity and mortality of cancer, because only a very small number of cancers are due to genetic factors, while the vast majority of which are caused by environmental factors. The WHO pointed out that at least one third of cancers can be prevented, and the prevention of cancer is the most economical and long-term strategy to control cancer. Currently, the unreasonable diet pattern and less physical activities are the leading causes of cancer. So a healthy diet helps to prevent cancer and reduces the risk of cardiovascular disease.

How to prevent it? Insisting on physical activity, maintaining a healthy body weight and a balanced diet can significantly reduce the risk of cancer.

Based on rigorous assessment, the World Cancer Research Fund states that most cancers are preventable. A healthy diet, active physical activity and healthy body weight will greatly reduce the risk of development of cancer. In 2007, a book titled "Food, Nutrition, Physical Activity, and the Prevention of Cancer: a Global Perspective" was jointly published by the World Cancer Research Fund and American Institute of Cancer Research. Based on this report, ten recommendations were put forward, which benefit the prevention of cancer as well as chronic diseases such as cardiovascular and cerebrovascular disease and diabetes, etc.

The ten recommendations are:

Recommendation 1: Be as lean as possible within the normal range of body weight.

Recommendation 2: Be physically active as part of everyday life.

Recommendation 3: Limit consumption of energy-dense foods and avoid sugary drinks.

Recommendation 4: Eat mostly foods of plant origin.

Recommendation 5: Limit intake of red meat and avoid processed meat.

Recommendation 6: Limit alcoholic drinks.

Recommendation 7: Limit consumption of salt and avoid mouldy cereals or pulses.

Recommendation 8: Aim to meet nutritional needs through diet alone.

Recommendation 9: Children should be breastfed.

Recommendation 10: Patients having cancer should follow the recommendation for cancer prevention.

9.7   Nutrition and infectious diseases

A healthy immune system can protect the body from infectious diseases, which acts as an integrated network consisted of immune cells and tissues throughout human body. This system works efficiently against invaders and destroy them. The nutrient fuels this immune system as the impetus to smooth its function. But this kind of fuel is not the same as we usually mentioned for energy–supply nutrients, which also includes some non–energy–supply nutrients such as vitamins and minerals, which can make the immune system work better and more smoothly. The recent studies have demonstrated that the malnourished patients have more infective and destructive viruses compared with the well–nourished patients. That means the protein or energy malnutrition and severe deficiencies of some nutrients can reduce the immune function. So, reasonable nutrition is a pivotal way to maintain the normal immune functions.

9.7.1   Nutrition and immunity

There is a vicious cycle consisted of malnutrition and infection. Malnutrition always rises the risk of infection; infection often depresses appetite and leads vomiting. Decreased appetite and vomiting cause more severe malnutrition, which increases the risk of infectious diseases.

9.7.1.1   Protein

Proteins are the material basis of the body's immunologically defense function. Proteins are important components of antibodies and various enzymes in vivo. Being in malnutrition, the structure and function of the tissues and organs are impaired.

Protein–energy malnutrition can cause an irreversible atrophy of the thymus, a reduction in the germinal centers of the lymph nodes, a reduction in the number of cells in the spleen and mesenteric lymph nodes.

Protein malnutrition mainly affects the number and function of T lymphocytes. It reduces total number of T lymphocytes in peripheral blood significantly and the antigen–induced proliferative response. Under this condition, IgA in secretion of the epithelial and mucosa and the lysozyme are significantly reduced, which will decrease the anti–infectious effect and lead to the spread of infection. Meanwhile, the lack of essential amino acids in the diet has an adverse effect on immune function with the inhibition of antibody synthesis and cell–mediated immune response.

9.7.1.2   lipids

Lipids also play an active role in immune regulation. In many developing countries, the intake of lipids is very low. Oleic acid, linoleic acid and arachidonic acid can inhibit the proliferation reaction of phytohemagglutinin and tuberculin–induced human lymphocytes. The lymphocyte membrane is affected by dietary fatty acids, which is important for the immune functions because the changes in membrane structure can affect the secretion and the transportation of immunoglobulins, membrane fluidity and permeability, cell–antigen binding, message delivery, and even cell proliferation. Intake of adequate $n-3$ fatty acids helps to suppress autoimmune diseases, which means that excessive fatty acid are prone to lipid peroxidation to affect the immune cell membrane structure and function to inhibit the cellular immune function. It is also important to note that because fat–soluble vitamins dissolve in lipids, the amount of lipids intake directly affects the level of some important fat–soluble vitamins which have an important effect on immune function, such as vitamins A and E. For example, the source of vitamin A is mainly fish oil and Vitamin A deficiency can lead to the decrease of immune function, thereby increasing the respiratory tract infections and diarrhea.

9.7.1.3 Vitamins

Vitamins are essential nutrients to maintain the body in good nutritional status. It contributes to many coenzyme, and is indirectly involved in immune cell proliferation and differentiation, as well as the DNA, RNA and antibody synthesis. Vitamin deficiency and imbalance will lead to the occurrence of some immune diseases with decreased immunity and damage.

(1) Vitamin A

The impact of vitamin A on immunity mainly includes two aspects: on T lymphocytes and B lymphocytes. Studies have found that vitamin A is an essential factor in T cell growth, differentiation and activation process. If vitamin A is deficient, lymphocyte proliferation will be decreased; late-onset hypersensitivity will be suppressed. Most important of all, vitamin A deficiency can impair the function of thymus and spleen. On the other hand, high doses of vitamin A can also cause damage to the immune system, weaken the inflammatory response and complement formation.

(2) Vitamin C

Vitamin C plays a main role in maintaining the immune system and is an important component of all living cells. It is involved in the synthesis of dopamine norepinephrine, and can promote antibody production and leukocyte phagocytic capacity, stimulate the vitality of T cells and B cells and enhance immune function. Vitamin C also plays an important role in maintaining complement activity and antibody production. In addition, neutrophils also need vitamin C. Vitamin C has anti-infective effect for maintaining the function of thymus reticular cells. Vitamin C deficiency will reduce the permeability of human blood capillary, which will make the invasion of pathogenic microorganisms easier. Most importantly, vitamin C acts as an antioxidant that prevents lipid peroxidation of lymphocyte membranes and maintains the integrity of the immune system.

(3) Vitamin E

Vitamin E is an essential component of all cell membranes, nuclear membranes and mitochondrial membranes and has important antioxidant functions as well as immune function. In T and B lymphocytes, lymphocytes have high levels of vitamin E, which is 10 times higher than that of red blood cells. Aging is synchronized with the decline of T, B lymphocyte immune function, while vitamin E can delay this process. Studies have found that after the supplement of vitamin E, people have an increased number of antibodies, increased spleen weight and the number of macrophages in the reticuloendothelial system. Vitamin E can prevent the synthesis of prostaglandin precursor by preventing the peroxidation of arachidonic acid causing the reduction of the synthesis of prostaglandin, which has the effect of immune-activity inhibition.

9.7.1.4 minerals

Although the amount of microelements in the body is very little, they play a broad and important role in the process of life process. Besides working on the metabolic and reproductive process, minerals also contribute to the process of immune function. The lack of some certain minerals can cause dysfunction of humoral, cellular specific immune responses and nonspecific immune.

(1) Iron

The immune system is very sensitive to iron. Iron deficiency will mainly cause the reduction of T cells and can inhibit the activation of T lymphocytes to produce macrophage migration inhibitory factor. Iron deficiency can also diminish the neutrophil bactericidal capacity and lead to increased infection.

（2）Copper

The deficiency of copper can reduce the number of mononuclear cells and T cells, which will weaken the ability of lymphocytes to respond to antigens. The immune function of copper mainly acts as an antioxidant coenzyme.

（3）Zinc

Zinc plays an important role in maintaining the structure and function of central immune organs (thymus, supracapsular space) and peripheral immune organs (lymph nodes, spleen and tonsils). The main mechanism of the effect of zinc on immune function is related to the formation of DNA and RNA polymerase. Zinc deficiency can lead to zinc-dependent enzymes such as thymidine kinase and deoxyribonucleic acid inactive, resulting in inhibition of DNA replication, RNA and protein synthesis, the decrease of the sensitivity of lymphocytes to antigens, and the reduction of lymphokine production. In addition, zinc can regulate the levels of cAMP/cGMP in cells to work on the proliferation of the immune cells. Zinc also works on the free radical metabolism and synergistic effect of other important microelements to transport and utilization.

（4）Selenium

Selenium is a cofactor of glutathione peroxidase/reductase and plays an important role in maintaining the balance of redox and clearing reactive oxygen species. It is generally believed that selenium deficiency decreases the content and activity of GSH-Px, diminishes its ability to decompose and eliminate peroxides, increases the reactive oxygen species and free radicals in tissues and body fluids, and impairs the resistance to infection. The optimal dose of selenium for the immune system is still unknown, but excessive intake of selenium can impair cellular and humoral immunity.

9.7.2   Nutrition support for infectious diseases

Malnutrition can weaken the immunity of patients and make people susceptive to a variety of infectious diseases. The infection can also affect the digestion and absorption of the nutrients, which cause the reduction of food intake and lead to further malnutrition. That is the formation of a vicious cycle as mentioned at the beginning of this section. In order to break the vicious cycle of malnutrition and immunodeficiency, it is very important to give nutrition support to infected people. Nutritional status is one of the important factors that determines the survival time and quality of life of infected patients. For example, such as AIDS patients, the nutritional support can promote the protein synthesis, provide the necessary nutrition for recovery of immune function.

Diet of patients with AIDS or other infectious diseases should be based on the principle of high energy, high protein and balanced foods, as well as increasing the fruits and vegetables, especially those riched in vitamin C, vitamin E, zinc and selenium in order to improve the immune function. Generally, patients with infectious diseases always have gastrointestinal dysfunction, thus the scientific and reasonable meals and meal times should be given.

Wang Ling, Zhao Qihong

Chapter 10

Nutrition Support

10.1 General application of nutrition support

Nutrition support is an important measure of clinical nutrition which focuses on the nutritional management of individual patients or groups of patients with established diseases to meet the best nutritional needs of individual patients and to prevent complications associated with nutrition, as well as to improve patient's prognosis and enhance the effectiveness of clinical therapy. To well manage nutrition support, appropriate nutritional evaluation is necessary. If the patient has a nutritional risk or malnutrition, he/she needs to be further observed or be provided for nutrition support in a right way, whether the support given, fits or not, the nutritional status needs to be re-evaluated. Therefore, nutrition assessment is very important both before and after the support is required. Based on the result of assessment, well-planned nutrition support could be offered to the patient, and during the supporting interval, re-evaluation could help the dietitians to make suitable adjustment for the supporting including both quantity and quality.

10.1.1 Assessment of nutritional risk for in-patient

In most cases, hospitalized patients have high risk of malnutrition under disease conditions and therefore extra nutrients and energy are required. When the patient is accompanied with digestive disorder or aging, along with therapeutic progress, such as surgery, chemotherapy, radio-therapy, and others, he/she might face less food intake (due to poor appetite or digestive tract dysfunction), which puts the patients at the risk of malnutrition or even induces under-nutrition. Assessment of nutrition risk could find the potential malnutrition status in the patients and help the dietitians make right decision to establish suitable nutritional supporting plan and prevent the situation getting worse. Good nutrition support is critical for the patients to tolerate some special clinical therapies. Nutrition risk screening is a good way to find out the potential nutrition risk for the patients. Nutrition screening is a simple, quick, and general procedure used by nursing medical or other staff, often at first contact with a patient, to detect significant risk of nutritional problems. There are several tools available for nutritional risk screening, such as malnutrition universal screening tool (MUST) and nutrition risk screening. Such as malnutrition universal screening tool (MUST) and nutrition risk screening (NRS) 2002. Once the high risk patients are screened out, their nutritional status evaluation should be followed to provide the appropriate indicators for nutritional support. It is suggested that nutrition risk screening should be conducted for all of the in-patients while they are admitted into the hospital. If the score of screening is high, further nutritional assessment should be followed.

10.1.2   Nutrition assessment of patients

Nutrition assessment is a more detailed, more specific evaluation of a patient's nutritional status, usually by an individual with some nutritional expertise (e. g. , dietitian, nutrition clinician, or nutrition nurse specialist). Assessment is carried out when serious problems are identified by the screening process based on detailed medical history, dietary history, physical examination and laboratory tests. It requires specific nutritional care plans to be developed for individual patients. In general, after evaluation of nutritional status, the dietitian should make a nutrition diagnosis for the patient.

10.1.3   Dietary management for in-patient

Dietary management for patient is a kind of nutrition intervention, which applies an appropriate intervention plan established according to the nutritional status and demands of individual patients. For example, an intervention plan for a patient with protein malnutrition should be made emphasizing on increasing dietary protein intake at the tolerable level of the patient. Patient nutrition is not a complete steady situation, but a dynamic process. Along with the alteration of patient's condition, nutritional status and demands are varied. Nutrition intervention for the patients should be appropriately re-arranged based on its effectiveness. To maximally meet patient's nutritional needs and achieve the best result of intervention, it is necessary to keep monitoring on patient nutritional status and make evaluation on the effectiveness of intervention. The nutritional intervention can be adjusted based on the result of evaluation.

For a large body of in-patients, dietary intervention presented as hospital diets is the major way in clinical nutrition practice. Hospital diet is an important therapeutic media in clinical practice. The design of patient diet should meet basal as well as disease requirement of the patients. Hospital diet is classified as basal diet (routine diet), experimental diet and therapeutic diet.

10.1.3.1   Basal diet

Basal diet is the fundamental for hospital diet and also named as routine diet. It is suitable for more than half of hospitalized patients. Its outlook of texture might be common food, soft food, semi-liquid, and liquid food.

(1) Common diet

It is similar to the common foods consumed by general population. The frequency and daily distribution of meals is almost the same as normal people. It is suitable for the patients without special requirement for diet, but with normal body temperature, oral cavity and gastrointestinal (GI) tract function. The dietary principle of common diet includes enough quantity and quality of food varieties, enough energy supply and proper cooking method.

(2) Soft foods

The texture of foods is soft and easy to be chewed and digested. It is suitable for the patients with light fever, difficulty of chewing, post surgery and aged patients. The dietary principle of soft food is also a balanced diet which supplies adequate nutrients to meet the patient's needs.

(3) Semi-liquid diet

It is a type of diet textured between liquid and soft diet. It is suitable for the patients with high fever, serious illness, weakness, chewing and swallowing difficulty, and the patients at rehabilitation stage of post-operation. The principles dietary are balanced diet and variety of foods. The protein intake is 40–60 g/d. Semi–liquid diet is easy to be digested. The meal frequency is five to six times a day and the meal volume is around 300 mL each time.

(4) Liquid diet

Liquid diet is an unbalanced diet and liquid like. This type of diet is suitable for the patients with high fever, serious illness, extremely weak, difficulty of chewing and swallowing, and post–operation. The dietary principles are liquid texture, high nutritional value, mild taste, and non–spicy. The meal frequency is six to eight times a day and the meal volume is around 250 mL each time. This kind of diet is not recommended for a long term use as it is an unbalanced diet. If it is necessary to have this kind of diet for a long period, it is better to select homogenized diets, elementary diets, or formulated drinks, and accompanied with parenteral nutrition. Some examples of this group of foods are fruit juice, vegetable juice, paste of lotus powder and rice–water. To avoid gas production, cow milk and soy milk are not allowed in this dietary group.

10.1.3.2 Experimental diets

Experimental diets are the diets taken for a special clinical purpose by adding or eliminating specific nutrient to assist diagnosis and evaluate the therapeutic effect.

(1) Glucose tolerant test diet

The diet is usually used to help diagnose diabetes and insulin resistance. In the most commonly per-formed version of the test, an oral glucose tolerance test (OGTT), a standard dose of glucose is ingested by mouth and blood glucose levels are checked two hours later.

The procedure is as following.

- A baseline blood sample is drawn.

- The patient is then given a solution having 75 g glucose to drink within a 5–minute time frame.

- Blood is drawn at intervals for measurement of plasma glucose. In general, the interval is 30 mi-nutes, which means at 0, 30 minutes, 60 minutes, 90 minutes and 120 minutes time points, blood is drawn for glucose test. For simple diabetes screening, the most important sample is the 2 hours sample and some-times, the 0 and 2 hours samples may be the only ones collected.

Interpretation of OGTT results: The interpretation of OGTT is shown in Table 10–1.

Table 10–1   WHO diabetes criteria–interpretation of OGTT

	Normal	IFG	IGT	DM
FPG level (mmol/L)	<6.1	≥6.1 and<7.0	<7.0	≥7.0
2 hrs Plasma Glucose level (mmol/L)	<7.8	<7.8	≥7.8	≥11.1

FPG: Fasting plasma glucose; IFG: impaired fasting glucose; IGT: impailed glucose tolerance; DM: diabetes mellitus.

(2) Experimental diet for creatinine clearance rate test

It is a test for renal function (Glomerular filtration rate) evaluation. It aims to test the clearance rate of endogenous creatinine by limiting the exogenous creatinine through special diet control. It is used in glomer-ulonepharitis and myasthenia gravis.

Procedure: Patient takes low protein diet (<40 g/d) without any meat for three continuous days. The quantity of main food should be no more than 300 g/d. The urine within the most recent 24 hours is collect-ed and its content of creatinine is quantified.

(3) Occult blood test diet

It is a diet specified for diagnosis of GI tract recessive bleeding. It is used to assist the diagnosis of gastric cancer, digestive ulcer with bleeding, and anemia with unknown reasons.

　　Procedure: It is not allowed to have meat, animal blood products, and green vegetables in the meals for three continuous days. Then the feces are collected for the test.

10.1.3.3　Therapeutic diets

　　Therapeutic diets are the diets constructed according to the patient's condition, by referring the routine diet, making some modifications on the dietary ingredients to approach the goal of treatment and rehabilitation. The dietary principle is balanced diet with complete nutrients except the ones should be eliminated.

　　(1) High energy diets

　　It is the diet containing high energy density to improve patient's malnutrition in a short period of time. It is suitable for the patients with tuberculosis, severe trauma, cancer, peri-operation period, malnutrition, and hyperthyroidism. The dietary principles is balanced diet with enough protein, carbohydrates, appropriate fat, and adequate vitamins and minerals. The quantity of daily energy intake is gradually increased at patient tolerable level, e. g. increasing 300 kcal/d and the snacks can be given between meals to increase energy intake. Plasma lipid profiles should be monitored to avoid lipid disorder.

　　(2) Low energy diets

　　It is the diet containing less energy than normal level. The goal of this diet is to reduce body fat storage, lose body weight, and decrease energy metabolic load. It is suitable for the overweight, obesity, and individuals need to reduce metabolic load, e. g. , T2DM, coronary heart disease (CHD), hypertension, and hyperlipidemia patients. The dietary principle is reducing daily energy intake. The energy reduced is between 500 and 1,000 kcal, but not lower than 800-1,000 kcal per day to avoid ketoacidosis. The dietary principles also include having enough protein which offers 15%-20% of total energy, more than half of the protein should be high biological value, having carbohydrates which supply more than 50% of total energy and limiting fine sugar intake, having enough essential fatty acid intake, but limiting total fat intake, having enough vitamins and minerals, but limiting sodium intake.

　　(3) High protein diet

　　It is a kind of diet with high protein content and suitable for malnutrition, severe burn, and chronic wasting diseases. The dietary principles are enough energy, high protein, e. g. , 90-120 g/d, but the protein still occupies less than 20% of total energy. The high biological value protein should be half to two thirds of the total protein in the diet. High protein diet is not suitable for the patients with liver dysfunction and renal failure.

　　(4) Low protein diet

　　It is a type of low protein diet, which aims to reduce liver and kidney metabolic load by decreasing nitrogen containing metabolites in the body. It is suitable for acute nephritis, renal failure, pre-hepatic coma. The dietary principles are restricting protein intake, e. g. , 20-40 g/d, having high quality protein to supply essential amino acid, keeping enough energy by increaseing carbohydrate proportion, and having enough other nutrients.

　　(5) Low fat diet

　　Low fat diet aims to improve patient's condition related to lipid disorder through restricting dietary fat intake. It is suitable for the patients with obesity, CHD, hyperlipidemia, hepatitis, pancreatitis, cholecystitis, enteritis, and short-bowel syndrome. The energy and total fat intake are based on the patient's condition. The dietary principle is low fat, in general cases, e. g. hypertension, CHD, and hyperlipidemia, which offers less than 25% of total energy from fat, and total quantity of fat intake is less than 50 g/d. For the cases of cholecystitis recovery period, daily fat intake should be less than 20% of the total energy, total fat intake should be less than 30 g/d. For the patients with acute pancreatitis and cholecystitis, the fat intake should be less than 15 g/d. The cooking is mainly at low fat measures, e. g. steaming, boiling, and stewing. Dairy products are low or non-fat.

(6) Low cholesterol diet

It is also a low fat diet, accompanied with low cholesterol daily intake (less than 300 mg/d). It is suitable to hyperlipidemia, hypertension, CHD, obesity, and gallstone. The dietary principle includes dietary fat supplying 20% –25% of total energy, less dietary cholesterol intake (less than 300 mg/d), avoiding animal brain, organ meat, egg yolk, and fish roe, increasing plant origin protein, e. g. , soy protein. It is better to have MUFA rich oil as cooking oil, e. g. , olive oil. Foods rich in vitamins, minerals, and dietary fiber are encouraged, e. g. , fruits, vegetables, beans, and soy products.

(7) Low sodium diets

It is a kind of diet to keep body water–electrolytes balance through restricting dietary sodium intake and then reducing water–sodium retention. It is classified into low salt, salt free diets, and low sodium diet. Low salt means that daily salt intake is 1–4 g. Salt free diet means that total dietary sodium intake is less than 1,000 mg per day. Low sodium diet means that daily total sodium intake is less than 500 mg. The diets are suitable to glomerular nephritis, heart failure, hypertension, pre–eclampsia, and cirrhosis hydroperitoneum. The dietary principle is limiting sodium containing seasonings, e. g. salt, soy source, monosodium glutamate, and baking soda, avoiding salty foods.

(8) Low fiber diet

It is a kind of diet with low dietary fiber and easily to be digested. Its goal is to minimize GI tract irritation, slow down bowl movement, and decrease the feces discharge. It is suitable to enteritis, typhoid fever, dysentery, GI tract bleeding, and esophageal varix. The dietary principle is that the diet should be soft and less dregs in texture with low fiber content. It is also nonirritant and easy to be swallowed. It is an unbalanced diet, therefore not suitable to be used for a long term.

(9) High fiber diet

It is a kind of high fiber diet made upon basal diet with extra dietary fiber added. Daily dietary fiber intake should be more than 25 g. The objective is to stimulate GI movement and help the feces discharge. It is suitable to constipation, foreign matter swallowing, obesity, CHD, hyperlipidemia, and diabetes. Dietary intake of fiber is no less than 25 g/d. Dietary principle is to increase the dietary fiber up to 40 g/d, to increase the intake of subterranean stem, leafy vegetables and beans, and drink more water to stimulate GI movement. Over loaded dietary fiber might influence the absorption of some minerals. Therefore, the mineral supplementation should be considered at this case.

(10) Low purine diet

This diet is special in low purine content. It is suitable to the gout and hyperuricemia. The dietary principle limits high purine food intake, e. g. choosing foods containing low levels of purines (less than 150 mg/100 g). For the cases of accompanied with obesity, total energy should have about 10% –20% deduction. Animal foods should be restricted and plant foods are encouraged. Daily protein intake is 50–70 g. Fat intake is 20% –25% of total energy. Since fructose can promote nuclear acid breaking down, honey and other fructose rich foods should be reduced. Vitamin B family and vitamin C can help urate dissolving, it is recommended to consume large amount fresh vegetables and fruits.

10. 1. 3. 4 The path of nutrition support

Nutrition support plays an important role in disease treatment and rehabilitation. The nutrition needs of patients are met through a variety of routes with different nutritional formulation components and administration of equipment. Generally, according to the administration methods, the nutrition support is classified into enteral nutrition and parenteral nutrition.

10.2   Enteral nutrition

The GI tract is always the preferred route of nutrition support. Enteral nutrition (EN) provides nutrients to the patients through oral or feeding tube. It offers physiologic, metabolic, safe, and less expensive nutrition support for patients. Compared with parenteral nutrition (PN), EN has following advantages on several aspects.

Physiology: ① Nutrients are metabolized and utilized more effectively via the enteral than the parenteral route; ②The GI tract and liver process enteral nutrients before releasing into systemic circulation; ③The GI tract and liver help to maintain the homeostasis of the amino acid pool as well as the skeletal muscle tissue.

Immunology: The intestine integrity is maintained by enteral nutrition through the prevention of bacterial translocation from the intestine, systemic sepsis, and potentially increased risk of multiple organ failure.

Safety: It can avoid the complications related to intravenous access.

Cost: the cost of enteral nutrition formula is less than parenteral nutrition formula.

10.2.1   Paths of enteral nutrition

Mouth: For the patients who are not able to have all nutritional needs by routine diet, it is encouraged to get nutritional support orally. The type of diet is largely dependent on patient original disease and current condition. Patients may choose suitable hospital diet (see the section of hospital diets).

Enteral feeding (also called the tube feeding): It is a method of providing nutrients into the GI tract through a tube. This method is used for nutritional support in patients who cannot ingest or digest sufficient amount of food but have adequate capacity of intestinal functional. Enteral feeding requires infusion of formulas through a tube into the upper GI tract. Feeding tubes can be divided into two categories: those entering the GI tract through the nose (nasogastric or gastroenteric tubes) and those entering through the abdominal wall (gastrostomy or jejunostomy tubes). The type of access for enteral feeding largely depends on the state of the upper GI tract and the duration of feeding. Generally, feedings for period less than 4 weeks can be provided through nasal tubes, whereas feedings for longer periods require more permanent tubes (gastrostomy or jejunostomy tubes). The nutrients are delivered into the digestive system in a liquid form. Patients who are unable to meet their needs with food and beverages by mouth alone and who do not have vomiting or uncontrollable diarrhea are suitable to be given tube feeding. There are four basic ways to connect the tube to either the stomach or the small intestine:

(1) A nasogastric (NG tube) passes through the nose, down the throat, and to the stomach.

(2) A nasoenteral (NE tube) passes through the nose, down the throat, through the stomach, and to the small intestine.

(3) A gastrostomy tube (G tube) passes through a small cut in the skin directly into the stomach.

(4) A jejunostomy tube passes through a cut in the skin directly into the small intestine.

Based on the patient's condition, the duration of feeding and other indications, physician can choose one of the four routes to give patient nutrition support under the dietitian's guidance.

The indications, advantages and disadvantages of the four tube feeding routes are listed in Table 10-2.

10.2.2　Formulas of enteral feeding

The enteral formula should be easily digested and absorbed. Some of the commonly used formulas are as follows.

(1) Mixed liquid

It is composed with cow milk, egg, sugar, oil and salt. It is in liquid form and an unbalanced high nutrient density diet.

(2) Blended diets or formulas

The blended formulations are a combination of table foods with added vitamins and minerals. The table food is ground using blender and then filtered using screen, making the food into homogenate with or without added vitamins and minerals. The indications of this diet include unconscious, well GI tract functioning, and inability of taking food by mouth. Its advantages include accurate quantity of macronutrients, feeding volume and the nutrients composition closing to normal diet. According to the patient condition and nutrition demands, one can produce well-balanced tube feeding diet at low cost. The disadvantages of these diets include inaccurate quantity of nutrients, especially the vitamins and minerals, and one of biggest problems is that the food is relatively thick and easy to block the feeding tube.

(3) High nitrogen formulas

They are designed to deliver a higher protein load to a patient without changing the overall caloric content. The calorie to nitrogen ratio is approximately $(120-130) : 1$.

(4) Modular diet formulas

They are individual nutrient components that are mixed to create an enteral formulation or to modify an existing formula. They present as separate nutrient units: fat, protein, or carbohydrate.

(5) Specialty formulas

Hepatic failure formulas: Patient with hepatic failure, their serum branched-chain amino acids (BCAA) levels are reduced and aromatic amino acids (AAA) levels are elevated. BCAA can inhibit AAA from crossing the blood-brain barrier, thus preventing them from acting as false neurotransmitters and inducing encephalopathy. The use of a high BCAA and low AAA formula is helpful to the hepatic failure patients.

Table 10-2　Enteral nutrition administration routes

Routes	Indications	Advantages	Disadvantages
Nasogastric (NG)	Intact gag reflex, no esophageal reflux Normal gastric empting Stomach uninvolved with primary disease	Easy tube insertion Larger reservoir capacity in stomach	Highest risk of pulmonary aspiration
Nasoenteral (NE)	Gastroparesis or impaired gastric empting Esophageal reflux Gastric dysfunction due to trauma or surgery	Reduced aspiration risk compared to NG	Potential GI intolerance (bloating, diarrhea) to goal TF infusion rate Tube displacement and potential aspiration

Continue to Table 10-2

Routes	Indications	Advantages	Disadvantages
Gastrostomy	Long term feeding; Normal gastric empting Swallowing dysfunction and subsequent impairment of ability to consume an oral diet Nasoenteric route unavailable Intact gag reflex, no esophageal reflux Stomach uninvolved with primary disease	Placed adjunct with GI Surgery No surgery needed for percutaneous endoscopic gastronomy Larger reservoir capacity in stomach	Potential risk of aspiration Potential infection at stoma site Potential skin excoriation from leakages of digestive secretions at stoma site Surgery needed for surgical gastrostomies
Jejunostomy	Long-term feeding High risk of aspiration Esophageal reflux Inability of upper GI tract Gastroparesis or impaired gastric empting Gastric dysfunction due to trauma or surgery	Reduced risk of aspiration Placed adjunct with GI Surgery No surgery needed for percutaneous endoscopic jejunostomy TF may be initiated immediately after injury	Potential GI intolerance to goal TF infusion rate Potential infection at stoma site Potential skin excoriation from leakages of digestive secretions at stoma site Surgery needed for jejunostomies

(6) Renal failure formulas

The goals of this diet are to reduce blood urea nitrogen production and slow the progression of renal disease. Renal failure formulas are low in protein, potassium, magnesium, phosphorous and sodium. To minimize the renal load, the nitrogen content in the formula is low and mainly from essential amino acids.

(7) Trauma formulas

Critically ill patients exhibit significant proteolysis and hydrolysis of muscle BCAA for energy. The patients may enter a period of negative nitrogen balance. A formula high in protein, especially BCAA might correct the negative nitrogen balance. This type of formula is also suitable for the postoperative patients and the patients with a large area of burn.

10.2.3　Indications and complications of enteral feeding

In general, EN is indicated in patients who cannot ingest adequate amounts of food but have adequate GI function to allow digestion and absorption of enteral formulas delivered into the GI tract through tubes. The indications include: ①Normal GI tract function, but unable taking food by mouth or unable to get enough nutrition by mouth alone, e. g., dysfunction of oropharynx or esophagus, skull injury, coma or delirious state, major burn, post-radiotherapy and chemotherapy; ②Close to normal GI tract function, but with other organ dysfunction: diabetes, hepatic failure, renal failure, and heart failure; ③GI tract abnormal: short bowl symptom, and GI fistula (can choose jejunostomy route by-pass the lesion site to apply EN).

10.2.3.1　Contraindications

The contraindications include: infants younger than three months of age because they are intolerant to the hyperosmotic formula due to the underdeveloped GI tract anatomy and function; severe GI tract pathological conditions, e. g., massive bowel resection, jejunum fistula, intestinal obstruction, severe acute pancreatitis, intractable vomiting or diarrhea, post-operation of gastric by-pass surgery.

10.2.3.2 Complications

The complications of EN can be minor, e. g. , nose bleeding, sinusitis, and a sore throat or life threatening, e. g. aspiration. The complications are sorted into four categories.

(1) GI tract: Nausea, vomiting, diarrhea. The common causes of diarrhea are cold formula, intestinal flora unbalance, lactase deficiency or health care associated infection.

(2) Metabolism: Water and electrolyte abnormalities, e. g. , dehydration, hypokalemia, hyperkalemia, hyponatremia, hypernatremia and hyperglycemia, even hyperosmotic nonketonic coma.

(3) Infection: Formula contamination and pulmonary aspiration.

(4) Mechanical: Mechanical injury (bleeding, ulcer) of nose, throat, esophageal, tube malposition and clogging.

10.2.4 Methods of EN administration

EN feedings are administered either in a continuous or intermittent basis. Continuous feedings are used to prevent and minimize the risk of aspiration. The indications are initiation of tube feeding, critically ill patients, intolerance of intermittent bolus feeding. Intermittent feeding may be used in medical stable patients who have adequate absorptive capacity to tolerate bolus feeding.

Monitoring: Tube feeding needs to be carefully monitored in order to prevent complications and assure the best supporting effect to the patients. Detailed information including name & brand of formula, volume, concentration, administrative velocity needs to be recorded. Making the head of bed at 30° or 45° angle may prevent aspiration. It is very important to ensure that the feeding tube is located in its position by suction of gastric residuals or X-ray test. The gastric residual should be checked every three to four hours. If it is more than two-thirds of total feeding volume left within four hours, the feeding velocity should be reduced or even stopped. The feeding tube needs to be replaced every 24 hours to prevent infection. The feeding tube needs to be flashed with water after each intermittent feeding to prevent clogging. Biochemistry tests including plasma glucose, blood urea nitrogen, lipids, protein and electrolytes should be measured daily or two to three times per week. White blood cell counts and total urine discharge within 24 hours should also be included in the monitoring.

10.3   Parenteral nutrition

Parenteral nutrition (PN) is feeding the patient intravenously, by passing the usual process of eating and digestion. PN is provided when the GI tract is nonfunctional because of an interruption in its continuity or impaired absorptive capacity. The patient receives nutritional formulas that contain nutrients such as salts, glucose, amino acids, lipids and vitamins. It is called total parenteral nutrition (TPN) when no food is given by other routes. PN has two administrative routes: central parenteral and peripheral parenteral routes.

10.3.1 Categories of parenteral nutrition

Central/total parenteral nutrition (TPN): TPN is indicated to the patients require long term (>10 days) supplemental nutrition, and could not receive all daily requirement through oral or enteral feedings. TPN delivers nutrients directly through central vein via catheter, generally through subclavian, jugular and femoral veins. The advantages of central vein paths are fast flow of blood stream and wider vessel cavity. It is good for large quantity and high concentration of liquid infusion. The disadvantages are complicated procedures (surgery needed) and serious complications (aerothorax, aeroembolism, and damages of blood vessels and nerves).

Peripheral parenteral nutrition (PPN) The nutrient solution is directly infused into peripheral vein and no need for the insertion and maintenance of a central venous catheter. Compared with TPN, it is easier to be conducted, less expensive, and has less chance of large vein damage. Its disadvantages include limited infusion quantity at a short period of time and some chances to cause peripheral phlebitis. If the patient needs large amount of nutrient infusion in a period of time or long time PN, it is suggested to choose TPN for nutritional support.

10.3.2　Parenteral nutrition solution requirements

10.3.2.1　Protein in the form of amino acids

There are balanced and unbalanced amino acid solutions depending on patient's states, e. g. , high BCAA solution for liver dysfunction patients and essential amino acid (EAA) solution for kidney dysfunction patients, whereas balanced amino acid solution with both EAA and non-EAA for patients without dysfunction of liver and kidney.

10.3.2.2　Fat as a lipid emulsion

It is a high energy density solution containing plant oil, emulsifier, and isosmotic agents. It provides essential fatty acids and energy.

10.3.2.3　Carbohydrate in the form of glucose (minor forms of fructose, maltose, and xylitol)

It provides about 70% –80% of total energy. To avoid hyperglycemia, the daily infusion should not be over 400 g.

10.3.2.4　Others

Water, electrolytes, vitamins and trace elements: Since our body cannot reserve water soluble vitamins, they must be added to the infusion solution. For long term PN, fat-soluble vitamins and trace elements should also be supplemented.

10.3.3　Indications and complications of PN

The indications of PN include the patients with severe digestive diseases, e. g. , GI tract obstruction, neonatal intestinal atresia, short-bowel syndrome, intestinal fistula, and intractable diarrhea, severe acute pancreatitis, during radiotherapy or chemotherapy, and high metabolic state, e. g. , major burn, severe trauma and septicemia.

10.3.3.1　Contraindications

The Contraindications of PN include severe abnormalities of water and electrolytes and high risk of complications.

10.3.3.2　Complications

(1) Catheter-related complications

They include pneumothorax, aeroembolism, catheter thrombus, damages of blood vessels and nerves in TPN, and peripheral phlebitis in PPN.

(2) Infections

Catheter-related infections include contaminations of the catheter, infusion solution, and the insertion site. The secondary infection can be caused by intestinal bacteria. TPN makes the intestine resting for a long time, which in turn reduces intestinal secretion, damages the intestinal structure, e. g. , thinner mucosa layer and shorter villi. The intestinal bacteria get chance to be in the blood circulation and cause global infection.

(3) Metabolic complications

Metabolic complications include carbohydrate disorder, e. g. hypoglycemia, hyperglycemia, hyperosmotic nonketonic coma, hyperlipidemia, water and electrolyte abnormalities, liver dysfunction. Hypoglycemia is common when giving a large dose of insulin while giving high glucose solution. Hyperglycemia is often occurred when giving high glucose solution within a short period of time, especially for the patient with diabetes or high risk of diabetes. Fast infusion of lipid emulsion can cause hyperlipidemia. The common electrolyte abnormalities include hypokalemia, hyperkalemia, hypocalcemia, and hypomagnesemia. High dosages of lipids, glucose, and amino acid can make hepatic tissue damage.

10.3.4　Monitoring

Vital signs including body temperature, BP and heart rate should be closely monitored. The quantity of infused solution and discharged urine should be recorded. The catheter should be in its location and its insertion area should be as clean as possible. The monitoring parameters of blood tests include liver function, renal function, plasma albumin, electrolytes, glucose, prothrombin time, white blood cell count and blood gas analysis. They may be tested several times a day or a few times a week depending upon the patient's state. In addition, patient's nutritional status should be evaluated during the PN process.

▶▶ *Summary*

Clinical nutrition consists of nutrition screening, evaluation, diagnosis, intervention, and monitoring/assessment of intervention. As an important intervention, nutrition support plays crucial roles in patient treatment and rehabilitation. Hospital diet is classified as basal diet (routine diet) , experimental diet, and therapeutic diet. Basal diet is the fundamental hospital diet. It is indicated to more than half of the hospitalized patients. Its texture might be common food, soft food, semi-liquid, and liquid food. Experimental diets are the diets designed for a special clinical purpose by adding or eliminating specific nutrients to assistant diagnosis and evaluate the therapeutic effect. Therapeutic diets are the diets constructed according to the patient's condition, by referring the routine diet, making some modifications on the dietary ingredients to approach the goal of treatment and rehabilitation. The dietary principles are balanced diet with complete nutrients except the ones should be eliminated.

The nutrition needs of patients are met through a variety of routes with different nutritional formulation components and administration of equipment. Generally, according to the administration methods, the nutrition support is classified into EN and PN. EN provides nutrients to the patients through oral or feeding tube. It offers physiologic, metabolic, safe, and less expensive nutrition support for patients. The advantages of EN include less expensive, less complications, easy to take care, and keeping GI tract functioning. The formulas of EN include mixed liquid, blended formulas, modular diet formulas, and specialty formulas. PN is feeding the patient intravenously, bypassing the usual process of eating and digestion. It includes central parenteral and peripheral parenteral nutrition. The formulas include amino acid solution, lipid emulsion, sugar, minerals, and vitamins. PN often causes severe complications, e. g. metabolic disorders and infections. The indications of PN should be carefully considered when selecting patients for PN. The nutritional support process should be closely monitored to prevent the complications.

Review questions

(1) How many types are hospital diets?

(2) Please state the types of basal diets and major indications.

(3) Please list five common therapeutic diets and their indications.

(4) What is the goal of nutrition support? How many types of nutritional support can you give?

(5) Why should we consider enteral nutrition as the first choice in nutritional support?

(6) What are the indications and complications of tube feeding?

(7) What are the indications and complications of PN?

Wang Ling

Chapter 11

Food Safety and Food Borne Diseases

▎ 11.1 Food safety

Food safety is a scientific discipline describing the handling, preparation and storage of food in ways that prevent food−borne diseases. This includes a number of routines that should be followed to avoid potential health hazards. In this way food safety often overlaps with food defense to prevent harm to consumers. The tracks within this line of thought are safety between industry and the market and then between the market and the consumer. In considering industry to market practices, food safety considerations include the origins of food including the practices relating to food labeling, food hygiene, food additives and pesticide residues, as well as policies on biotechnology and food and guidelines for the management of governmental import and export inspection and certification systems for foods. Considering market to consumer practices, the usual thought is that food ought to be safe in the market and the concern is safe delivery and preparation of the food for the consumer.

Food can transmit disease among people as well as serve as a growth media of bacteria that can cause food poisoning. In developed countries there are intricate standards for food preparation, whereas in less developed countries the main issue is simply the availability of adequate safe water, which is usually a critical item.

11.1.1 Concepts of food safety

The concept of Food Safety has its broad and narrow sense. The broad food safety sense mainly refers to its legal definition as followings.

The legal definition of food safety in Article 105 of Food Safety Law of the People's Republic of China stipulates that the food is nontoxic, harmless and compliant with reasonable nutritional requirement, and will not cause any acute, chronic and potential hazards to human health. The legal definition of food safety prescribes the quality safety and nutritional indexes of food.

World Health organization (WHO) considers food safety as the public health problems caused by the toxic and hazardous substances in food. These substances refer to chemical or physical toxic rather than general materials and mainly focus on the public health problem but not on an individual person. It is a scientific discipline describing handling, preparation, and storage of food in ways that prevent food–borne illness. In November 2017, WHO has launched new guidelines on use of medically important antimicrobials in food–producing animals, recommending that farmers and the food industry stop using antibiotics routinely to promote growth and prevent disease in healthy animals. These guidelines aim to help preserve the effectiveness of antibiotics that are important for human medicine by reducing their use in animals.

11.1.2　Concept distinction

11.1.2.1　Food safety and food hygiene

Food hygiene are the conditions and measures necessary to ensure the safety of food from production to consumption.

In 1996, WHO distinguished food safety from food hygiene in its Guidelines for Strengthening National Food Safety Programs. Food safety is defined as a guarantee that will not cause damage to the consumer when it is produced and/or consumed by its intended use. Food safety emphases that food should not contain substances or materials that may damage or threaten human health. Food hygiene means all the conditions that must be created and the measures must be taken to ensure food safety and suitability at the whole food chain. The former one means the goal and the latter is the measure and guarantee to achieve it.

11.1.2.2　Food safety and food security

The Food Security concept presented by the Food and Agriculture Organization (FAO) of the United Nations and can be understood as food safety, food security and food security strategy. The new concept of food safety adopted by the FAO World Security Council in April 1983. The ultimate goal of food safety is to ensure that all people can buy and receive the basic food they need at any time. From this point of view, food safety is a systematic project which requires the active participation of the whole society in order to achieve a comprehensive solution. Therefore, food safety should be mainly considered from the political, economic, agricultural and food supply aspects.

Food Security covers both the food supply–demand balance and nutritional balance. From the macroscopic sense, the meaning of food security highly overlaps with food safety. In fact, food safety and food security have both a measurement of food shortage and malnutrition boundaries to a certain level. It becomes a food safety and security issue, when food pollution and nutritional imbalance reach to a certain degree.

11.1.3　Characteristics

11.1.3.1　The importance

Food safety is a worldwide public health problem that affects both human health and socioeconomic development. Food safety incidents can easily afflict large population, if taken advantage of by malicious people, it could have serious consequences. The ties between food safety, the national economy and international trade are more and more popular. Food safety and food standards have been widely used as the important methods of trade and technical barriers.

11.1.3.2　The complexity

The influential factors of food safety are complex and diverse. Nowadays, around the world, people with poor awareness of environmental protection and bad environment quality are likely to be attacked by frequent food–borne diseases. Furthermore, the threat of the pollution from farming and animal husbandry is becoming more and more serious.

11. 1. 3. 3 The particularity

The particularity of food safety is that, unlike other acute infectious diseases, it won't be effectively controlled by the development of economy, the living standards, the improvement of sanitation conditions and the long-term planned immunization. In contrast, new food safety issues will continue to emerge as the mechanization and centralization of food production, the widespread use of chemicals and novel technologies, the advanced testing tools, the growing awareness and the demand of public health.

11. 1. 3. 4 The relativity

The absolute safety of food is impossible, the so-called relative safety of food is that a food or ingredient will not lead to the actual certainty of health damage if it is used in the reasonable mode of consumption and the amount of normal consumption. Therefore, if conducting food safety analysis, we should proceed from the reality of food composition, food science and technology to clearly provide nutritious food with good quality food, and try our best to minimize any possible risk with the current test methods in order to protect the consumers.

11. 2　Food contamination

Food contamination is generally defined as foods that are spoiled or tainted because they either contain microorganisms, such as bacteria or molds, or toxic substances that make them unsafe for consumption.

Food contamination can be classified into three categories.

Biological contamination, including bacteria and bacterial toxins, molds and mildew toxins, intestinal viruses, parasites and worm eggs, insects, etc.

Chemical contamination, including pesticides, heavy metals, polycyclic aromatic hydrocarbons, N-nitroso compounds, food additives, harmful substances migrated from food containers or food packaging materials, and produced in the process of food processing.

Physical contamination, including pollutants such as seed, debris and dust from food production, processing, storing, transporting and selling processes.

Also, a special kind of physical contamination, radioactive contamination should be paid attention to the pollution caused in mining, smelting, production and application of the natural radioactive material and accidents.

11. 2. 1　Biological contamination of food and its control

Microorganisms caused food contamination can be divided into three categories according to the pathogenic ability to human body: ①Pathogenic microorganisms are bacteria and viruses that can cause infection, such as pathogenic bacteria and its toxins. ②Conditional pathogenic microorganisms are disease-causing microbes under certain conditions, which are not pathogenic in normal conditions. ③Non-pathogenic microorganisms. In general, microorganisms which are important to food safety are bacteria, fungi or molds, each of which has many diverse forms and many environmental and nutrient requirements.

11. 2. 1. 1　Classification of food biological contamination

(1) Bacteria and their toxins

Bacterial contamination of food materials is a major cause of health problems. The contamination bacteria gain entry into the body of the consumers and infect them. In some cases, they produce toxins, which cause severe illness to the consumers even in absence of the bacteria. Enterobacteriaceae, Staphylococcus, Vibrio, Pseudomonas, Xanthomonas, Micrococcus, Bacillus, Clostridium, Flavobacterium, Halobacterium, Halococcusand Lactobacillus are some of the bacterial pathogens that are commonly found in food. Bacterial infection through food is characterized by several symptoms like nausea, vomiting, diarrhea, fever, headache and fatigue.

(2) Yeasts

Yeasts are the other type of microorganism contaminating food. They are larger than most bacteria and contain their genetic material in a nucleus. Yeast can usually grow under more adverse conditions than bacteria. Thus they can withstand a lower water content or higher sugar and salt, and can grow under somewhat reduced oxygen conditions. However, yeasts are easily killed by heat during pasteurization.

(3) Molds

Molds are the hardest of the microorganisms that can grow on food. Molds generally need oxygen to grow and thus are usually seen only on the surface of food. Waxing the top of homemade jams is a way to prevent mold growth. Molds are the most resistant microorganisms to the reduced water content and can grow in conditions of high salt or sugar content. Some molds produce toxic substances that can have a great effect on consumer health. This mold, Aspergillus flavus, produces a toxin – aflatoxin – that kills ducklings when present in their feed even in small doses. The toxin can also cause liver cancer if consumed in low doses over a long period of time. Contamination can occur when cottonseed, cereal grains, and peanuts are not dried enough before being held in silos or grain elevators, especially when there is a lot of rain around harvest time.

The FDA has set a maximum of 20 $\mu g/kg$ of food or 20 parts per billion (ppb) for aflatoxin. This means that in one billion pounds of food there cannot be more than 20 pounds of the toxin distributed in it. Based on animal studies, the FDA confirms that this amount will cause no harm to human. Any food with aflatoxin greater than this level is considered to be adulterated and subject to seizure and destruction. Mixing a batch of cereal grains of high levels with one of low level to achieve less than 20 ppb in the final batch is also illegal. Milk has a lower action level of 0.5 ppb.

(4) Others

Bacteria, molds and their toxins are the most common and serious pollution factors to food. However, food biological contamination caused by viruses also aroused people's concern, such as rotavirus, Norwalk virus, hepatitis A virus and avian influenza virus. Parasites and their eggs can also contaminate food directly or indirectly through water or soil which polluted by feces. In addition, insects contamination are mainly produced by mites, moths and flies.

11.2.1.2　Environmental factors controlling the growth of microorganisms

To prevent growth or destroy the microbes, several environmental factors should be considered in processing of foods: temperature, oxygen level, acidity, availability of water and nutrients.

(1) Temperature

Each microorganisms has an optimum temperature range for growth. Above or below this range growth cannot occur. For pathogens, temperature below 7 ℃ and above 63 ℃ is adequate to prevent their growth. Thus, any process with temperature within these limits has a potential hazard to health.

(2) Oxygen level

As with temperature, each microorganisms has a particular requirement for oxygen. Some require O_2 while others are killed or inhibited in its presence.

(3) pH

Most organisms can grow only in a specific pH range just as most have a specific temperature range; pH control can be used to prevent or slow down decay in many foods.

(4) Water availability

Removing water can control microbial growth. Different organisms have different resistances to water removal. The availability of water from food to the environment or to an organism is called water activity or equilibrium relative humidity (ERH). The water activity (a_w) scale arises from 0 to 1. Multiplying by 100 converts it to the equilibrium relative humidity (% ERH). From the standpoint of microbial growth, all foods below an a_w of 0.6 or 60% ERH are safe. Thus, when drying foods we try to remove enough water to below this level.

(5) Nutrients

The availability of nutrients such as carbohydrates, protein and some minerals also affect microbial growth. Generally, the richer nutrients in food, the more suitable for microorganisms to grow in.

11.2.1.3 Food preservation against biological contamination

The basic principle of food preservation is to control the temperature, water, hydrogen, ion concentration and osmotic pressure of food or use other antibacterial measures to kill microorganisms or reduce its ability to grow. Among the modern processes of food preservation are refrigeration and freezing, heating, drying and dehydration, irradiation, and the addition of chemical preservatives.

(1) Refrigeration and freezing

The principle behind refrigeration and freezing for preservation of foods is to slow down microbial growth as well as chemical and biochemical reactions by lowering the environmental temperature. In general, for every 10 ℃ lowering of temperature, shelf life of most food increases by 2−5 times in the refrigerated temperature range.

(2) Heating

Heating can damage microbial enzymes, liposome and cell membrane. Common methods include pasteurization, pressure sterilization, ultra−high temperature (UHT) for short time sterilization and microwave sterilization. Liquids such as milk are commonly pasteurized. pasteurization is now a widely used process that kills microbes (mainly bacteria) in drink and canned food. Pasteurization of milk was suggested by Franz von Soxhlet in 1886. In the early 20th century, Milton Joseph Rosenau established the standards (i. e. low temperature, slow heating at 60 ℃ (140 ℉) for 20 minutes) for the pasteurization of milk. Previous pasteurization methods used temperatures below boiling, since at very high temperatures, micelles of the milk protein casein irreversibly aggregate or curdle. Latest methods use higher temperature with short time. Among the pasteurization methods listed below, the two main types of pasteurization used today are high−temperature, short−time (HTST, also known as "flash") and extended shelf life (ESL):

HTST milk is forced between metal plates or through pipes heated on the outside by hot water and the milk is heated to 72 ℃ (161 ℉) for 15 seconds. Milk simply labeled "pasteurized" is usually treated with the HTST method.

UHT, also known as ultra−heat−treating, processing holds the milk at a temperature of 140 ℃ (284 ℉) for four seconds. During UHT processing milk is sterilized and not pasteurized. This process lets consumers store milk or juice for several months without refrigerator. The process is achieved by spraying the milk or juice through a nozzle into a chamber filled with high−temperature steam under pressure. After the temperature reaches 140 ℃ the fluid is cooled instantly in a vacuum chamber, and packed in a pre−sterilized airtight container. Milk labeled "ultra−pasteurized" or simply "UHT" has been treated with the

UHT method.

ESL milk has a microbial filtration step and lower temperatures than UHT milk. Since 2007, it is no longer a legal requirement in European countries (for example in Germany) to declare ESL milk as ultra-heated; consequently, it is now often labeled as "fresh milk" and just advertised as having an "extended shelf life", making it increasingly difficult to distinguish ESL milk from traditionally pasteurized fresh milk.

A less conventional, but US FDA-legal, alternative (typically for home pasteurization) is to heat milk at 63 ℃ (145 ℉) for 30 minutes.

(3) Drying and dehydration

Drying refers to naturally decreasing food water such as in the sun or in the wind. With the aid of all kinds of technical methods to reduce water content in food can be known as dehydration.

(4) Food irradiation

Food irradiation is the process of exposing foodstuffs to ionizing radiation. Ionizing radiation is the energy that can be transmitted without direct contact to the source of the energy (radiation) being capable of freeing electrons from their atomic bonds (ionization) in the targeted food. Irradiated food does not become radioactive. The radiation can be emitted by a radioactive substance or generated electrically. Nowadays, food irradiation preservation is mainly used in food sterilization, insecticidal, inhibition of vegetable germination and delaying fruit ripe to extend the food storage period.

(5) Other food preservation methods

Food can be soaked in sugar, salt and vinegar to prolong the storage period. And the addition of chemical preservatives or fermentation could also be considered as useful food preservation methods.

11.2.2　Chemical contamination of food and its prevention

Chemicals can end up in food either intentionally added for a technological purpose (e. g. , food additives), or through environmental pollution of the air, water and soil. Chemicals in food are a worldwide health concern and are a leading cause of trade obstacles. There are many kinds of chemical contaminants, including toxic metals, non-metals, organic and inorganic compounds. Chemical pollution of food is complex and diverse, involving a wide range of aspects. Chemicals usually do not change the appearance of contaminated food, but stably exist, which results in difficulties to be eliminated from certain food. Importantly, chemical pollutants can bio-accumulates and concentrates along with food chain and finally exert great harm to humans.

11.2.2.1　Contamination of toxic metals and prevention

Toxic metals contaminating food is very common. The use of pesticides, industrial waste emissions, food processing and storage, transportation and sales, the high natural environment background value can all cause heavy metal contamination of food. The well-known heavy metals that cause food pollution and harm to human health including lead, cadmium, mercury and arsenic.

(1) Lead

Lead (Pb) can persist in the environment, including soils and water polluted by industrial waste emissions, leading to Pb contamination of plant and animal-derived food. However, agricultural pesticides containing lead, food containers and utensils, and lead salt stabilizer in machinery, pipeline and PVC used in food processing would also pollute our food. Lead is mostly absorbed through the digestive tract. Generally, children absorb Pb more efficiently than adults. Lead can accumulate in human body for a long time, mainly damage the hematopoietic system, nervous system and kidney.

(2)Mercury

Mercury (Hg) releaseing mainly arises from humans activities, such as the emission of industrial wastes from metal processing. Inorganic Hg reaches aquatic environments and is converted into methyl mercury (MeHg) by sediment bacteria, and then bioaccumulated and biomagnified through the aquatic food chain. Eventually, fish at the topmost trophic levels contain the highest concentrations of MeHg. Inorganic mercury absorption rate is low, more than 90% excreting from feces, so it usually has moderate toxicity to human body. However organic mercury especially methyl mercury, with the higher rate of absorption, easily accumulated in the body exerts great harm to the health. The long−term intake of food contaminated by methyl mercury can cause methyl mercury poisoning. Several large−scale poisoning incidents occur in Japan, resulting from local residents consumed fish highly contaminated by Methyl mercury. Methyl mercury poisoning is mainly manifested by the damage of nervous system; in addition, methyl mercury also has teratogenic and embryonic toxicity.

(3)Cadmium

Cadmium (Cd), as an important chemical raw materials, is widely used in industrial production. Therefore, industrial wastes emission containing Cd is an predominant way of food pollution. Besides, food packaging materials and containers can also pollute food. Cd is mainly absorbed through the digestive system, and distributes mostly in the kidney, followed by the liver. Cadmium poisoning mainly damages the kidney, bone and digestive system, as well as showing mutagenic and carcinogenic toxicity.

(4)Arsenic

Industrial waste, organic arsenic fungicides, raw materials used in food processing, chemicals and additives, as well as food containers and packaging materials contaminated by arsenic (As), can cause As contamination of food. The organic arsenic does much more serious damage to human than inorganic arsenic. Once absorbed into the blood through the digestive tract, it mainly accumulates in the liver, kidney, spleen, lung, skin, hair, nails, bones and other organs and tissues. Acute arsenic poisoning is mainly manifested as gastroenteritis symptoms and chronic poisoning mainly undermines the central nervous system.

For the toxic metal contamination of food, it is important to limit the industrial waste emissions so as to cut off the source of pollution; meanwhile to take mandatory measures such as the development of constricting standard of toxic metals in food, strengthened supervision and inspection to prevent food being contaminated by poisonous metals.

11.2.2.2 Pesticide and veterinary drug residues and prevention

Pesticide and veterinary drug residues are also important sources of chemical contamination of food.

(1)Pesticide and pesticide residues contamination

According to the chemical composition and structure, pesticides can be categorized into organochlorine pesticide (e. g. , dichlorodiphenyldichloroethene, DDT), organophosphorus pesticide (e. g. , methamidophos, internal phosphorus), carbamate pesticides, pyrethroid and so on. Pesticide residues in food mainly come from agricultural application, environmental pollution, and biological enrichment. Organochlorine pesticides most easily bioaccumulate in the body and are very resistant to degradation. The acute toxicity is mainly manifested in the nervous system, liver and kidney damage, while chronic toxicity is mainly in liver, blood and nervous system. Organophosphorus pesticides are more toxic. The effect of acute poisoning appears as nerve conduction dysfunction; while chronic poisoning mainly involves in serious nerve system damage, together with blood system and visual damage.

(2)Veterinary drugs contamination

Veterinary drugs include a variety of chemicals, such as antibiotics (sulfonamides, furans) , antiparasitic agents, and even hormones. Veterinary drug residues in food mainly come from drug abuse, illegal use of drugs and feed additives as well as eliminated drugs. Human exposure to veterinary drugs via food may be given rise to acute toxicity, chronic toxicity and teratogenic, carcinogenic, and mutagenic toxicity. At the same time, veterinary drugs can induce allergic reactions, and destroy intestinal flora balance. Abuse of antibiotics contributes to the production of drug-resistant bacteria strains.

(3) Prevention against food pesticide and veterinary drug contamination

Prevention measures include: to adopt the comprehensive management measures and strengthen the administration of the production, operation, application of pesticides and veterinary drugs; to improve and strictly enforce the Maximum Residue Limits (MRLs) standards; to introduce reasonable process to eliminate the residues; to innovative crop cultivation technology and improve animal rearing environment so as to reduce the use of pesticide and veterinary drugs.

11.2.2.3   N-nitroso compounds contamination and Prevention

(1) Source of N-nitroso compounds

Agricultural fertilizer, pickled vegetables, animal food preservatives and abuse of color protection agents act as the main source of N-nitroso compounds in food. Human exposure to N-nitroso compounds through food arises acute toxicity undermining the liver, bone marrow and lymphatic system; meanwhile leading to teratogenic, carcinogenic, and mutagenic toxicity.

(2) Prevention against food N-nitroso compounds contamination

There're several ways to prevent N-nitroso compounds contamination. Firstly, substituting nitrogenous fertilizer with molybdenum fertilizer; secondly preventing food from microbial contamination; and then limiting strictly the amount of nitrate or nitrite in food processing; lastly establishing appropriate food allowance standards and strengthening monitoring.

11.2.2.4   Contaminants formed during food production and cooking processes

A variety of chemicals are produced in the food production process or during cooking, because of the mutual reactions of components in food. These include polycyclic aromatic hydrocarbons, which mainly come from smoked and grilled meat. The priority to prevent harmful compounds in food processing and cooking procedure is to improve the processing technology of food and to choose healthy cooking methods, such as steaming.

11.2.2.5   Contaminants from the package or packaging process

Food containers and packaging materials contact with food directly in the process of food production, processing, packaging, and transportation. Toxic chemical substances (dioxins, acrylonitrile, vinyl chloride monomer, etc.) in containers and packaging materials may migrate to food, and give rise to food contamination. In order to prevent this kind of food contamination, it is of great significance to strengthen the safety supervision and management of food containers and packaging materials. The packaging materials should be with good grade and used in proper ways.

11.2.3   Physical contamination and prevention

11.2.3.1   Food impurity contamination and prevention

(1) Common impurity contamination in food

Common impurity contamination can come from the production, storage and transportation of food, such as dirt, sand and hair. However, nowadays, another common impurity contamination is food fraud. Food fraud is a kind of process in which non-food substances are intentionally added into food, mostly lower the raw material cost. The food safety concern caused by food fraud has attracted more and more attention. There are many kinds of food impurities, which not only destroy seriously the order of the market economy, but also damage the economic interests of the consumers, damage the physical and mental health of the residents, and even causes casualties.

(2) Prevention of food impurity contamination

In order to minimize food impurity contamination at a society level, we should strengthen the supervision and management of food production, storage, transportation, sales process, implement good manufacturing practices (GMP), improve the processing technology and testing methods, constitute strict food hygiene standards, enforce the "food safety law" and crack down food fraud.

11.2.3.2 Food radioactive contamination and prevention

(1) Radioactive contamination of food

The radioactive pollutants in food can be divided into natural radioactive pollution and artificial radioactive pollution, and the former in food accounts for greater proportion. Plant food is contaminated by natural and artificial radionuclide from environmental pollution (water, soil and air). When radioactive substances in the air deposited on plants, soil or water, they might enter the food chain. While radionuclides can be finally accumulated in animals' body via the food chain, which results in the pollution of animal food. Among so many kinds of radionuclides, ^{90}Sr and ^{137}Cs have long half-life and are easy to accumulate through food chain. Radionuclides in food mainly influence the immune system, reproductive system, and even exert carcinogenic, teratogenic and mutagenic effect. In general, food stuffs available on markets are unlikely to be contaminated with very high levels of radioactive substances. The chance of acute health effect is not common. If people are exposed to high dose of radiation, radiation sickness with acute symptoms like nausea, vomiting, extreme tiredness, hair loss, skin burns and diminished organ function will occur and immediate medical attention is required. In addition, the prolonged consumption of radioactively contaminated foodstuffs may increase the risk of cancer in exposed persons.

(2) Prevention of radioactive contamination of food

Codex Alimentarius Commission has established guideline levels for different radionuclides in foods destined for human consumption and traded internationally, which have been contaminated following a nuclear or radiological emergency. These guideline levels apply to food after reconstitution or as prepared for consumption. As far as generic radiological protection of food consumers is concerned, when radionuclide levels in food do not exceed the corresponding guideline levels, the food should be considered as safe for human consumption. The guideline levels are defined for two separated categories "infant foods" and "other foods" due to the fact that, for a number of radionuclides, the sensitivity of infants could pose a problem. For routine work, on one hand, paying enough attention to health supervision and management to prevent food contamination by radioactive substances; on the other hand, we should always be prepared for radioactive emergencies response.

11.3　Food-borne diseases

Food-borne diseases encompass a wide spectrum of illnesses and becoming a growing public health problem worldwide. They are mostly the result of ingestion of food stuffs contaminated with microorganisms or chemicals. The contamination of food may occur at any stage in the process from food production to consumption ("farm to fork") and result from environmental contamination, including pollution of water, soil or air.

The most common clinical presentation of food-borne disease takes the form of gastrointestinal symptoms. For example, food-borne and water-borne diarrheal diseases are problems for every country in the world. Diarrhea is the most common symptom of food-borne illness and other serious consequences including kidney and liver failure, brain and neural disorders, reactive arthritis, cancer and even death.

11.3.1   Global burden of food-borne diseases

11.3.1.1   Basic elements of food-borne diseases

WHO defines food-borne disease as "syndromes that are acquired by eating food that contain sufficient quantities of poisonous substances or pathogens", that is, pathogenic substances enters the body by means of food transmission and causes toxic or infectious illness. According to WHO, food-borne diseases have three basic elements: food is the media of disease transmission; pathogenic agents that cause food-borne diseases are virulence factors in food; and clinical features are acute toxic or infectious manifestations. Food-borne diseases mainly include the most common diseases as followings: food poisoning, food-borne enteric infections, food-borne parasitic diseases and toxic diseases caused by toxic and harmful contaminants in food. Food poisoning in the context of food-borne disease occurs frequently. With the deep insight of food-borne diseases, the scope of which keeps expanding, such as food-borne allergic diseases and chronic degenerative diseases caused by food nutrition imbalance (cardiovascular and cerebrovascular diseases, Cancer, diabetes, etc.).

11.3.1.2   Global situation of food-borne diseases

In both developed and developing countries, food-borne diseases are serious threats to health, especially for children, pregnant women and the elderly. Precise information on the burden of food-borne diseases can adequately inform policy-makers and allocate appropriate resources for food safety control and intervention efforts. On December 3 of 2015, WHO launched a program to estimate the global burden of food-borne diseases. A report, resulting from the WHO Food-borne Disease Burden Epidemiology Reference Group (FERG), provided the first estimation of global food-borne disease incidence, mortality, and disease burden in terms of Disability Adjusted Life Years (DALYs).

According to the report, the most frequent causes of food-borne diseases worldwide were diarrhoeal disease agents, particularly norovirus and Campylobacter spp. Food-borne diarrhoeal disease agents that caused 230,000 (95% UI 160,000-320,000) deaths, were Salmonella Typhi, Taenia solium, hepatitis A virus, and aflatoxin particularly non-typhoidal Salmonella enterica (NTS) which causes diarrhoeal and invasive disease. The global burden of food-borne disease by these 31 hazards was 33 (95% UI 25-46) million DALYs in 2010; 40% of the food-borne disease burden was among children under five years of age. There were considerable differences in the burden of food-borne disease among subregions delimited on the basis of child and adult mortality. The highest burden per population was observed in Africa (AFR) (AFR D and AFR E subregions), followed by South-East Asia (SEAR) (SEAR B and SEAR D subregions) and Eastern Mediterranean (EMR) D subregion.

11.3.2   Causes of food-borne diseases

The pathogenic factors causing food-borne diseases are varied and could be summarized into three categories: biological factors, chemical factors and physical factors.

Biological factors include bacteria and their toxins, parasites and protozoa, viruses and rickettsia, toxic animals and their toxins, and mycotoxins. Bacteria and their toxins are the most important pathogens of food-borne diseases.

Chemical factors include residues of pesticides and veterinary drugs; unqualified food production tools, containers, packaging materials and illegal additives; toxic and hazardous chemicals such as cadmium, lead, arsenic and azo-compounds; may be produced during food processing, such as greasy polymers produced by repeated heating of fats; polycyclic aromatic hydrocarbons (PAHs) produced from baked or smoked animal foods; nitrite produced in the process of food pickling and so on.

Physical factors mainly refers to the irrational emissions of waste and accidental leakage of radioactive materials in mining, smelting, national defense, production activities and scientific experiments. These radioactive substances contaminate food through all aspects of the food chain, causing chronic damage to the body and long-term injury effects.

11.3.3 Classification of food-borne diseases

Generally, food-borne diseases are classified into four major categories as below based on the pathogens, bacteria and their toxins, fungi and their toxins, parasites and virus contamination. They are the most common kinds of food-borne disease and usually be called 'food poisoning'.

According to Food Safety Law of the People's Republic of China, Food Poisoning refers to the non-infectious acute and subacute diseases arising from the intake of food with biological or chemical toxic and hazardous substances or mistake toxic and hazardous substances. Acute gastroenteritis caused by overeating, food-borne intestinal infections (e. g. , typhoid fever) and parasitic diseases (e. g. , trichinosis and cysticercosis), and diseases characterized by chronic poisoning (such as carcinogenic, teratogenic, mutagenic) due to once, large amount or long-term small amount intake of toxic or harmful substances, are not included in the category of food poisoning.

11.3.3.1 Food-borne diseases caused by pathogenic organisms or intoxications

(1) Infections caused by bacteria or intoxications

Infections caused by bacteria or intoxications are a kind of food poisoning caused by ingestion of food containing bacteria or bacterial toxins.

(2) Food-borne mycotoxins and alimentary mycotoxicosis

Food-borne mycotoxins and alimentary mycotoxicosis refer to food poisoning caused by food contaminated with fungi and their toxins which cannot be destroyed by normal cooking heat treatment.

(3) Infections caused by parasites

Infections caused by parasitic refer to a kind of intestinal parasitic disease with relatively short incubation period, in which susceptible individuals ingest food contaminated by pathogens such as parasites, larvas or eggs.

(4) Infections caused by viruses

Infections caused by viruses are food poisoning caused by the ingestion of food containing viruses.

11.3.3.2 Intoxications caused by toxicants from animal foods

The diseases are the food poisoning caused by ingestion of animal-origin toxic foods. There are two main types of food that cause animal food poisoning: animal foods containing toxic ingredients naturally and animal foods containing a large amount of toxic ingredients produced under certain conditions.

11.3.3.3 Intoxications caused by toxicants from plant foods

Intoxications caused by toxicants from plant foods refer to the food poisoning which due to the ingestion of plant origin toxic food, such as nuts containing cyanide glycosides, toadstool and beans, etc.

11.3.3.4 Intoxications caused by toxicants from chemical foods

This kind of food-borne diseases is caused by ingestion of chemical toxic food, such as organophosphorus pesticides, tetramine, and nitrite.

11.3.4   Characteristics of food-borne diseases

Food-borne diseases have three basic characteristics. First, food is the vector that carries and transmits pathogens. Second, the pathogenic factor are various pathogens, toxins, chemicals or nuclide contained in the food. Third, the main clinical characteristics of food-borne diseases are acute or subacute poisoning or acute infection.

Infections caused by bacteria or intoxications are the most common type of food poisoning, which has high morbidity, low mortality and obvious seasonal character of incidence. Food-borne mycotoxins and alimentary mycotoxicosis have high morbidity, high mortality, and obvious seasonal and regional character of incidence. Food-borne virus infections can be transmitted through food and water, and it can be propagated in the intestines after entering the human body. Intoxications caused by toxicants from animal foods have high morbidity and high mortality. The characteristics of intoxications caused by toxicants from plant foods vary with the types of food that causes poisoning. Intoxications caused by toxicants from chemical foods have high morbidity and mortality, while seasonal and regional characters are not obvious.

11.3.5   Control of food-borne diseases

11.3.5.1   Prevention

Food-borne diseases, especially those caused by bacteria, viruses, parasites and fungi, are preventable. The education in safe food handling is a key measure for prevention, including containing antimicrobial resistance. WHO launched the Five Keys to Safer Food Programme to assist the Member States in promoting safe food handling behaviors and educating all food handlers, including consumers, with tools easy to adopt and adapt.

(1) Five key principles if WHO to prevent food-borne diseases are as followings.

1) Prevent contaminating food with pathogens spreading from people, pets, and pests.

2) Separate raw and cooked foods to prevent contaminating the cooked foods.

3) Cook foods for the appropriate length of time and at the appropriate temperature to kill pathogens.

4) Store food at the proper temperature.

5) Do use safe water and safe raw materials.

To ensure the same understanding in practice along the full chain, WHO has developed five addilional Keys materials directed to rural people who grow fruits, vegetables and fish for their own use or for sale on local markets. WHO's objective is to target those who usually do not have access to food safety education despite the important role they play in producing safe food for their community.

(2) Five additional Keys materials directed by WHO to rural people are as followings.

1) Keep clean.

2) Separate raw and cooked.

3) Cook thoroughly.

4) Keep food at safe temperatures.

5) Use safe water and raw materials.

11.3.5.2   Management and control

To establish a national even international public health contingency response mechanism, a disease monitor and data collection network and an ascertaining network of laboratories are of great importance for emergency response and management of food-borne diseases.

When a food poisoning occurs, the patients should be treated as soon as possible. For acute poisoning caused by chemical substances and some toxic animals and plants, patients should be given emetic, gastric lavage and catharsis promptly, and receive special treatment drugs and detoxification drugs. For patients poisoned by biological pathogenic factors, symptomatic treatments should be provided and different treatment plans should be taken based on different pathogenic factors as well as the close attention to the health changes in people with the same dietary history, and giving medical observation and prophylactic medication if necessary.

The targeted compulsory measures should be taken immediately for patients with definite causes of food poisoning, such as cutting off contaminated water, banning sales and consumption of contaminated food, and ordering producers and traders to recall the food that caused poisoning have been sold out. Suspicious food should be sealed up for safekeeping temporarily, prohibited sales and consumptions, and then processed after sampling and inspection.

For food-borne diseases caused by drinking water contamination, the management of water sources should be strengthened and the water source, water supply, storage and disinfection facilities should be inspected and improved to ensure the sanitation of drinking water. Water sources should be disinfected and tested before they can be used.

For infectious diseases that can be transmitted through food such as hepatitis A, cholera, etc., the defense measures should be made with terminal disinfection to the contaminated sites of patients.

Xu Yajun

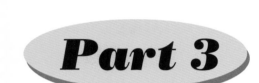

Part 3

Occupational Environment and Health

Chapter 12

Introduction to Occupational Health

12.1 Introduction

Occupational health is a multifaceted and multidisplinary field concerned by protecting the health of workers from diseases and injuries. This field involves the improvement of the work environment and the promotion of the health of workers in general. The relationship between the work environment and the health of workers is complex, which is influenced by many factors. The health outcome could be caused by work, modulated by work or unrelated to work.

12.1.1 Introduction to occupational health

The field of occupational health is concerned with "identification and control of the risks arising from physical, chemical, and other workplace hazards in order to establish and maintain a safe and healthy working environment. These hazards include chemical agents, such as toxic metals or solvents, physical agents, such as loud noise or vibration, and machinery hazards, such as electricity or dangerous machinery. " In addition to identifying and controlling job-related risks, occupational health specializes in "the recognition, diagnosis, treatment, and prevention of illnesses, injuries resulting from hazardous exposures in the workplace". The field maintains an interdisciplinary approach, which includes the application of medicine, epidemiology, toxicology engineering, and management to occupational health issues in an organizational context. In addition, the field is closely aligned with the traditional concerns of preventive medicine and public health. Linked with occupational health is occupational medicine, the branch of medicine that deals with the diagnosis, treatment, and prevention of occupational diseases and injuries occur at work or in specific occupations, that is, diseases directly caused by exposure to workplace hazards.

The international concept ualization and development of occupational health occurred during the 20th century. Key influences were the establishment of the International Commission for Occupational Health, in 1906, and the establishment of the Industrial Labor Organization (ILO), after the Second World War. The International Labor Organization convention 161 (1985) described the components of workplace occupational health provision. Concepts of occupational health have developed subsequently, influenced by the definition of the World Health Organization (WHO). Health is a positive affirmation of physical, mental, and social well–being, not merely the absence of disease. There has also been the recognition that occupational health has a positive contribution to making the performance of enterprises and to the well–being of the communities in which they are based. The WHO concept of health, environment, and safety management in enterprises describes comprehensive occupational health as the long–term maintenance of the working ability of employees, taking into account occupational, environmental, social, and lifestyle determinants of health. More recently, the WHO healthy workplace model has portrayed a healthy workplace as "one in which workers and managers collaborate to use a continual improvement process to protect and promote the health, safety and well–being of all workers and the sustainability of the workplace" by considering four discrete, albeit linked areas. These include: health and safety concerns of the physical work environment; health, safety, and well–being concerns in the psychosocial work environment, including work organization and workplace culture; personal health resources in the workplace (support and encouragement of healthy lifestyles by the employer); and ways of participating in the community to improve the health of workers, their families, and members of the community. According to the Twelfth Session of the Joint ILO/WHO Committee on Occupational Health (1995), occupational health has three key objectives: the maintenance and promotion of workers' health and working capacity; the improvement of working environment and work to become conducive to safety and health; the development of work organization and working cultures in a direction which support health and safety at work, and in doing so also promote a positive social atmosphere and smooth operation, and may enhance the productivity of the undertaking. A new paradigm for occupational health has emerged that extends the classical focus on what might be termed "health risk management", that is, the focus on workplace hazards and risk to health–to include the medical aspects of sickness absence and rehabilitation, the support and management of chronic non – communicable diseases, and workplace health promotion.

To continue the development of occupational health, to strengthen the supervision and management of workers is needed, especially in some representative industries with high risks, such as coal mines, the pharmaceutical industry, and pesticide manufacturers. Many efforts are needed to promote research on the prevention and control of occupational health; motivate the government to improve regulations and standards; perfect the diagnosis of occupational diseases and improve the reporting system; as well as train health professionals. Furthermore, new occupational risks, such as ergonomic factors and job stress, as well as the traditional hazards, will need attention simultaneously.

12.1.2 History of occupational health

Occupational health emerged as an important issue for humanity beginning with ancient societies. Occupational hazards have been noted since the classical period of human history, which spanned approximately 500 BCE to 500 CE in the time of the ancient Greeks and Romans. In addition to theorizing about the cause of disease, the important contributions were the recognition of the hazards of chemicals used in the production of metals. Hippocrates (460–370 BCE) recognized the toxic properties of lead. Pliny the Elder (23–79 CE) noted that the toxic properties of sulfur and zinc and he invented a mask constructed from the bladder of an animal for protection against dusts and metal fumes. During the early and late Renaissance periods, Paracelsus (1493—1541) elaborated some of the crucial principles of toxicology. Agricola (1494—1555) wrote about the dangers that affected workers in trades such as metal working. Ramazzini (1633—1714), who is often called the father of occupational medicine, created elaborate descriptions of the manifestations of occupational diseases among many different types of workers. He is also considered as a pioneer in the field of ergonomics and wrote De Morbis Artificum Diatriba (Diseases of Workers), published in

1,700, which highlighted the risks posed by hazardous chemicals, dusts, and metals used in the workplace. Percival Pott (1714—1788) described the occurrence of scrotal cancer among chimney sweeps. Alice Hamilton (1869—1970) created awareness of phosphorus necrosis of the jaw (phossy jaw) and called attention to industrial plumbism. By doing this, Hamilton is regarded as the mother of occupational medicine.

12.1.3 Significance of the occupational environment in health

Occupational health is significant to society in view of the large percentage of the population that is currently employed and the numerous waking hours that the typical employed person spends on the job. Given the scale of the workforce, occupational health constitutes a major public health issue. Also, occupational health issues can extend beyond the time of active employment. In particular, retired persons may be afflicted by the sequelae of work-related conditions acquired when they were actively employed.

Occupational health hazards and job-associated injuries affect workers in all countries around the world. The international significance of occupational health reflects the working conditions for many adults and child labor in developing countries. Occupational illnesses and injuries contribute substantially to global morbidity and mortality. Migration of persons in search of employment has become a global phenomenon. Immigrant workers often experience increased risks of injuries and disease from their employment in host countries. The number of work-related deaths that occurs worldwide is estimated at approximately 2 million annually, with disease likely to be the cause of most of these deaths. This figure is likely to be a major underestimate of the actual number of deaths. Exposures to occupational hazards are important determinants of morbidity worldwide. Regarding occupational morbidity, five major occupationally associated risk factors are classified as workplace carcinogens, airborne particulates, hazards for injuries, ergonomic stressors for back pain, and noise. These five risk factors contribute to a large percentage of the overall global burden of disease from lung cancer, leukemia, pneumoconiosis, chronic obstructive pulmonary disease, asthma, injuries, back pain and hearing loss.

12.2 Occupational environment and health

12.2.1 Occupational hazards and exposure

Occupational hazards are dangers to human health and well-being which are associated with specific occupations. Occupational hazards can be classified into three types of hazards according to the sources. For purpose of hazard control and disease prevention, hazards are classified largely on the basis of their physical and chemical characteristics, since these characteristics determine the route of exposure. Workers may be exposed to contaminants by inhalation, absorption through the skin, ingestion, or injection. Inhalation and skin absorption are the primary routes of exposure for most materials in the occupational environment. Environmental agents can be classified as physical hazards, chemical hazards, and biological hazards. Physical hazards include noise, vibration, ionizing and non-ionizing radiation, and temperature extremes, etc. The materials such as toxic metals, pesticides, toxic gases are classified as chemical hazards. Biological hazards refer to exposure to infectious or immunologically active agents such as molds, fungi, and bacteria.

12.2.2 Occupational disease

An occupational disease is any chronic ailment that occurs as a result of work or occupational activity.

It is an aspect of occupational safety and health. An occupational disease is typically identified when it is shown that it is more prevalent in a given body of workers than in the general population, or in other worker populations.

Under the law of workers' compensation in many areas, there is a presumption that the specific diseases are caused by the worker being in the work environment and the burden is on the employer or insurer to show that the disease came about from another cause. Diseases compensated by national workers compensation authorities are often termed occupational diseases in a narrow sense. However, many countries do not offer compensations for certain diseases like musculoskeletal disorders caused by work (e. g. , in Norway). Therefore, the term "work-related diseases" is utilized to describe diseases of occupational origin. This term however would then include both compensable and non-compensable diseases that have occupational origins.

Some well-known occupational diseases include occupational lung diseases, occupational skin diseases, occupational cancer, etc. Occupational lung diseases include asbestosis among asbestos miners and those who work with friable asbestos insulation, as well as black lung (coal worker's pneumoconiosis) among coal miners, silicosis among miners, quarrying and tunnel operators and byssinosis among workers in parts of the cotton textile industry. Occupational asthma renders a vast number of occupations at risk. Bad indoor air quality may predispose for diseases in the lungs as well as in other parts of the body. Occupational skin diseases are ranked among the top five occupational diseases in many countries. Occupational skin diseases and conditions are generally caused by chemicals and having wet hands for long periods while at work. Eczema is by far the most common, but urticaria, sunburn and skin cancer are also of concern. Contact dermatitis due to irritation is inflammation of the skin which results from a contact with an irritant. It has been observed that this type of dermatitis does not require prior sensitization of the immune system. There have been studies to support that past or present atopic dermatitis is a risk factor for this type of dermatitis. Common irritants include detergents, acids, alkalies, oils, organic solvents and reducing agents. The acute form of this dermatitis develops on exposure of the skin to a strong irritant or caustic chemical. This exposure can occur as a result of accident at a workplace. The irritant reaction starts to increase in its intensity within minutes to hours of exposure to the irritant and reaches its peak quickly. After the reaction has reached its peak level, it starts to heal. This process is known as decrescendo phenomenon. The most frequent potent irritants leading to this type of dermatitis are acids and alkaline solutions. The symptoms include redness and swelling of the skin along with the formation of blisters. The chronic form occurs as a result of repeated exposure of the skin to weak irritants over long periods of time. Clinical manifestations of the contact dermatitis are also modified by external factors such as environmental factors (mechanical pressure, temperature, and humidity) and predisposing characteristics of the individual (age, sex, ethnic origin, pre-existing skin disease, atopic skin diathesis, and anatomic region exposed). Another occupational skin disease is glove-related hand urticaria. It has been reported as an occupational problem among the health care workers. This type of hand urticaria is believed to be caused by repeated wearing and removal of the gloves. The reaction is caused by the latex or the nitrile present in the gloves. Other diseases of concern include overuse syndrome among persons who perform repetitive or forceful movements in constrictive postures, carpal tunnel syndrome among persons who work in the poultry industry and information technology, computer vision syndrome among persons using information technology for hours and lead poisoning affecting workers in many industries that processe or employ lead or lead compounds.

12. 2. 3   Preventive aspects of occupational diseases

Occupational health deals with all aspects of health in the workplace and has a strong focus on primary prevention of hazards. The health of the workers has several determinants, including risk factors at the workplace leading to cancers, accidents, musculoskeletal diseases, respiratory diseases, hearing loss, circulatory diseases, stress related disorders and communicable diseases and others. The primary prevention is the most effective to control occupational hazards.

12.2.3.1   Material substitution

Elimination or reduction of extreme toxic materials, such as asbestos as an insulating material, or benzene in solvents, adhesives and gasoline, is well established. However, these substitutions have the risk of replacing one hazard with another. For example, the replacement of benzene with another chemical, such as toluene or xylene, with similar solvent properties, may reduce the risk of exposure to a carcinogen, but increase the hazard of exposure to a neurotoxin.

12.2.3.2   Industrial process modification

The application of engineering control technology to modify the design of industrial processes is a very effective method of intervention to reduce exposure. Many common industrial processes, such as material handling procedures, can be redesigned to minimize the release of contaminants. The control of potential hazards at the design stage is more efficient than redesign of existing systems.

12.2.3.3   Isolation

This approach can be implemented by enclosure to isolate a source from the working environment or by isolating the workers from a contaminated environment. Both approaches may be part of a comprehensive exposure−control strategy; however, containment of the source is generally preferable.

12.2.3.4   Ventilation

There are two general types of ventilation: dilution ventilation and local exhaust ventilation. Although they are frequently used together, the two of ventilation are very different in design and performance. Most workplaces require local ventilation to capture contaminants at or near their source and remove them from the work environment.

12.2.3.5   Personal protective equipment

Personal protective equipment is at the lowest level of the hierarchy of exposure control methods. These devices are intended to provide a barrier between workers and contaminated environment, which include equipment to protect the eyes, (safety glasses, goggles, and face shields); the skin (gloves, aprons and full body suits made of impervious materials); and the respiratory tract (a wide variety of respiratory protective devices).

12.2.3.6   Education and training

Worker education and training are essential components of effective programs of primary prevention and exposure control. Any of the control strategies could exert function best when workers understand the physical and chemical hazards associated with their work, as well as methods for controlling these hazards.

12.3   Trends and challenges of occupational health

12.3.1   Globalization and occupational health

Globalization of the world economy and global outsourcing are contemporary trends with important implications for the workplace. Examples of function that can be outsourced include manufacturing, information technology services, and customer support. Companies headquartered in the economically advanced countries are able to gain economic advantages by relocating some of their activities to less developed regions, where wages and other costs are lower. This outsourcing trend and growing importance of supply chains has implications for the working conditions and health and safety of workers of supplier and contracting companies. In developing country, standards for occupational health may be less rigorous than their counterparts in the developed world. Related to globalization of economic activities is the integration of regional economies, which also affect the worker's health.

WHO is implementing a Global Plan of Action on Workers' health 2008—2017 endorsed by the World Health Assembly in 2007 with the following objectives: devising and implementing policy instruments on workers' health; protecting and promoting health at the workplace; improving the performance of and access to occupational health services; providing and communicating evidence for action and practice; and incorporating workers' health into other policies.

12.3.2　New technologies in occupational health

New technologies such as nanotechnologies hold much potential for supporting groundbreaking progress in diverse field such as medicine, energy production, and products for the consumer. It is possible that nanomaterials may affect human health adversely, although the potential adverse health effects of manufactured nanomaterial exposure are not yet fully understood and exposures in humans are mostly uncharacterized.

A growing employment field known as "green jobs" promises opportunities in the sustainable, low-carbon sector. The "green jobs" includes jobs that help to protect ecosystems and biodiversity; de-carbonize the economy; and minimize or altogether avoid generation of all forms of waste and pollution. Although green jobs can contribute greatly to society, it will be necessary to assure the health and safety of the workers who are likely to be employed in this new industry. For example, one category of green jobs focuses on the development of renewable energy sources and devices for increased energy efficiency, in which the workers were exposed to the risk from electrical shocks and falling from working at heights. One of important task for occupational health is to identify hazards associated with green jobs and develop methods for controlling them. Another green economy is recycling operation which helps to preserve scarce resources. Electrical and electronic waste is one of the fastest-growing categories of waste. This waste stream contains precious metals and toxic chemicals, which markedly impact the human health.

12.3.3　Occupational health in different groups of population

Child labor was common in England during the 19th century. Currently, it is a problem of particular concern for developing countries. In these countries, poor children are often forced to leave school to work and support their families. They may be exposed to hazardous materials and deleterious chemicals, and at great risk of injuries. Children are more vulnerable to injury and the effects of toxic chemicals due to their behaviors and developmental stages.

Globally, participation of women in the workforce has increased steadily, especially in rapidly industrializing Asian countries. Women who work in factories and in health-care facilities may be exposed to toxic chemicals and radiation. The impact of such exposures upon reproductive function is a vital area of concern for occupational health. Many female workers also experience high stress since they need to manage their households in addition to working outside of the home.

Many industrialized countries are facing the challenges of an aging workforce. The number of older workers (persons 55 years of age and older) is increasing. Occupational injuries and illnesses among older workers tend to be less frequent than among younger workers, however, older workers' injuries and illnesses are more serious. Comprehensive health promotion and health protection programs need to be developed for them. In the United States of America, it is projected that by 2020, 25% workforce will be aged $\geqslant$ 55 years. In Europe, it is predicted that a combination of reducing birth rates and rising life expectancy will halve the ratio between people of working age and people over the age of 65 years by 2060. Asia will also have to address this emerging issue. Japan is considered the World's oldest country, and by 2040, it is predicted to have the highest median age of its population. In addition, China, Hong Kong, and Singapore are reported to be the fastest aging among the countries of the region. In absolute numbers, China and India have the largest older populations. WHO has developed an active aging policy framework. Active aging is defined as the process of optimizing opportunities for health, participation, and security in order to enhance quality of life as people age. Work is recognized as an important component of active aging, and WHO has stated that, throughout the world, if more people would enjoy opportunities for dignified work (properly remunerated in adequate environments, protected against workplace hazards) earlier in life, people would reach old age able to participate in the workplace. The workplace and occupational health has an important role, therefore, in promoting the health and well-being of workers, via the adoption of the WHO healthy workplace model, and in becoming part of mainstream healthcare for the purposes of treating and supporting people with non-communicable diseases. WHO considers workplace health programs as one of the best options for prevention and control of non-communicable diseases (NCDs) and for mental health. Such programs can help achieve the WHO objective of reducing the avoidable deaths of NCDs and the burden of mental ill health, and to protect and promote health at the workplace as stipulated in the Global Plan of Action on Workers' health 2008—2017.

Immigrant workers become a numerical majority in some countries, especially in the developed countries. Some groups of immigrant workers may be at increased risk for hazardous occupational exposures and worsening conditions; many of these exposures are greatly underestimated.

12.3.4 The strategic perspectives for occupational health

The global action plan of WHO Plan asserts that the health of workers is determined not only by occupational hazards, but also by social and individual factors, and access to health services. It raises concern that there are major gaps between and within countries in the exposure of workers and local communities to occupational hazards and their access to occupational health services. The function of occupational health services has been to protect workers from workplace hazards. These may lead to workplace injuries, cancer, and hearing loss, as well as respiratory, musculoskeletal, cardiovascular, reproductive, neurological, skin, and mental ill health disorders. Globally, exposures to carcinogens are estimated to cause 8% lung cancer, the most frequent cause of cancer. Occupational exposures to airborne particulates probably cause 12% of deaths due to chronic obstructive pulmonary disease. There are also deaths due to silicosis, asbestos related diseases, and other pneumoconiosis. However, in high-income countries, morbidity due to conditions such as low back pain and common mental health disorders has become the focus of occupational health services. The workplace has been identified as a key setting for addressing the rising incidence and prevalence of mental ill health. The growing evidence of the global impact of mental illnesses is demonstrated by the finding that 5 of the 10 leading causes of disability, worldwide, are mental health problems. Mental illness is considered to be as relevant in low-income countries as in wealthy ones, cutting across age, gender, and social strata. In China, 20% of the working population was found to suffer from mental health problems. The workplace is an appropriate environment in which to raise awareness of mental health and to use good mental health practice to influence attitudes toward mental ill health. The "hidden epidemic" of occupational disease comprises the established diseases, such as the pneumoconiosis and asbestos–related diseases, in addition to emerging conditions. Technological, social, and organizational changes in the workplace, as well as rapid globalization, have seen the emergence of new risks and challenges. Musculoskeletal and mental health disorders will require new approaches to stem the increasing incidence. There will be a need for better data to inform prevention strategies. Challenges to be overcome in this regard include: the lack of knowledge and experience in diagnosis, recognition, and report of occupational diseases; inclusion of small–and medium–sized enterprises in national reporting schemes; changing working populations as a result of migration; and the long latency of occupational diseases. Further analysis of the global burden of disease reveals that the incidence and prevalence of non–communicable diseases pose the greatest challenge to both public and occupational health. Thus, future occupational health practice will be based on a holistic biopsychosocial approach to the promotion of health, well–being, and work ability. The strategic implication of the paradigm shift from a "labor approach" to a "public health approach" is that there will be a move away from a consideration of occupational health toward a focus on worker's health. This means that occupational health practitioners will be concerned with not only employed workers, that is, those under some form of employment contract, but also self–employed and informal workers. Interventions will extend to families and communities, and will not be restricted to actions at the workplace. The promotion and maintenance of health and well–being will involve a consideration of all health determinants and will not be restricted to work–related health issues. Importantly, the health of workers will not be seen as only the responsibility of employers, but also of the wider stakeholder group, including health, work, and environment authorities, insurance companies, and other healthcare practitioners. Many companies have now developed health and well–being strategies that encourage healthy behaviors at work and at home, and promote participation in physical activity challenges. The activity–tracking devices is made to download data to mobile phones. The outputs may be used for both motivational purposes and construction of organizational risk profiles. Improvements in the profiles may attract lower insurance premiums for companies. Social media may be used to develop online communities and to facilitate activity challenges. This will redefine the remit and roles of occupational health practitioners and may necessitate searching for a new term to describe the role and function of the discipline.

▶▶ *Summary*

Occupational health is concerned with protecting the health of workers from diseases and injuries associated with hazardous work–related exposures. This field involves the improvement of the work environment and the promotion of the health of workers in general. Occupational health hazards have been observed since the classical period of human history. Occupational diseases and injuries are significant concerns for the most countries. The primary prevention is the most effective to control occupational hazards.

Practice questions:

(1) Define the following terms: occupational health, occupational exposures, and work–related disease.

(2) What is the significance of adverse health outcomes associated with work?

(3) State five adverse health outcomes that have been linked to the work environment.

Meng Xiaojing

Chapter 13

Occupational Hazards

13.1　Introduction

Throughout the world, most adults spend much of their waking hours at work. Work provides a number of economic and other benefits. At the same time, occupational workers face a variety of hazards including chemicals, biological agents, physical factors, adverse ergonomic conditions, psychosocial factors, and so on. Occupational hazard as a term refers to the source or situation experienced in the workplace with a potential harm to an exposed person. Occupational hazards are dangers to human health and wellbeing which are associated with specific occupations. Occupational hazard signifies both long-term and short-term risks associated with the workplace environment and is a field of study within occupational safety and health and public health. Short term risks may include physical injury, while long-term risks may be increased risk of developing cancer, heart disease, and other chronic diseases. About 2.9 billion workers across the globe are exposed to hazardous risks at their workplaces.

Exposure to occupational hazards can adversely affect the human body. Adverse effects range from a-symptomatic physiological and bio-chemical changes to symptoms of illness, to diagnosed diseases, and finally to death. For some risk factors, there is a very clear connection between the exposure and the disease. For example, the primary route of exposure to airborne particulates, gases and vapors is inhalation, whereby these agents gain access to the respiratory system and are either deposited (in the case of particulates) or enter the circulatory system (gases and vapors). Diverse risk factors cause more than one type of outcome of interest. For example, exposure to asbestos can result in malignant conditions of the lung and the pleura, malignant conditions of the peritoneum, and nonmalignant conditions of the lung (asbestosis). Some exposures, such as occupational noise, are well characterized. Others have not been well characterized or are multi-faceted, but the disorders they caused are clear (such as occupational injuries).

13.2　Chemical hazards

Chemical hazards are a subtype of occupational hazards that are dangerous to human health. These compounds in the form of solids, liquids, gases, mists, dusts, fumes and vapors exert toxic effects by inhalation (breathing), absorption (through direct contact with the skin) or ingestion (eating or drinking). Airborne chemical hazards exist as concentrations of mists, vapors, gases, fumes or solids. Some are toxic through inhalation and some of them irritate the skin on contact; some can be toxic by absorption through the skin or through ingestion and some are corrosive to living tissue. Exposure to chemicals in the workplace can cause acute or long-term detrimental health effects. The degree of risk from exposure to any given substance depends on the nature and potency of the toxic effects and the magnitude and duration of exposure.

13.2.1 Productive toxicants

13.2.1.1 Metal and metalloid

A large number of metals and metalloids are used in the industry. Metals can exist as elemental metals, or in the ionic or organic forms with each form having its own specific toxicity. Exposure to metals and the metalloids usually takes the form of inhaling metal-containing dust, inhaling fumes from molten metal or inhaling or ingesting salts of the element. The industrial physician should be aware of the toxic effects of lead, mercury, arsenic, cadmium, manganese, beryllium, chromium, zinc and others. The toxic health effects depend upon the duration and the dose or concentration of exposure.

13.2.1.2 Irritant gases

Toxic gases can be classified according to their physiological action into: asphyxiating and irritant gases. Irritant gases can be inhaled or absorbed through the mucosal surfaces. Water-soluble irritant gases (e. g., chlorine, ammonia, sulfur dioxide, hydrogen chloride) dissolve in the upper airway and cause mucous membrane irritation. Less soluble gases (e. g., nitrogen dioxide, phosgene, ozone) are more likely to damage the lower respiratory tract, even lead to pulmonary oedema.

Irritant gases are capable of causing an inflammatory response of the mucous membranes of the eyes, nose, throat, and lungs. Irritant gas exposures predominantly affect the airways. Examples of common irritant gases are ammonia, chlorine, formaldehyde, hydrogen sulfide (and other reduced sulfides), oxides of sulfur or nitrogen, and acid gases.

13.2.1.3 Asphyxiating gases

An asphyxiating gas is the most common cause of chemical poisoning. Asphyxiating gases reduce the body's ability to absorb, transport, or utilize inhaled oxygen. In other words, by their specific toxic action they render the body incapable of utilizing the supply of adequate oxygen to the tissues. These gases have in common the characteristic that they interfere with oxygen or energy metabolism in cells. They are classified as either simple or chemical asphyxiants on the basis of the mechanism of toxicity. Examples include carbon dioxide, helium, nitrogen, nitrous oxide, aliphatic hydrocarbon gases such as butane, ethane, methane, and propane, and noble gases such as argon, helium, neon, and radon. Carbon monoxide is a toxic gas that acts by binding to haemoglobin and preventing haemoglobin from delivering oxygen to tissues in the body.

13.2.1.4 Organic solvent

Organic solvents are organic liquids in which other substances can be dissolved without changing their chemical composition. Organic solvents are used routinely in commercial industries. They are used in the extraction of oils and fats in the food industry, the chemical industry, paint, varnishes, enamel, degreasing process, dry cleaning, printing and dying in the textile and rayon industries. Organic solvents are usually volatile. Their vapors may be inhaled or adsorbed from skin contact. Inhalation and dermal absorption are important approaches of toxic exposure. These solvents include aromatics (such as benzene and toluene) and halogenated hydrocarbons (such as trichloroethylene, perchloroethylene and carbon tetrachloride). Other commonly used solvents are the alcohols, xylene and ether. Exposures often involve mixtures of solvents.

13.2.1.5   Aromatic amino and nitro compounds

Aromatic amino-and nitro-compounds represent one of the most important classes of industrial and environmental chemicals containing at least one amino or nitro group attached directly to an aryl moiety. With the great expansion of the dye and explosives industries necessitated by war production, increasing numbers of workers are called upon to manufacture, or to handle many aromatic amino and nitro compounds. Aromatic amino and nitro compounds, including the aniline, Trinitrotoluene (T. N. T.), phenyl-hydrazine and phenylhydroxylamine are of great importance in those industries. Their toxic responses are often similar due to a common metabolic intermediate. In most operations, it may well be that inhalation and ingestion are the most important modes of entry, while in warehouse, where the concentration of air-borne T. N. T. is very low the skin may be the most important portal of entry. Many aromatic amines have been shown to be potent carcinogens, mutagens, skin sensitizers, and/or hematotoxicants capable of inducing methemoglobinemia.

13.2.1.6   Polymers

Polymers are molecules that consist of a long, repeating chain of smaller units called monomers. They have the highest molecular weight among any molecules, and may consist of billions of atoms. Both synthetic and natural polymers play essential and ubiquitous roles in everyday life. There are two types of polymers: natural and synthetic polymers. Natural polymeric materials such as shellac, amber, wool, silk and natural rubber have been used for centuries. A variety of other natural polymers exist, such as cellulose, which is the main constituent of wood and paper.

The list of synthetic polymers includes synthetic rubber, phenol formaldehyde resin, neoprene, nylon, polyvinyl chloride (PVC or vinyl), polystyrene, polyethylene, polypropylene, polyacrylonitrile, PVB, silicone, and many more.

13.2.1.7   Pesticides

Pesticides are biologically active chemicals designed to control insect, animal, and plant pests. They are classified into several groups, according to their chemical composition. Their toxicity varies widely and depends on the compound, of which the major functional classes are insecticides, including organochlorines, organophosphates, and carbamates, and herbicides. Pesticides are widely used in homes and gardens, schools, parks and agricultural fields. The pesticide exposed occupational groups considered were both agricultural and non-agricultural. Agricultural occupational groups included farmers, farm workers, pesticide mixers and loaders, agricultural pesticide applicators, crop duster pilots, and flaggers for crop duster pilots. Non-agricultural pesticide exposed groups considered are nursery and greenhouse workers, chemical lawn care workers, golf course workers, park maintenance workers, and landscape maintenance workers. Occupational exposures to these chemicals are through dermal and inhalational routes, while non-occupational exposures usually occur by accidental ingestion.

13.2.2   Productive dusts

13.2.2.1   Introduction

If the work atmosphere is dusty, dusts will inevitably be inhaled. Dust particles below five microns in diameter are called respirable particles since they have the chance to reach the alveoli. The respiratory tract has certain defense mechanisms against dusts, but when the environment is very dusty, a significant amount of dusts can be retained in the lungs. Dusts are generated and released into the atmosphere during operations of handling, crushing, grinding, colliding, exploding, and heating organic or inorganic materials such as rock, ore, metal, coal, wood and grain.

Dusts are classified into inorganic and organic dusts or soluble and insoluble dusts. Inorganic dusts consist of silica, mica, coal, asbestos dust, etc. ; organic dusts include cotton and the like. The soluble dusts dissolve slowly, enter the systemic circulation and are eventually eliminated by body metabolism. The insoluble dusts remain, more or less, permanently in the lungs. They are mainly the cause of pneumoconiosis. The most common dust diseases are silicosis and anthracosis.

13.2.2.2   Silica

Silicon (Si) is the second most common element in the Earth's crust. The compound silica, also known as silicon dioxide (SiO_2), is quite common and found in many rocks, such as granite, sandstone, gneiss and slate. Silica occurs in 3 forms: crystalline, microcrystalline (or cryptocrystalline) and amorphous (non-crystalline). Quartz is the most common form of crystalline silica. Exposure occurs in mining and quarrying operations, stone cutting and shaping, foundry operations, glass and ceramics manufacture, sandblasting and manufacture of abrasive soaps which may produce fine to ultrafine airborne silica dusts. Breathe in the dusts causes silicosis, a severe disease that can scar the lungs.

13.2.2.3   Silicates

Silicates are SiO_2 combined with an appreciable portion of cations. Myriad silicate anions can exist, and each can form compounds with many different cations. Approximately 30% of all minerals are silicates and 90% of the Earth's crust is made up of silicates, SiO_4^- based material. They are classified based on the structure of silicate groups, which contain different ratios of silicon and oxygen. Talc, asbestos, and mica are examples of silicates. Asbestos fiber is a naturally occurring, fibrous silicate mineral which is resistant to heat and many chemicals. In addition to mining and extraction, exposure to asbestos occurs in its use for insulation, in the making of asbestos clothes, in the manufacture of asbestos cement pipes and other products, vinyl floor tiles and in brake and cloth lining. Asbestos fibers, when inhaled, will cause diffuse interstitial fibrosis of the lungs, pleural thickening and calcification.

13.2.2.4   Coal dust

Coal dusts are fine powdered form of coal, which is created by the crushing, grinding, or pulverizing of coal. Because of the brittle nature of coal, coal dusts can be produced during mining, transportation, or by mechanically handling coal. It is a form of fugitive dusts. Coal dusts are relatively inert and not as fibrogenic as in silica dust. Coal dusts that enter the lungs can neither be destroyed nor removed by the body. Occupational exposure to coal dusts leads to anthracosis or coal workers' pneumoconiosis (CWP), which has enormous social, medical and economic importance of many countries in the world where coal mining is a major industry. About 10% of the workers who are working in coal mine for more than 20 years are having CWP.

13.2.2.5   Other dusts

Other types of pneumoconiosis can be caused by inhaling dusts containing aluminum, antimony, barium, graphite, iron, kaolin, and among others. There is also a type called mixed-dust pneumoconiosis. Byssinosis, which caused by exposure to cotton dust, is sometimes included among the pneumoconioses, although its pattern of lung abnormality is different from the pneumoconioses listed here.

13.3   Physical hazards

13.3.1   Introduction

Physical hazards are a set of occupational hazards that can cause harm with or without contact. Examples of physical agents include adverse weather conditions, noise, vibration, electromagnetic radiation, and electricity etc. These factors act singly or in combination.

13.3.2   Adverse weather conditions

Temperature extremes are found in many occupations and pose a danger to workers. Heat is a common health hazard in industries. Heat stress can cause heat stroke, exhaustion, cramps, and rashes. Heat can also fog up safety glasses or cause sweaty palms or dizziness, all of which increase the risk of other injuries. Workers near hot surfaces or steam also are at risk for burns. Dehydration may also result from overexposure to heat. Cold stress also poses a danger to many workers. Overexposure to cold conditions or extreme cold can lead to hypothermia, frostbite, trench foot, or chilblains.

Pressure above or below atmospheric pressure in the workers' surroundings is associated with health risks in certain occupations, such as undersea diving and aviation. Conditions in the workplace may expose the worker to unusually high or low pressures. Examples are decompression sickness and high altitude sickness.

13.3.3   Noise

Sound is propagated in the form of waves, each of which can be described in terms of frequency measured in hertz (Hz) and intensity as expressed in decibels (dB). Human ear can hear sounds ranging in frequency from 20 Hz to 20,000 Hz. Noise is unwanted sound and one of the most common of all the occupational hazards. Each year in the US, twenty-two million workers, such as mine workers, are exposed to higher levels of noise that could potentially harm their health. These noise levels are potentially hazardous to their hearing and can produce other adverse effects as well. Workers are exposed to noise in textile and glass industries, ship building, aeroplane manufacture, engineering industries, manufacture of boilers and pressure vessels and power plants. Noise can be continuous or impulse and is especially prevalent in the manufacturing industries.

13.3.4   Vibration

Vibration, either whole-body vibration or segmental vibration, occurs when a particular body part is affected by vibrations from tools. Workers exposed to whole vibrations include tractor drivers, transport workers, workers involved in drilling for petroleum and those in the textile industry. Whole body vibrations cause various ailments related to congestion of pelvic and abdominal organs. Segmental vibrations affect workers using pneumatic or electrical vibrating tools in mining, road construction, shoe manufacture and sawing.

13.3.5   Ionizing and non-ionizing radiation

Ionizing radiation include electromagnetic ionizing radiation (like X-rays and gamma-rays, radiation), and particle radiation (like alpha, beta and neutrons). Ionizing radiation is used in medicine, industry, agriculture, research and atomic warfare. Both types cause ionization or excitation of atoms which leads to tissue destruction.

Nonionizing radiation consists of electromagnetic radiation of longer wavelengths when the energy level is too low to ionize atoms but sufficient to cause physical changes in cells. Ultraviolet radiation is the most common form and exposure occurs in welding, metal cutting and carbon arc. Infrared radiation exposure occurs in front of furnaces, in steel mills, in the glass industry, in blacksmiths and in chain manufacture.

13.3.6　Other factors

Illumination is one of the physical factors. Adequate lighting should be provided either by natural or artificial means, avoiding shadows and glare and observing appropriate colors and contrast. Poor or defective illumination leads to eye strain, fatigue and increased accident rates. Defective illumination in miners leads to miner's nystagmus (rapid, involuntary movement of the eyes).

13.4　Biological hazards

13.4.1　Introduction

Occupational infections are defined as infections caused by exposure to biological agents, such as bacteria, viruses, fungi and parasites at the workplace. These can occur following contact with infected persons and animals or their tissues, secretions, or excretions. Occupational infection itself may be the result of the infection itself (such as pneumonia), toxins produced by the pathogen (as is the case with tetanus), the result of damage done by the pathogen (as in hepatitis) or the result of the body's defenses against the pathogen (as in tuberculosis). Some infections can be transmitted from one person to another and are said to be transmissible, or "contagious". Occupations that deal with plants or animals or their products, or with food and food processing may expose workers to biological hazards. Laboratory and medical personnel also can be exposed to biological hazards. Outdoor workers at risk for these hazards include farmers, foresters, landscapers, groundskeepers, gardeners, painters, roofers, pavers, construction workers, laborers, mechanics, and any other workers who spend time outside. Almost any infection could occur as a result of occupational exposure but certain occupations carry a higher risk than others. These include agricultural workers, health care workers and laboratory personnel, workers involved with animals and animal products and outdoor workers in general where there may be exposure to excreta of infected animals.

13.4.2　Bacteria

The common pathogenic bacteria include mycobacterium tuberculosis, bacillus anthracis, and brucella. Pulmonary tuberculosis is caused by Mycobacterium tuberculosis (Koch's bacillus) and is transmitted occupationally by droplet infection, contact with infected material from humans (sputum) or animals.

Brucellosis is caused by brucella which can infect cattle, sheep and pigs. The disease causes recurrent abortion in animals and is present in the placenta, in animal secretions, in milk and in urine. Exposed workers are veterinarians, workers in agriculture and animal husbandry, shepherds and laboratory and slaughterhouse workers. Most occupational cases occur through the contact with infected animals or their secretions and products.

Anthrax is caused by Bacillus Anthracis and essentially an animal disease. Exposed workers are those in agriculture and animal husbandry, slaughter houses, tanneries and those working in the manufacture of goods from wool, hair, bones and leather.

13.4.3　Virus

Health care workers who are likely to come in contact with the blood and body fluids of infected persons with viral hepatitis B and viral hepatitis C are at great risk of virus infection. The exposure to patient's body fluids via contaminated glassware and other contaminated equipment, such as needles, provides an opportunity for contact with mucous membranes or parenteral inoculation.

Transmission of the acquired immunodeficiency syndrome (AIDS) agent, the Human immunodeficiency virus (HIV), occurs only through sexual contact, perinatally from an infected mother and through contaminated blood or blood products. These viruses are not transmitted through casual, non-intimate workplace contact or social encounters, such as eating in restaurants or using public transportation or bathroom facilities.

13.4.4　Other microorganism

There are other biological risks caused by protozoal and parasitic microorganism (like Malaria, Hookworms, tapeworms) and Fungi (such as ornithosis, tnea-infections, psittacosis, and coccidiomycosis).

13.5　Social, psychological and ergonomic hazards

13.5.1　Introduction

Psychosocial hazards are occupational hazards that affect someone's social life or psychological health. Psychosocial hazards in the workplace include occupational burnout and occupational stress, which can lead to burnout. The capacity to adapt to different working environments is influenced by many factors such as education, cultural background, family life, social habits and what the worker expects from employment. The health effects of psychological hazards can be classified into psychological and behavioral changes, including hostility, aggressiveness, anxiety, depression, alcoholism, drug addiction, absenteeism.

Except psychosocial hazards, occupational disorders due to ergonomic hazards are common. Ergonomics is primarily aimed to optimize, first and foremost, the comfort, as well as the health, safety and efficiency, of the worker. Applying ergonomic principles however, is not only beneficial to workers. The benefits to employers are equally significant and are both visible and measurable in terms of increased efficiency, higher productivity, reduction in work time lost due to illness or injury and decreased insurance costs.

13.5.2　Psychosocial factors

Psychosocial factors are job satisfaction, service condition, leadership, type of work, communication, payment, welfare state, trade union activity, incentives, etc. In modern occupational health, importance is given to the condition in which people work, their attitude toward their job, their hopes and fear. Stress can be considered to be a psychological reaction to an imbalance between demand on the worker and the workers' ability to do the job to a satisfactory degree of comfort or expectation. Burnout is a popular term for a debilitating psychological condition in which the worker feels tired, disappointed, unfulfilled and anxious. It occurs in some workers after prolonged periods of stress and a feeling of frustration or lack of accomplishment.

The psychosocial hazards arise from the workers' failure to adapt to an alien psychosocial environment. Psychosocial factors include social characteristics such as patterns of interaction within family or occupational groups, cultural characteristics such as traditional ways of solving conflicts, and psychological characteristics such as attitudes, beliefs and personality factors. Frustration, lack of job satisfaction, insecurity, poor human relationships, and emotional tension are some of the psychosocial factors which may undermine both physical and mental health of the workers. The increasing stress on automation, electronic operations and nuclear energy may introduce newer psychosocial health problems in industry. Psychosocial hazards are therefore assuming more importance than physical or chemical hazards.

13.5.3 Ergonomic factors

Ergonomics is the study of the complex relationships between people, physical and psychological aspects of the work environment (e. g. , facilities, equipment and tools), job demands and work methods. It is a field which integrates knowledge derived from the human sciences (in particular anatomy, physiology and psychology) to match jobs, systems, products and environments to the physical and mental abilities and limitations of workers. A properly designed workplace and work process leads to greater efficiency, more productivity, fewer injuries, fewer musculoskeletal problems, less fatigue, less spoilage of work product, better quality and more satisfied workers. Ergonomics stresses fitting the job to the worker as compared to the more usual practice of obliging the worker to fit the job. Much of ergonomics is devoted to improving the human-machine interface so that the worker is able to operate equipment efficiently and with minimal strain. Some problems arise from poorly designed job tasks. Many ergonomic problems including increased assembly line speeds, added specialized tasks, repetitive motion, eye strain and heavy lifting problems, can cause ergonomic hazards resulting from technological changes.

13.6 Occupational carcinogens

13.6.1 Introduction

Occupational cancer is cancer caused by exposure to carcinogens that fall under Group 1 of the International Agency for Research on Cancer (IARC) in the workplace.

IARC classifies the agents into five groups. Group 1: Proven human carcinogens (based on epidemiological studies among workers with long exposure); Group 2A: Probable human carcinogens (evidence from animal studies which are relevant to human exposure); Group 2B: Possible human carcinogens (evidence of significant increase in cancer incidence in more than one animal species or strains); Group 3: Agents are not classifiable as carcinogenic to humans; Group 4: Agents probably not carcinogenic to humans.

Carcinogens can be divided into three major categories: chemical carcinogens, physical carcinogens, and oncogenic viruses. The IARC has classified 203 chemical or biological agents or exposure situations as known or probable human carcinogens. It covers 120 agents, mixtures or exposure circumstances as Group 1 (carcinogenic to humans), including various chemical compounds, pharmaceuticals and bacterial and viral infections. Of them many are encountered in occupational settings, e. g. , asbestos and cadmium. An additional 83 agents, mixtures or exposure circumstances have been classified as Group 2A (probably carcinogenic to humans). Those with occupational significance include diesel fumes and benzidine-based dyes. Although IARC classifies agents according to their overall carcinogenicity, specific cancer sites are also considered. Some well-established occupational cancers include mesothelioma caused by asbestos, and liver angiosarcoma caused by vinyl chloride monomers and arsenic.

13.6.2   Chemical carcinogens

Human cancers caused by occupational exposure to chemical carcinogens have largely been identified. The common chemical carcinogens include polycyclic aromatic hydrocarbons (PAHs), aniline and homologs, aromatic amino and nitro compounds, chromates, compounds of nickel, arsenic and inorganic arsenic compounds, beryllium and beryllium compounds, cadmium compounds, nickel compounds, crystalline forms of silica, and especially asbestosfibers. There are also substances of variable or unclear chemical makeup that are considered carcinogens, such as coal tar pitch volatiles and coke oven emissions. Chemical carcinogenesis is a prolonged process and occupational cancer has commonly taken 20 or more years from first exposure to become apparent, and this time−lag contributes to the difficulties experienced in linking cause and effect. Occupational causes of cancer have been much simpler to identify when there has been a greatly increased risk of workers developing a particular form of cancer, or when the cancer caused has been one that is very uncommon in the general population. For example, past conditions in those parts of the chemical industry using certain aromatic amines led to a 30−fold increased risk of workers developing bladder cancer. Mesothelioma of the pleura and peritoneum, and haemangiosarcoma of the liver, are normally very rare forms of cancer but have arisen in workers exposed to asbestos fibers and vinyl chloride, respectively.

13.6.3   Physical carcinogens

Physical carcinogens include ultraviolet rays from sunlight and ionizing radiation from radioactive materials in industry and in the general environment. The Main Source of UV Radiation is the sunlight, the other are UV Lamp and Welders. In human, excessive exposure to UV rays can cause various forms of skin cancer like squamous cell, carcinoma basal cell carcinoma and malignant melanoma. Ionizing Radiation includes all kinds of X−rays, alpha, beta rays and radioactive isotope problems and neutrons may also cause cancer. Most frequently, radiation induces leukemia also known as blood cancer.

13.6.4   Other carcinogens

A number of viruses are suspected of causing cancer in humans, and are frequently referred to as oncogenic viruses. Examples include human papillomaviruses, the Epstein−Barr virus, and the hepatitis B virus, all of which have genomes made up of DNA. Human T−cell leukemia virus type I (HTLV−I), which is a retrovirus (a type of RNA virus), is linked to tumor formation in humans. Although exposure to such agents is not primarily occupational, there are groups of individuals exposed to them because of their work, for example, hospital workers exposed to hepatitis B virus.

13.7   New and emerging risks

Changes in work processes and work organization have resulted in new occupational health risks and new occupational diseases. Working environments are constantly changing along side the introduction of new technologies, substances and work processes, together with changes in the labor market, and with new forms of employment and work organization. These changes bring new opportunities as well as new risks for workers and employers, which in turn demand political, organizational, technical, and regulatory initiatives to ensure high levels of safety and health at work. The new and emerging risks are generally identified as follows.

Risks previously unknown are caused by new processes, new technologies, new types of workplaces, or social or organizational change. For example, nanotechnology is a key technology of the 21st century with far-reaching implications for science, industrial development and new product design. However, despite the potential adverse effects on human health, the toxicology of these nanostructured materials (nanotoxicology) has not been investigated sufficiently. Due to the small size, engineered nanomaterials (ENMs) have unique properties that improve the performance of many products. A key issue of ENMs is the unknown human risks of the applied nanomaterials during their life cycle, especially for workers exposed to ENMs at the workplace. Workers in nanotechnology may be exposed to novel properties of materials and products causing health effects that have not yet been fully explored.

Globalization and growth of the service sector result in more competition, increase of economic pressures, more restructuring and downsizing, more precarious work, and an increase in job insecurity, as well as increased intensification and time pressures at work. The number of workers who work in temporary employment is increasing.

Important emerging physical risks are physical inactivity and the combined exposure to a mixture of environmental stressors that multiplicatively increase the risks of musculoskeletal disorders (MSDs), the leading cause of sickness absence and work disability. Important emerging psychosocial risks are job insecurity, work intensification, high demands at work, and emotional demands, including violence, harassments and bullying. Additionally, work-life balance may also be considered as risk. Emerging dangerous substances are due to technological innovation.

▶▶ *Summary*

The potential risks to life or functioning of an individual is inherently associated with his occupation or work environment. When work is associated with health hazards, it may cause occupational disease, be one of the multiple causes of other diseases or may aggravate existing ill-health of non-occupational origin. Exposures to occupational hazards, which encompass chemical, physical, biological, ergonomic and psychosocial hazards contribute to the morbidity and mortality of many diseases.

Harmful chemical compounds in the form of solids, liquids, gases, mists, dusts, fumes and vapors exert toxic effects by inhalation (breathing), absorption (through direct contact with the skin) or ingestion (eating or drinking). Airborne chemical hazards exist as concentrations of mists, vapors, gases, fumes or solids. Some of them are toxic through inhalation and others irritate the skin on contact; some can be toxic by absorption through the skin or through ingestion and some are corrosive to living tissue. The degree of worker risk from exposure to any given substance depends on the nature and potency of the toxic effects and the magnitude and duration of exposure. Physical hazards include excessive levels of noise, vibration, extremes of weather conditions, and ionizing and non-ionizing electromagnetic radiation. Biological hazards exist in exposures to bacteria, viruses, fungi and other living organisms that can cause acute and chronic infections by entering the body either directly or through breaks in the skin. Ergonomic hazards usually result from technological changes or poorly designed job tasks, such as increased assembly line speeds, added specialized tasks, increased repetition, heavy lifting problems and poorly designed tools or work areas. Psychosocial factors include boring, repetitive tasks, production pressure, stress, low pay and lack of recognition.

Practice questions:

(1) What're occupational hazards?

(2) How to classify the occupational hazards?

Yan Zhen

Chapter 14

Occupational Diseases

14.1 Introduction

14.1.1 Definition of occupational diseases

An "occupational disease" is any disease contracted primarily as a result of an exposure to risk factors arising from work activity (from World Health Organization). The definition, however, has two main mandatory elements in common: the causal relationship between exposure in a specific working environment or work activity and a specific disease; and the fact that the disease occurs among the group of exposed persons with a higher frequency rate than in the rest of the population, or in other worker populations. Many occupational diseases are unique to the hazards encountered in certain workplaces and do not, or rarely, exist apart from workers. The disease must occur as a natural incident of a particular occupation. Silicosis, for example, simply does not occur unless the patient has been exposed to silica dusts and this almost never occurs except in the workplace.

The causal relationship is established on the basis of clinical and/or pathological data, occupational background and job analysis, identification and evaluation of occupational risk factors and of the role of other risk factors. As a general rule, the symptoms are not sufficiently characteristic to allow an occupational disease to be diagnosed without the knowledge of the physical, chemical, biological and/or other risk factors encountered in the exercise of an occupation. Occupational diseases are entirely preventable if hazards in the workplace are eliminated or controlled.

The World Health Organization detailed information (including diagnostic criteria) on disease with occupational origin in the 11th revision of its International Statistical Classification of Diseases and Related Health Problems (ICD-11), which will come into effect on 1st January 2022. Reportable occupational diseases refer to the occupational diseases mentioned in national lists as part of national laws or administrative provisions liable for compensation and subject to prevention measures. Reported occupational diseases are reportable diseases already passed through legally required reporting process. However, the list of reportable occupational diseases, as well as the related compensation systems, differs from country to country, making comparisons considerably more difficult.

Under the law of workers' compensation in many jurisdictions, there is a presumption that specific disease are caused by the worker being in the work environment and the burden is on the employer or insurer to show that the disease came about from another cause. Diseases compensated by national workers compensation authorities are often termed occupational diseases. However, many countries do not offer compensations for certain diseases like musculoskeletal disorders caused by work (e. g. , in Norway). Therefore, the term of work-related diseases is utilized to describe diseases that can be caused, worsened or jointly caused by working conditions. Work-related diseases have multiple causes, where factors in the work environment may play a role, together with other risk factors, in the development of such diseases. A case of work-related illness does not necessarily refer to recognition by an authority whereas occupational diseases have a specific or a strong relation to the occupation, generally with only one causal agent while work-related diseases have a complex etiology. Among their multiple causal agents, factors arising from the work and/or working environment play a role in the development of such diseases.

An occupational disease is different from an injury caused by an accident at the workplace, although both are covered under workers' compensation. An injury happens suddenly, such as when a worker catches an arm in a machine or slips and falls at work. By contrast, occupational diseases often develop slowly and silently over a number of months or years. Because symptoms can appear gradually, you might be unaware that a disease is developing until it's too late.

14.1.2　Characteristics of occupational diseases

The cause of occupational disease is often overlooked by health care providers. This is due to several special characteristics of occupational disease that may obscure its occupational origin. The main characteristics of occupational diseases are:

(1) The clinical and pathological presentation of most occupational diseases is identical to that of non-occupational diseases; e. g. , asthma (excessive airway narrowing in the lungs) due to airborne exposure to toluene diisocyanate is clinically indistinguishable from asthma due to other causes.

(2) Occupational disease may occur after the termination of exposure. An extreme example would be asbestos-related mesothelioma (a cancer affecting the lung and abdomen) which can occur 30 or 40 years after the exposure.

(3) The clinical manifestations of occupational diseases are related to the dose and timing of exposure; e. g. , at very high airborne concentrations, elemental mercury is acutely toxic to the lungs and can cause pulmonary failure, while at lower levels of exposure, elemental mercury has no pathologic effect on the lungs but can have chronic adverse effects on the central and peripheral nervous systems.

(4) Occupational factors can act in combination with non-occupational factors to produce disease; e. g. , exposure to asbestos alone increases the risk of lung cancer five-fold; and the long-term smoking of cigarettes increases the risk of lung cancer between 50 and 70 fold.

14.1.3　Diagnostic principles of occupational disease

Occupational illnesses and injuries are conditions that are caused or exacerbated by exposures or stressors in the workplace. The key criteria for diagnosing an occupational disease in any individual are:

(1) There must be sufficient indications for occupational exposure. Evidence on exposure may be obtained through taking the occupational history, results of occupational hygiene measurements taken at the workplace, biological monitoring results, and/or records of incidents of over-exposure.

(2) The time interval between exposure and effect must be consistent with what is known about the

natural history and progress of the disease.

(3) The clinical features must fit in with what is known about the health effects following exposure to the specified agent. The symptoms and signs should fit, and this may be supported in some cases by suitable diagnostic tests.

(4) Exposure must precede health effects. However, in some conditions such as occupational asthma, a past history of childhood asthma and/or asthmatic attacks occurring before occupational exposure, does not automatically rule out the possibility of a workplace agent causing subsequent asthmatic attacks.

(5) The differential diagnosis must be considered. There are non-occupational conditions that have similar clinical features as occupational diseases, and a physician will have to take this into account before diagnosing or excluding an occupational disease.

14.1.4　Methodology for recognition of occupational diseases

The causal relationship is established on the basis of clinical and pathological data, occupational background and job analysis, identification and evaluation of occupational risk factors and of the role of other risk factors. Epidemiological and toxicological data are useful for determining the causal relationship between a specific occupational disease and its corresponding exposure in a specific working environment or work activity. In the case of frequent illnesses with a low etiological fraction (when work is only one of the many causes), epidemiological research among large groups of workers is more valuable than individual reports.

As a general rule, the symptoms are not sufficiently characteristic to enable an occupational disease to be diagnosed as such without the knowledge of the pathological changes engendered by the physical, chemical, biological or other factors encountered in the exercise of an occupation. Epidemiological studies are facilitated by the fact that links are relatively easy to establish between records of health outcomes with past occupational exposure data. It is possible in epidemiology to examine the consequences of an occupational and environmental exposure in the manner in which it actually occurs in humans, not the artificial manner in which laboratory studies of animals are done. The issue of dose, route of exposure, concomitant exposures and host factors are also directly assessed.

The recognition of a disease as being occupational is a specific example of clinical decision-making or applied clinical epidemiology. Deciding on the cause of a disease is not an "exact science" but rather a question of judgment based on a critical review of all the available evidence, which should include a consideration of the following.

(1) Strength of association. The greater the impact of an exposure on the occurrence or development of a disease, the stronger the likelihood of a causal relationship.

(2) Consistency. Different research reports have generally similar results and conclusions.

(3) Specificity. Exposure to a specific risk factor results in a clearly defined pattern of disease or diseases.

(4) Temporality or time sequence. The exposure of interest preceded the disease by a period of time consistent with any proposed biological mechanism.

(5) Biological gradient. The greater the level and duration of exposure, the greater the severity of diseases or their incidence.

(6) Biological plausibility. From what is known of toxicology, chemistry, physical properties or other attributes of the studied risk or hazard, it makes biological sense to suggest that exposure leads to the disease.

(7) Coherence. A general synthesis of all the evidence (e. g. , human epidemiology and animal stud-

ies) leads to the conclusion that there is a cause−effect relationship in a broad sense and in terms of general common sense.

(8) Interventional studies. Sometimes, a primary preventative trial may verify whether removing a specific hazard or reducing a specific risk from the working environment or work activity eliminates the development of a specific disease or reduces its incidence.

▶▶ *Summary*

Occupational disease is defined as any disease contracted as a result of an exposure to risk factors arising from work activity. Reportable occupational diseases refer to the occupational diseases mentioned in national lists as part of national laws or administrative provisions. The diagnosis of occupational disease will need to entail the detailed occupational and medical history, clinical examination for specific symptoms and signs, and workplace evaluation to exposure and exclude other non−occupational causes.

Practice questions:

(1) What is 'Occupational Disease'?

(2) What are diagnostic principles of occupational disease?

Yan Zhen

14.2　Occupational poisoning

14.2.1　Metal and metalloid poisoning

14.2.1.1　Lead Poisoning

Lead poisoning is a syndrome of intoxication caused by increased levels of the heavy metal lead in the body. Lead has no known physiologically relevant role in the body. However, once it is deposited in the body, it would have severe effects on human body.

(1) Characteristics

Lead (Pb) is a heavy, soft, blue−gray metal characterized by high density and corrosion resistance. Its melting point and boiling point are 327.5 ℃ and 1,740 ℃, respectively. The color of the lead compounds-presents diversity. For example: lead tetra oxide, Pb_3O_4, is brown. Lead's characteristic properties include high density, softness, ductility and malleability. Lead is widely used in building construction, lead−acid batteries, bullets and shot, weights, as part of solders, fusible alloys, and as a radiation shield.

(2) Exposure

1) Occupational exposure: In adults, occupational exposure is the main cause of lead poisoning. People can be exposed to lead compounds when they work in facilities that produce a variety of lead−containing products; these include radiation shields, ammunition, and ceramic glazes. In addition, lead miners and smelters, glass manufacturers, battery manufacturers and recyclers, and plastic manufacturers are at risk for lead exposure.

2) Environmental exposure: Residual lead in soil contributes to lead exposure in urban areas. Plant can accumulate lead in the body and its fruit. Eating foods grown in contaminated soil can give a lead hazard. Lead from the atmosphere or soil can end up in groundwater and surface water. It is also potentially in drinking water, e. g. , from plumbing and fixtures that are either made of lead or have lead solder.

3) Pharmacogenic exposure: Lead is commonly incorporated into herbal remedies such as China Zhang-dan, and so on. These are the risks of blood lead and health, because they contain lead.

(3) Pathomechanism

1) Absorption: In the occupational environment, lead and its compounds are mainly in the form of powder (smoke) dust and enter into the human body through the respiratory tract, and only a small amount of lead compounds are taken in by the digestive tract.

2) Distribution: After absorption, lead mainly distributes in bones, blood, brain, liver, kidney, and can cross placenta. Because fetal blood brain barrier is open, fetal brain is easy to be damaged by lead. After lead is absorbed from the lungs or the gastrointestinal tract, it enters the blood stream. At first, lead attaches to proteins in the blood that carry it to different tissues or organ systems in the body, such as liver and kidney. Most of the lead present in the blood is bound to the red blood cell. Doctors can tell how much lead a person has been exposed to by measuring the levels of lead in the blood. It's very important to remember that lead cannot be destroyed or changed to something else in vivo. The amount of lead stored in the body has been described as the "body burden" of lead. Among adults, over 95% of the total body stores of lead are found in bone. For children, about 70% of lead is stored in bone.

3) Excretion: The body gets rid of lead in the urine and through the gastrointestinal tract. However, many people (and most occupationally exposed workers) are unable to get rid of as much lead as they take in. That is why the "body burden" of lead increases over the decades. Until late in life, most persons are steadily getting more and more lead in their tissues. Only among the elderly, for example those 70 or 80 years old, the body lead burden begin to get less. Lead can be released from the bone when the person has a disease and take in some acidic medicine, for example osteoporosis, or sometimes during pregnancy and lactation (breast feeding).

4) Inhibition of the heme synthesis: The primary cause of lead's toxicity is its interference with a lot of enzymes because it binds to sulfhydryl groups found on many enzymes.

One of the main causes for the pathology of lead is that it interferes with the activity of an essential enzyme called delta-aminolevulinic acid dehydratase, or ALAD, which is important in the biosynthesis of heme. Lead's interference with heme synthesis results in anemia.

5) Inhibition of the release of neurotransmitters: It interferes with the release of glutamate, an important neurotransmitter in many functions including learning. It is reported that lead exposure decreased the amount of NMDA receptors in part of the brain. In addition, lead has been found in animal studies to cause cell death in brain.

(4) Signs and symptoms

Lead poisoning can cause a variety of symptoms and signs which vary depending on the individuals and the duration of lead exposure.

1) Acute poisoning: Absorption of large amounts of lead in a short time can cause acute poisoning. In acute poisoning, typical neurological signs are pain, muscle weakness, paraesthesia, and symptoms associated with encephalitis. Gastrointestinal symptoms are abdominal pain, nausea, vomiting, diarrhea and constipation.

2) Chronic poisoning: Chronic poisoning usually presents with symptoms affecting multiple systems, but is associated with three main types of symptoms: gastrointestinal, hematological, and neurological. Signs of chronic exposure include loss of short-term memory or concentration, depression, nausea, wrist drop, abdominal pain, loss of coordination and numbness and tingling in the extremities. Fatigue, problems with sleep, headaches, and anemia are also found in chronic lead poisoning. A blue line along the gum, with bluish

black edging to the teeth, known as Burton line is another indication of chronic lead poisoning.

(5) Diagnosis

Diagnosis of lead poisoning is based on the clinical signs, and detailed and reliable occupational exposure of lead compounds.

1) The main clinical signs: Constitutional findings may include headaches, irritability, fatigue, difficulty sleeping, difficulty learning or concentrating, aggressive behavior, stomachache, constipation, vomiting, nausea, weight loss, anemia, unusual paleness.

2) The blood lead levels: The main tool in diagnosing and assessing the severity of lead poisoning is laboratory analysis of the blood lead levels (BLL). Blood lead levels are an indicator mainly of recent or current lead exposure, not of total body burden. The National Institute for Occupational Safety and Health (CDC/NIOSH) reference blood lead level in adults is 10 μg/dL.

(6) Treatment

The main therapy for lead poisoning is to remove lead from the body by chelation therapy. The chelating agents used for treatment of lead poisoning are edetate disodium calcium ($CaNa_2EDTA$) and dimercaprol (BAL) which are given by injection. All of $CaNa_2EDTA$ and dimercaprol can form complexes with lead ions and be excreted in the urine.

(7) Prevention

In most cases, lead poisoning is preventable by avoiding exposure to lead. Prevention strategies can be divided into: individual (measures taken by a family); preventive medicine (identifying and intervening with high-risk individuals) and public health (reducing risk on a population level).

14.2.1.2　Mercury Poisoning

(1) Characteristics

Mercury is a silver and white liquid metal. The gravity of mercury is 13.59 grams per cubic centimetre. Its melting point and boiling point are −38.9 ℃ and 356.6 ℃, respectively. At room temperature, it can evaporate to become steam. Metal mercury surface tension is large. After spills on the ground, mercury can form a lot of small bead and increase the evaporation surface area. The mercury vapor can be adsorbed on the wall, ceiling, etc.

(2) Exposure

Those workers who are involved in mercury mining and smelting, the manufacture and maintenance of electrical equipment factory can be exposed to mercury steam or mercury compounds.

(3) Pathomechanism

The metallic mercury vapor enters the body through the respiratory tract, and the absorption rate of mercury vapor can reach more than 70% in lung tissue. It is difficult for metallic mercury to enter the body through digestive tract and the skin, but mercury salt and organic mercury are easily absorbed by the digestive tract.

1) Distribution: Mercury in the blood can be transformed to mercury ions by oxidation, and then distributed in the body's tissues and organs with the blood circulation and accumulated in the kidney, mainly in renal cortex. Mercury is fat-soluble, so it is easy to pass through the blood-brain barrier into the brain. Once mercury is ionized by oxidation in the brain and it loses fat-solublility, hard to be cleared from brain tissue.

2) Excretion: Mercury is excreted mainly through the kidney, and a small amount of mercury compounds discharged with saliva, sweat or milk.

3) Intoxication mechanism: The intoxication mechanism of mercury remains unclear. It is thought that mercury ions have strong affinity with thiol (—SH). Due to the important role of —SH in diverse proteins,

the binding of Hg with —SH can change the structure and function of proteins, leading to loss of protein function. However, this notion does not fully explain the characteristics of mercury toxicity.

(4) Signs and symptoms

Acute poisoning: Clinical symptoms of acute mercury poisoning are generally acute, including fever, dizziness, headache and other symptoms of tremor, which are mainly caused by pneumonia, renal injury and mild gingivitis. Symptoms of mild poisoning present as oral-gingivitis or acute bronchitis; moderate poisoning can be manifested as interstitial pneumonia or significant proteinuria; severe poisoning can cause renal failure or severe poisoning encephalopathy.

Chronic poisoning: Chronic mercury poisoning results in neural syndrome in the early phase. With the development of the disease, irritability syndrome, oral gingivitis and oral-tremor occur. Mild poisoning presents nerve syndrome, oral gingivitis, fingers, tongue and eyelid tremor or proximal renal tubular dysfunction; moderate poisoning can show character, mood changes or upper limb coarse tremor and obvious renal damage. The patients with severe poisoning show toxic encephalopathy.

(5) Diagnosis

Diagnosis of elemental or inorganic mercury poisoning is based on the history of exposure, clinical findings, and elevated concentrations of mercury in the body, especially whole-blood and urine.

(6) Treatment

It is crucial to identify and remove the source of mercury. Removal of clothes, washing skin with soap and water, and moving the patient to a clean area are needed. In addition, chelation therapy for inorganic mercury poisoning can be done with dimercaptosuccinic acid (DMSA), 2,3-dimercapto-1-propanesulfonic acid (DMPS), or dimercaprol (BAL), respectively.

(7) Prevention

Mercury poisoning can be prevented (or minimized) by eliminating or reducing exposure to mercury and mercury compounds. Use of proper ventilation and personal gas mask is needed in mercury contamination atmosphere. Special medical surveillance of mercury exposure workers should include a neurologic and physical examination and mercury detection in urine.

14.2.2　Irritant and asphyxiating gas poisoning

Irritant gas is a set of harmful gases which induce irritant effect on the eyes, the respiratory tract mucosa and skin. Asphyxiating gas is a set of harmful gas which mainly causes the asphyxia of cells after being inhaled with gaseous form. For example, CO, HCN, CH_4.

14.2.2.1　Irritant gas poisoning

(1) Definition and Characteristics

Most of the irritant gases are corrosive. This kind of gases can leak from the corrosive pipeline and containers, and result in pollution of the environment and acute poisoning. It is needed to obey the operating rules in order to avoid acute poisoning.

In addition to ammonia (alkali forming compounds), ozone (strong oxidant) and cadmium oxide (metal oxide), most of the stimulant gases are acid forming gases. Although there are many kinds of them, chlorine, ammonia, phosgene, nitrogen oxides, hydrogen fluoride, sulfur dioxide and sulfur dioxide are common ones.

(2) Pathomechanism

Common toxic effect of irritant gases on human body is characterized on the eyes, respiratory mucosa and skin irritation, and result in local damage. The extent of damage and the site of action is closely related to, and mainly depends on the concentration of irritant gases, exposure time and water solubility. The gas with high solubility mainly damage the eyes and upper respiratory tract mucosa; the gas with low solubility easily reaches and damages the deep respiratory tract. For the gases with moderate solubility, they damage the eyes and upper respiratory tract in low concentrations, and may invade the respiratory tract deep at high concentrations. Pulmonary edema is the most serious damage caused by the irritant gas poisoning.

(3) Signs and symptoms

1) Acute poisoning

● Irritation: Photophobia, tears, runny nose, sore throat, cough, chest tightness and conjunctival and pharyngeal hyperemia. Inhalation of high concentrations of irritant gases can cause laryngeal spasm or edema, even die of asphyxia.

● Poisoning bronchitis and pneumonia: Patients appear paroxysmal cough, chest tightness, chest pain and shortness of breath, a little dry rales and moist rales in the lung. X−ray detection shows increased lung texture, unclear edge of lung texture and the focal large high density shadow in the lungs.

● Toxic pulmonary edema: The clinical process can be divided into four phases. The stimulation period: after inhalation of high concentrations of irritant gas, irritation symptoms occur in the eyes and upper respiratory tract mucosa; the latent period: the symptoms disappear or relieve, but the disease is still in progress. Close attention should be paid to the occurrence of lung edema. The incubation period generally lasts 2−12 hours, a few up to 24−72 hours. Pulmonary edema period: sudden coughing, chest tightness, breath with difficulty, coughing with large pink frothy sputum will take palce. There are a lot of moist rales in the lung. Chest X−ray shows lung markings, thickening and different sizes of shadows, such as butterfly shape. The recovery period: the symptoms and signs gradually diminish or disappear. If the treatment is received in time, the symptoms generally disappear in 3−4 days.

● The occurrence of toxic pulmonary edema depends on the toxicity, water solubility, concentrations of irritant gases, contact time and the body's stress ability.

● Acute respiratory distress syndrome (ARDS): ARDS is an acute respiratory failure characterized by progressive respiratory distress and hypoxemia. Severe pulmonary edema is one of the important causes of ARDS. The mortality of this disease can reach as high as 50%.

2) Chronic poisoning: Chronic conjunctivitis, rhinitis, pharyngitis, bronchitis and dental acid erosion can be caused by chronic exposure to low concentrations of irritant gases.

(4) Diagnosis

The diagnosis is based on the acute contact history of the irritant gases and the clinical manifestations of the respiratory system damage.

(5) Treatment

Active prevention and treatment of pulmonary edema is the key to the rescue of irritant gas poisoning.

1) On−site treatment: The patient should be quickly removed from the poisoning site and the contaminated skin cleaned with a large amount of clean water. Those who show symptoms of irritation should undergo symptomatic treatment, rest in bed, avoid physical activity, and be observed for at least 12 hours. Those exposed to nitrogen oxides should be observed 24−72 hours.

2) Rational oxygen therapy: The concentration of oxygen should not exceed 60%. If severe pulmonary edema or ARDS occurr, positive pressure ventilation should be continuously given.

3) Hormone therapy: Short course usage of glucocorticoid at adequate dosage should be administrated to reduce pulmonary capillary permeability in the early period. 200−600 mg of hydrocortisone can be injected intravenously daily or alternatively 20 − 40 mg dexamethasone intravenously or intramuscularly. The latent

period should be 20 mg of dexamethasone.

4) Maintaining airway patency: Aerosol inhalation of broncho spasmodic agents and antifoaming agents should be performed, such as dimethyl−silicon oil (defoaming). If necessary, tracheotomy should be carried out. The patients should be prescribed to inhale weak base (4% sodium bicarbonate) or weak acid (2% boric acid or 5% acetic acid) to neutralize acid or alkaline irritant gases.

5) Maintaining the balance of water, electrolytes and acid−base: The volume of fluid replacement is based on the principle of no aggravation of pulmonary edema. Proper use of diuretics or dehydrating agents can be recommended. Meanwhile, control of infection, prevention and treatment of complications are also critical.

14.2.2.2   Carbon monoxide poisoning

(1) Characteristics

Carbon monoxide (CO) is colorless, tasteless, odorless, non−irritating gas, with a specific gravity of 0.967, slightly soluble in water and easy to dissolve in ammonia water.

(2) Exposure

In industrial production, the incomplete combustion of carbon containing substances can produce CO. Such as coke, steel and iron making in metallurgical industry, and various kinds of boilers.

(3) Pathomechanism

CO mainly enters the body through the respiratory tract and combines with hemoglobin (Hb) to form carboxyhemoglobin (HbCO) in the blood, which leads Hb lose capacity for carrying oxygen. The affinity of CO combined with Hb is 240 times stronger than oxygen combined with Hb. The dissociation rate of HbCO is 3,600 times slower than that of oxygenated hemoglobin (HbO_2). In addition, HbCO also affects the dissociation of HbO_2, resulting in hypoxemia and hypoxia.

(4) Signs and symptoms

1) Acute poisoning: Patients with mild poisoning can appear severe headache, dizziness, weakness, nausea, vomiting or mild, moderate disturbance of consciousness, but no coma, HbCO concentration is higher than 10%. The patients with moderate poisoning may have disturbance of consciousness, and mild to moderate coma, and HbCO concentration is above 30%. Patients with severe poisoning can appear serious disorder of consciousness, cerebral edema, shock or severe myocardial damage, pulmonary edema, respiratory failure and so on. HbCO concentration is higher than 50%. CO poisoning patients' skin and mucosa shows cherry −red disco loration.

2) Delayed encephalopathy: After recovery from acute CO poisoning some patients show sudden spirit, consciousness disorder or extrapyramidal dysfunction (Parkinson disease), pyramidal nerve damage (such as hemiplegia, positive pathologic reflex or urinary incontinence), focal cerebral cortex dysfunction (such as aphasia, blindness) in about 2−60 days of "latent period".

(5) Diagnosis

The diagnosis is based on the acute exposure history of CO, the clinical manifestations and HbCO concentrations in the blood.

(6) Treatment

The poisoning patients should be quickly moved to fresh air, loosened the collar, kept warm and the state of consciousness paid closely attention. According to the degree of poisoning, oxygen is given with the appropriate approach. Mild poisoning patients can undergo atmospheric oxygen inhalation and symptomatic treatment. Moderate and severe poisoning patients should actively receive hyperbaric oxygen. It is very important to prevent cerebral edema and delayed encephalopathy for severe poisoning.

In patients with delayed encephalopathy, hyperbaric oxygen, glucocorticoids, vasodilators, or anti-Parkinson drugs, and other symptomatic measures should be used with supportive treatments available.

14.2.2.3 HCN poisoning

(1) Characteristics

Hydrogen cyanide is a colorless gas with bitter almond flavor, easily soluble in water and ethanol, diethyl ether and other organic solvents. The aqueous solution is hydrocyanic acid.

(2) Exposure

It is widely used in electroplating industry, such as copper plating, chromium plating, nickel plating. In metallurgical industry, gold and silver are extracted from ore by cyanidation process. It is used as raw material for synthesis of acetonitrile, acrylonitrile and butyronitrile in chemical industry.

(3) Pathomechanism

HCN mainly enters the body through the respiratory tract, and high concentrations of liquid hydrocyanic acid can be absorbed through the skin. HCN rapidly dissociates into cyanide ion (CN—), which combines with a variety of intracellular enzymes containing iron, copper, zinc and other metal ion and inhibits enzyme activity. CN— has the highest affinity with ferric ion (Fe^{3+}), can quickly combine with mitochondrial oxidation of cytochrome oxidase Fe^{3+}. Therefore, the enzyme loses electron-transfer ability, resulting in mitochondrial respiratory chain interruption. The cells cannot use oxygen, causing intracellular suffocation. Under this situation, blood oxygen saturation is high, but can't be used by cells, causing HCN poisoning, the patients' skin and mucous membrane appear bright red.

CN— can combine with sulfur under the action of thiocyanate synthetase in the body to form a low toxicity and stable thiocyanate which is discharged from urine.

(4) Signs and symptoms

Acute poisoning: Inhalation of high concentrations of HCN could result in no sign sudden collapse and "shock-like" death due to breath stopping. The clinical course of HCN inhalation poisoning with low concentrations could be divided into four stages. ①Prodromal stage: There is a smell of bitter almonds in exhaled breath. The the patients' main symptoms include irritation of the eyes, the throat and the upper respiratory tract, and then nausea, vomiting and tremor, and a bright red color with skin and mucosa. ②Dyspnea stage: Difficulty in breathing, rapid pulse, becoming smaller and then expansion with both sides of the pupils, a bright red color gradually becoming purple with skin and mucosa. ③Spasm stage: Tonic and clonic convulsions, and even opisthotonos, incontinence, loss of consciousness. ④Paralytic period: The whole body muscle paralysis, the reflex disappears, the breath becomes shallow and slow, and finally the death happens due to the breath and the heartbeat stopping.

Chronic effects: Chronic exposure to low concentrations of HCN can cause chronic inflammation of the eye and upper respiratory tract, such as chronic conjunctivitis, rhinitis and pharyngitis, and neurologic syndrome.

(5) Diagnosis

The diagnosis is based on the acute exposure of HCN gas and the clinical manifestations.

(6) Treatment

HCN poisoning is developing very rapidly, so the rescue should quickly use the antidote.

On-site treatment: Quickly move the patients from the poisoning site to the fresh air, clean the contaminated skin thoroughly, replace the contaminated clothes, and give the antidote as soon as possible.

Detoxification treatment: Sodium nitrite-sodium thiosulfate therapy: ①The patient should immediately receive 3% sodium nitrite through slow intravenous injection, followed with 25%-50% sodium thiosulfate using the same needle. Blood pressure should be closely monitored during treatment period. ②Application of N, N–Dimethyl–4–aminophenol, 4–DMAP) : 4–DMAP is a new type of methemoglobin formation agent for sodium nitrate substitution since 4–DMAP generates methemoglobin more quickly than sodium nitrite, which has no effect on smooth muscle expansion, does not cause a drop of blood pressure.

14.2.3   Organic solvent poisoning–Benzene poisoning

14.2.3.1   Characteristics

Benzene (C_6H_6) is a colorless oily liquid at room temperature. It has a characteristic "aromatic" sweet odor. It is highly volatile with a boiling point at 80.1 ℃. Benzene is slightly soluble in water and is easy to dissolve in organic solvents, such as ethanol, chloroform and ethyl ether.

14.2.3.2   Exposure

In industrial production, benzene is widely used in a common raw material in organic chemical synthesis, solvent, extractant and diluent, etc.

14.2.3.3   Pathomechanism

Benzene enters the body in the form of benzene vapor mainly through the respiratory tract, only a little benzene is absorbed through the skin. About 50% of benzene is discharged by respiratory tract in the original form, 10% of benzene stored in lipid rich tissues in the original form. 40% of benzene shows ring oxidation in liver microsomal cytochrome P450 metabolism, resulting in the formation of hydroxylation of hydroquinone or catechol. The phenolic metabolites of benzene can be excreted with urine sulfate or glucuronic acid. Therefore, the content of phenol in the urine and the benzene content in breath can be used as a biomarker for recent benzene contact. The acute toxic effect of benzene presents as the anesthetic effect of the central nervous system, while the chronic toxic effect is mainly on the hematopoietic system, but its pathogenesis is not clear.

14.2.3.4   Signs and symptoms

(1) Acute benzene poisoning

The acute manifestation of benzene poisoning is mainly the symptoms of central nervous system. Mild poisoning can cause dizziness, headache, nausea, vomiting and gait stagnation, sometimes accompanied by mucosal irritation and mild disturbance of consciousness. Severe benzene poisoning can occur as morderate, severe unconsciousness and even failure of respiratory and circulatory function. The levels of blood benzene and urine phenol are increased.

(2) Chronic benzene poisoning

Chronic benzene poisoning mainly damages the hematopoietic system. The earliest and most common abnormal manifestation is the continuous decrease in white blood cell counts in peripheral blood, mainly neutrophilia, but lymphocytes are relatively increased, followed by thrombocytopenia. Mild benzene poisoning shows neuroid syndrome and easy infection and/or bleeding tendency. White blood cell count is generally less than 4×10^9/L or neutrophil below 2×10^9/L, and platelet count below 60×10^9/L. In moderate benzene poisoning, the white blood cell count is lower than 3×10^9/L or neutrophil is lower than 1.5 $\times10^9$/L, and the platelet count lower than 40×10^9/L. Severe benzene poisoning can appear whole blood cell decrease or aplastic anemia, myelodysplastic syndrome or leukemia. There are many kinds of leukemia caused by benzene, and they are more common in acute myelogenous leukemia.

14.2.3.5   Diagnosis

The diagnosis of benzene is based on the exposure of benzene and the clinical manifestations.

14.2.3.6 Treatment

In the case of acute benzene poisoning, the patient should be quickly moved to the fresh air place, immediately replace the contaminated clothes, clean the contaminated skin with soapy water, and keep warm. The patients with acute benzene poisoning can be intravenously injected with glucuronic acid and vitamin C, but adrenaline is prohibited. The patients with chronic benzene poisoning have no special detoxification drugs. The focus of treatment is to restore the damaged hematopoietic function and give symptomatic treatment.

14.2.4 Aromatic amino-compounds and nitro-compound poisoning

14.2.4.1 Aniline poisoning

(1) Characteristics

Aniline ($C_6H_5NH_2$) is a colorless oily liquid. It has a special odor. It can be browned after a long-term placement. Its melting point is -6.2 ℃, the boiling point is 184.3 ℃, and the steam density is 3.22 g/L. It is slightly soluble in water and soluble in benzene, ethanol and ethyl ether.

(2) Exposure

Exposure to aniline may occur in aniline synthesis, printing and dyeing, dyestuff manufacturing, rubber, plastic, spice and pharmaceutical industries.

(3) Pathomechanism

Aniline can enter human body through the respiratory tract and the skin, with the latter as the main cause of occupational poisoning. The liquid and vapor of aniline can be absorbed through skin, and the absorption rate increases with the rising concentrations of gas and its humidity. Inhalation of aniline through the respiratory tract can also cause occupational poisoning.

The intermediate products of aniline metabolites have greater toxicity in vivo, such as phenyl hydroxylamine. N-hydroxybenzenamineis oxidized to p-aminophenol, which can combine with sulfate or glucuronic acid and be discharged from urine. Therefore, urine amino phenol is related to blood methemoglobin. A small amount of original aniline is excreted from the respiratory tract. N-hydroxybenzenamine has a strong oxidizing ability and can make the hemoglobin to methemoglobin, causing tissue hypoxia. It can also cause inner integument protein denaturation of red blood cells and Heinz body formation, and cause hemolytic anemia.

(4) Signs and symptoms

1) Acute poisoning: The patients with mild aniline poisoning appear cyanosis on lips, tongue, ear, finger (toe) and nail, and accompanied by dizziness, headache, chest tightness, fatigue and other symptoms. Blood methemoglobin concentration is 10% -30%. The patients with moderate aniline poisoning show obvious skin and mucosa cyanosis, which is accompanied by mild hemolytic anemia or chemical cystitis, mild liver and kidney damage, with mildly elevated Heinz bodies and blood methemoglobin concentration in 30% -50%. The patients severe aniline poisoning may present severe cyanosis of skin and mucosa, obvious disorder of consciousness or hemolytic anemia, severe liver and kidney damage and significant increasement of Heinz body. The concentration of methemoglobin in blood reaches 50% and urine colour becomes dark brown.

2) Chronic poisoning: The patients with chronic aniline poisoning have neural syndrome, accompanied by hepatomegaly, abnormal liver function, anemia and contact dermatitis.

(5) Treatment

The patients with acute benzene poisoning should be quickly removed from the exposure site the contaminated cloth should be replaced and the skin should be washed with soapywater (not hot) or 75% alcohol. Those patients whose blood methemoglobin concentration is in 30% –40% should be given special anti-dote of methylene blue.

14. 2. 4. 2   Trinitrotoluene poisoning

(1) Characteristics

Trinitrotoluene(TNT) has six isomers. It is a colorless or yellowish crystal. Its melting point is 82 ℃ and boiling point 240 ℃. It is extremely hard to dissolve in water and easily dissolved in organic solvents such as acetone,benzene and toluene.

(2) Exposure

Trinitrotoluene is widely used as an explosive in the construction of national defense,mining and tunneling.

(3) Pathomechanism

TNT enters human body through skin and respiratory tract. Under the production conditions,TNT dusts are easily absorbed through the skin. The higher the temperature,the greater the skin absorption rate. Therefore,the absorption of skin is the main cause of occupational TNT chronic poisoning.

TNT is mainly metabolized in liver microsomes and mitochondria,and its original form and metabolites are excreted from urine. The content of 4−amino−2,6−two nitro toluene and TNT in urine can be used as a contact biomarker.

The toxic mechanisms of TNT have not been fully elucidated. It is believed that TNT can be reduced to nitro anion radicals in the body and produce a lot of ROS by free radical chain reaction,which causes peroxidation reaction of lipid,DNA,protein and other biological macromolecules and damages the cell structure and protein function.

(4) Signs and symptoms

1) Acute poisoning: Occupational acute TNT poisoning is rare.

2) Chronic poisoning: Chronic exposure to TNT mainly damages the liver and eye lens. Toxic cataract is an early and typical sign of TNT poisoning. The patients with mild TNT poisoning show hepatomegaly and abnormal liver function. The patients with moderate TNT poisoning present large liver,toughening and abnormal liver function or splenomegaly. The patients with severe TNT poisoning may have cirrhosis or aplastic anemia.

(5) Treatment

There is no special detoxifying medications for the damage to the liver and eye lens. Generally,the corresponding treatment programme is made according to the condition of the disease,and the drugs that are harmful to the liver are forbidden or used carefully.

14.2.5   Polymer poisoning–vinyl chloride poisoning

14. 2. 5. 1   Characteristics

Under normal pressure vinyl chloride is a colorless gas and slightly aromatic. The vapor density is 2. 15 g/L. It is slightly soluble in water and easily soluble in ethanol and ether,and carbon tetrachloride.

14. 2. 5. 2   Exposure

Vinyl chloride is mainly used as monomer for the production of poly vinyl chloride (PVC). People expose to vinyl chloride during synthesis process,including converter,fractionating tower,storage tank,compressor and polymerizer,especially in polymerization kettle cleaning,repair and accident.

14. 2. 5. 3   Pathomechanism

Chloroethylene mainly enters the body by inhalation through the respiratory tract. Liquid chloroethylene can be partially absorbed by the skin when the skin is contaminated.

The chloroethylene inhaled through the respiratory tract is mostyly distributed in the liver and kidney, followed by skin and plasma. Most of its metabolites are discharged from urine.

Vinyl chloride metabolism pathway is related to its concentrations. Inhaled vinyl chloride at low concentrations, is mainly metabolized by alcohol dehydrogenase pathway in the liver and hydrolysed to 2-chloride ethanol, and ultimately forms chloroacetaldehyde and chloroacetic acid. Inhaled vinyl chloride at high concentrations, when the metabolic pathway of alcohol dehydrogenase reaches saturation, it is mainly metabolized by Hepatic Microsome Cytochrome P450, and produce high activity intermediate oxide metabolites of vinyl chloride, spontaneous rearrangement of oxidized vinyl chloride results in the formation of chloroacetaldehyde.

14.2.5.4　Signs and symptoms

(1)Acute poisoning

Acute vinyl chloride poisoning presents the anesthetic effect on the central nervous system. Mild poisoning is associated with headache, dizziness, fatigue, chest tightness, malignant, lethargy, instability of gait and so on. The patients should be moved to fresh air space. Symptoms can disappear. Severe poisoning can lead to disturbance of consciousness, acute lung injury and even brain edema, which can cause persistent coma or even death.

(2)Chronic poisoning

Long term exposure to vinyl chloride has many adverse effects, such as neurasthenia syndrome, peripheral neuropathy, acral osteolysis, liver enlargement, liver dysfunction, and thrombocytopenia.

14.2.5.5　Treatment

(1)Acute poisoning

The poisoning patients should be quickly moved to the fresh air place immediately, take off the contaminated clothes, clean the contaminated skin with clean water, be kept warm and rest in bed.

(2)Chronic poisoning

It is beneficial to give the patients liver protection and symptomatic treatment. The splenectomy is feasible the surgical indication. Once acromegaly osteolytic disease is diagnosed, the patients should stop exposing vinyl chloride as soon as possible.

14.2.6　Pesticide poisoning

14.2.6.1　Definition and classification

Pesticides are any substances used to prevent, destroy, repel, or mitigate insects, rodents, nematodes, fungi, or other organisms considered pests.

Classification by target organism: Herbicides, algicides, avicides, bactericides, fungicides, insecticides, miticides, molluscicides, nematicides, rodenticides and virucides.

Classification by chemical structure: Many pesticides can be grouped into chemical families. Prominent insecticide families include organochlorines, organophosphates, and carbamates. Organochlorine pesticides are a kind of synthetic chemical pesticides. Their physical and chemical properties are stable, both the persistence and bioaccumulation are strong, and they are also difficult to degrade naturally in environment, so they can be threats to ecosystems and human health through evaporation, migration, food chain transfer, biomagnification and other paths. For example, DDT (dichlorodiphenyltrichloroethane) is the first synthetic organochlorine pesticide. It was banned in China in 1989 due to its persistence in the environment.

Organophosphate pesticides degrade rapidly by hydrolysis upon exposure to sunlight, air, and soil, although small amounts can be detected in food and drinking water. Their ability to degrade makes them an attractive alternative to the persistent organochloride pesticides. Although organophosphates degrade faster than the organochlorides, they have greater acute toxicity, posing risks to people who may be exposed to large amounts.

14.2.6.2　Exposure

People can expose to pesticides through a large number of different routes at work place, at home, at school and eating food.

(1) Occupational exposure

Pesticide poisoning is an important occupational health issue because pesticides are used in a large number of industries, which puts many different types of workers at risk. Extensive use of pesticides puts agricultural workers in particular at increased risk for pesticide poisoning. Different job functions contribute different levels of exposure. Most occupational exposures are caused by absorption through skin such as the face, hands, forearms, neck, and chest. This kind of exposure is sometimes enhanced by inhalation in settings including spraying operations in greenhouses and other closed environments.

(2) Accidental and suicidal exposure

Suicides with agricultural pesticides represent a major hidden public health problem accounting for approximately one-third of all suicides worldwide. It is one of the most common forms of self-injury in the Global South. The World Health Organization estimates that 300,000 people die from self-harm each year in the Asia-Pacific region alone. Most cases of intentional pesticide poisoning appear to be impulsive acts undertaken during stressful events, and the availability of pesticides strongly influences the incidence of self-poisoning.

(3) Residential exposure

When thinking of pesticide poisoning, one usually does not take into consideration the contribution by household. This form of pesticide use would contribute to the third type of poisoning, which is caused by long-term low-level exposure. As mentioned before, long-term low-level exposure affects individuals from sources such as pesticide residues in food as well as contact with pesticide residues in the air, water, soil, sediment, food materials, plants and animals.

14.2.6.3　Pathomechanism

(1) Organophosphate pesticides

Organophosphates affect the nervous system by disrupting the enzyme acetylcholinesterase that degrades acetylcholine, a neurotransmitter. In detail, cation sites of organophosphates combine with the anionic sites of acetylcholinesterase, and form complex. Then, the complex degrades into choline and acetyl-acetylcholinesterase. Acetyl-acetylcholinesterase dehydrates into acetylcholinesterase and acetic acid. Organophosphates combine with the hydroxy site of acetylcholinesterase, and form phosphorus acylation cholinesterase, leading to the inhibition of the activity of acetylcholinesterase.

(2) Carbamate pesticides

Carbamate pesticides affect the nervous system by disrupting the acetyl-acetylcholinesterase that regulates acetylcholine, a neurotransmitter. The enzyme effects are usually reversible.

(3) Organochlorine insecticides

They were commonly used in the past, but many have been removed from the market due to their toxic health and environmental effects and persistence in the environment (e.g., DDT and chlordane).

(4) Pyrethroid pesticides

These pesticides were developed as a synthetic version of the naturally occurring pesticide pyrethrin, which was found in chrysanthemums. They have been modified to increase their stability in the environment. Some synthetic pyrethroids are toxic to the nervous system. Pyrethroid is a kind of synthetic pesticides, which molecular structure consists of two parts, chrysanthemum acid and alcohol.

14.2.6.4　Signs and symptoms

The signs and symptoms of acute intoxication with organophosphates and carbamatea are best characterized on the neurophysiologic basis by grouping them according to the affected class of cholinergic receptor.

Muscarinic symptoms: this kind of symptoms can appear at the early stage and mainly present as nausea, vomiting, abdominal pain, diarrhea, drooling, sweating, blurred vision, small pupil, increased respiratory secretions, bronchospasm, etc. In severe cases, pulmonary edema and urinary incontinence can occur. The above symptoms are usually the first symptoms.

Nicotine like symptom: whole body tight feeling, poor flexibilit, chest pressure feeling, muscle bundle trembles, heartbeat and blood pressure rising, breathing muscle paralysis.

There are some variabilities in parasymathetic nervous system manifestations because they are opposed by the sympathetic nervous system that has preganglionic cholinergic innervation. Thus the heart rate may be slow, normal, or fast and the pupils may be small, normal, or large depending on which system predominates. In most organophosphate−poisoned patients, 90% of them have at least muscarinic manifestations, 40% of them have both muscarinic and nicotinic manifestations, and 30% of them have muscarinic and CNS manifestations. The number of systems involved increases with the severity of intoxication. Mild poisoning is usually manifested as mild muscarinic signs and symptoms only. The death of acute organophosphate poisoning is usually due to respiratory failure. Bronchorrhea or pulmonary edema, bronchoconstriction, and respiratory muscular paralysis all contribute to respiratory failure. Seizures are not uncommon in cases of severe poisoning.

14.2.6.5　Diagnosis

Most pesticide−related poisoning have signs and symptoms that are similar to common medical conditions, so a complete and detailed environmental and occupational exposure history is essential for correctly diagnosing a pesticide poisoning. A few additional screening questions about the patient's work and home environment, in addition to a typical health questionnaire, can indicate whether there was a potential pesticide poisoning. If one is regularly using carbamate and organophosphate pesticides, it is important to obtain a baseline cholinesterase test. If one has had a baseline test and is suspected to have a poisoning later, comparison of the current cholinesterase level with the baseline level will help identify the extent of the problem.

14.2.6.6　Treatment

Specific treatments for acute pesticide poisoning are often dependent on the pesticide or class of pesticide responsible for the poisoning. However, there are basic management techniques that are applicable to most acute poisonings, including skin decontamination, airway protection, gastrointestinal decontamination, and seizure treatment. Decontamination of the skin is performed while other life−saving measures are taking place.

After clothing removed, the patients should be showered with soap and water, and the hair shampooed to remove chemicals from the skin and hair. The eyes are rinsed with water for 10−15 minutes. The patients are intubated and oxygen administered, if necessary. In more severe cases, pulmonary ventilation must be supported mechanically. Activated charcoal is sometimes administered as it has been shown to be successful with some pesticides. Studies have shown that it can reduce the amount absorbed if given within 60 minutes.

14.2.6.7   Prevention

Accidental poisonings can be avoided by proper labeling and storage of containers. When handling or applying pesticides, exposure can be significantly reduced by protecting certain parts of the body, such as underarms, face, scalp, and hands. Using chemical-resistant gloves has been shown to reduce contamination by 33% -86%.

To aid prevention of acute pesticide poisoning, concerning both accidental death and suicides, the governments should promulgate measures to control accessibility. Concerning long-term low-level exposure, which people are exposed from sources such as pesticide residues in food and products, an individual could choose to purchase organic food. Buying organic food and organic products would reduce the intake of pesticides.

▶▶ *Summary*

Occupational disease, a health problem which caused by exposed to harmful factors in workplace, has its own certain characteristics. In China, occupational diseases are classfied into 10 categories, including 132 kinds. Such as lead poisoning, mercury poisoning, irritant gas poisoning. The diagnosis of occupational disease should be undertaken by the medial organizations authorized by the public health government at province level or above. The prevention of occupational disease should follow the principle of tertiary prevention.

Practice questions:

(1) Define the following terms: lead poisoning, mercury poisoning, irritant gas, asphyxiating gas, pesticide.

(2) State the clinical manifestations and pathogenesis of lead poisoning, mercury poisoning, irritant gas poisoning, asphyxiating gas poisoning, pesticide poisoning, aniline poisoning, trinitrotoluene poisoning and benzene poisoning.

(3) Describe the treatment of pesticide poisoning, aniline poisoning, trinitrotoluene, poisoning lead poisoning and HCN poisoning.

Zeng Huaicai

14. 3　Pneumoconiosis and other occupational respiratory diseases

14.3.1　Introduction

Occupational lung disease such as pneumoconiosis is work−related respiratory diseases that were observed in ancient times in the writings of Hippocrates and in the records of Song Dynasty. Till now, pneumoconiosis is still the most seriously occupational disease in China and many developing countries. Most of occupational respiratory diseases are gradually disabled lung function and are not easily diagnosed. Especially, the earlier stage of pneumoconiosis shows non−classic symptoms. Besides, most of occupational respiratory diseases could not be cured. Therefore, preventive measures are very important.

14.3.1.1　Productive dusts

Productive dusts are defined as the long−term suspended particulate matter at workplace, which could pollute working environment and impair workers' health leading to varieties of occupational respiratory diseases such as pneumoconiosis.

Occupational dusts exposure can occur in varieties of settings, including mining, metallurgy and manufacturing, fur processing, textile industry, and agriculture. Depending on physical and chemical characteristics, productive dusts can be classified into inorganic and organic dusts. The inorganic dusts include mineral dusts (such as quartz, asbestos, talc, coal), metallic dusts (such as lead, manganese, iron and beryllium) and artificial dusts (such as silicon carbide, cement and glass fiber). The organic dusts include animal origin (such as fur, silk, bone, keratin), plant origins (such as cotton, linen, cereal, sugarcane, tobacco, wood dust) and artificial dusts (such as resin, rubber, fibers). Besides, in most cases, two and more types of dusts are mixed at the workplace which are called as mixed dusts such as coal dust with silica.

(1)Physical and chemical features

The adverse effects of productive dusts on workers' health can be determined by physical and chemical properties of dusts. The amount of dusts deposited on the airways that can reflect the severity of dust−induced diseases are depending on concentrations, exposure time, and frequency of dusts at the workplace. More deposited dusts on the airways means increase risk of respiratory diseases. The different chemical components of dusts can induce different harmful effects on workers, such as fibrosis, irritant, intoxication and allergic lesions. Lung fibrosis is produced by free crystalline silica. Occupational poisoning can be found in the workers exposed to metallic dusts and some other metallic dusts can induce allergic asthma or pneumonia.

(2)Dust dispersion

Dust dispersion is defined as a system in which particles are dispersed in a gas phase. Dust dispersion is classified according to the two parameters in relation to the gas phase, the size and weight of the dust particles are in relation to the particles of the gas phase. The former is called as quantity of dust dispersion, the latter is called as quality of dust dispersion. Dust dispersion can be used to predict inhalation and deposition of dust particles in the respiratory system, which is closely related with adverse effects of dusts on health. Higher dust dispersion leads to lower dust settling velocity and longer suspending time, which means that more dusts can be inhaled by workers. Furthermore, higher dispersed particles have larger specific surface area which means more adsorption and reactions on the surface of the particles.

(3) Dust size distribution

In many situations, we don't need to know the exact size, shape and density of dusts. Therefore, aerodynamic equivalent diameter (AED), not geometric diameter, is introduced to predict where in the respiratory tract such particles deposit. Aerodynamic equivalent diameter of an irregular particle is defined as the diameter of a sphere of density 1 g/cm^3 or 1,000 kg/m^3 with the same settling velocity as the irregular particles. It is therefore related to Stock diameter (d_p) as: AED (μm) = $d_p\sqrt{Q}\sqrt{Q}$ (d_p: Stock diameter, Q: relative density.). Generally speaking, particles with the AED less than 15 μm can be inhaled into respiratory tract and cause health problems, of which, most of the particles with the diameter between 10 and 15 μm deposited in the upper tract are defined as inhalable dust. Inhalable particles less than 5 μm can penetrate in the deep of the lung, called as respirable dusts.

(4) Dust hardness

Mechanical damage of respiratory mucous membrane by dusts is determined by the hardness of dusts. Hard dusts with bigger sizes and irregular shapes may be responsible for mechanical damage to respiratory tract, if inhaled in the alveoli, this phenomena is hard to be observed due to humid microenvironment.

(5) Dust solubility

The site and the extent of adsorption of particles in the respiratory system are determined by water solubility of these particles, since soluble dusts are more easily absorbed into blood. For example, soluble toxic dusts such as lead and arsenic compounds can be dissolved in upper respiratory tract and cause acute heavy metal poisoning. On the contrary, the toxicity of inertial dusts such as flour powder is lower due to its slight solubility and blockage of the airways. The other condition is the insoluble silica dust stay in the lung and cause long-term toxicity.

(6) Dust charge

Dust particles can be charged through material crushing, interactive friction or absorbed charged ions. The charge amount of particles is determined by size, density, temperature and humidity at the workplace. 90% –95% of suspended dusts in the air are charged particles. In general, charged particles are more liable to be intercepted and settled down in the airways. The same charged particles repel with each other, increasing the dust stability in the air, on the contrary, the dusts with opposite charges can attract each other to result in electrostatic deposition.

(7) Dust explosibility

Some combustible dusts such as coal (35 g/m^3), sugar (10.3 g/m^3), flour and sulfur (7 g/m^3) have explosibility, when they are dispersed in air at the time of ignition, which need to be confined.

(8) Dust radioactivity

Natural radioactive thorium (^{232}Th) with a half-life of 1.4×10^{10} years, come from rare earth dusts, and can emit α radiation, increasingthe risk of lung cancer.

14.3.1.2   Impacts of dust deposition and clearance

Dust deposition mechanisms in human respiratory system are determined by inertial impaction, settlement, diffusion, interception, and electrostatic deposition. Inertial impaction and settlement are triggered by dusts with bigger size more than 1 μm. Small particles with diameters less than 0.5 μm are deposited in the bronchioles and alveoli through Brownian movement. For fibrous dusts, interception is the major way to settle down. In the meantime, dusts inhaled into airways are expelled or eliminated in the three ways: interception of respiratory tract, mucociliary escalator, and macrophage phagocytosis. By means of these three clearance ways, majority of dusts inhaled can be expelled outside of body in 24 hours. Only 1% – 3% of dusts may stay in the airways. But, if the respiratory system were damaged due to long-term dust inhalation, the clearance mechanism would not work and lung diseases occur.

(1) Interception of dusts in respiratory tract

Dusts can be intercepted in the nasal passages, pharynx and tracheobronchial trees after inertial impaction, diffusion and electrostatic deposition. Dusts deposited in the airways can trigger smooth muscle contraction to narrow the airway area which could reduce airflow and increase dusts deposition. Deposited dusts can be expelled by cough and sneeze.

(2) Mucociliary escalator

Mucous secreted by goblet cells located in the upper respiratory tract can form a mucous layer to cover respiratory surface. This mucous layer helps trap dust particles. Beyond that, small hairs called as cilia covering the respiratory tract can swing rhythmically to transport dusts adhesion to mucous layer toward the laryngopharynx upwards and outwards, and then, the dusts are eventually either spat swallowed into the digestive system. This process is called mucociliary escalator.

(3) Macrophage phagocytosis

Dusts penetrated into the alveoli can be recognized and engulfed by alveolar macrophage. Most of dust cells can be expelled outside of body by ameboidism movement through the mucociliary system. Nevertheless, a small number of dust cells are damaged by dusts, and the disintegrated dust cells are engulfed into alveolar macrophage repeatedly till the macrophage get exhaustion. In addition, dust and dust cells can penetrate lung hilum and bronchial lymph nodes into lymphatic circulation, eventually into blood circulation to reach other organs.

14.3.1.3　Health effects

Dusts produced either by mechanical or construction processes are inhaled and deposited in the airways over times. The respirable dusts can penetrate into the deepest site of the lung and repeated exposure can lead to permanent lung diseases. Depending on the type of dusts, the diseases resulted from occupational dust exposure are described below:

(1) Pneumoconiosis

This is one of a group of interstitial lung diseases caused by inhaling certain kinds of dust particles that deposited deeply in the lung causing inflammation and fibrosis, and one of the most serious occupational diseases in the worldwide. The disease appears in different forms, depending on the type of dusts. Based on clinical manifestations, X-ray radiography, pathological autopsy and experimental research, pneumoconiosis can be classified into five types.

1) Silicosis: caused by inhalation of dust containing high concentrations of free silica.

2) Silicatosis: caused by inhalation of silicate dusts such as asbestos, talc and mica.

3) Carbon pneumoconiosis: caused by inhalation of coal, graphite, carbon black, activated carbon.

4) Mixed dust pneumoconiosis: caused by inhalation of free silica dusts combined with other dusts.

5) Metallic pneumoconiosis: inhalation of metallic dusts such as aluminum dust.

Classification and Lists of Occupational Diseases in China issued in 2013 covers a 12 pneumoconiosis: silicosis, asbestosis, coal workers pneumoconiosis, graphite pneumoconiosis, carbon black pneumoconiosis, talc pneumoconiosis, cement pneumoconiosis, mica pneumoconiosis, aluminosis, Welder's pneumoconiosis, Founder's pneumoconiosis, and Pottery worker's pneumoconiosis.

(2) Organic dust induced diseases

Organic dusts such as raw cotton and bagasse dust contain many biological materials that can trigger reactions in the body, which may be an allergy response leading to asthma-like breathing difficulty. For example, byssinosis resulting from raw cotton and other textile shows chest tightness, breathing difficulties, wheezing and cough, usually at the beginning of a workweek and relieves as the workweek progression, therefore called Monday Fever.

(3) Thesaurosis of metal dusts and hard metal pneumoconiosis

Some metal dusts such as tin, iron, stibium, barium inhaled and deposited in the lung may cause foreign body granuloma. The other heavy metal dust such as tungsten, titanium and cobalt may cause hard metal pneumoconiosis which is similar to the clinical presentation of hypersensitive pneumonitis.

(4) Other respiratory system diseases

Productive dusts are inhaled and deposited in the alveoli or air sacs in the lung. The presence of the dusts in the lung can cause inflammatory reaction that can turn the normal elastic lung wall into fibrous scar tissue, over time, can cause the lung to lose elasticity and impair lung function. Therefore, besides pneumoconiosis, productive dusts may cause trachitis, bronchitis, pneumonitis, asthmatic rhinitis, bronchial asthma, chronic obstructive pulmonary diseases, compensatory emphysema, pulmonary heart diseases, and bacterial infection (tuberculosis).

(5) Mechanical stimulation

Productive dusts stimulate respiratory mucous membrane, lead to dilatation and congestion of the capillaries, increas secretion of mucous gland, which help to intercept more dusts. Over time, respiratory tract mucosal hypertrophy results in dystrophy of epithelial cells and atrophic respiratory diseases. Moreover, dusts may clog hair follicles leading to obstructive seborrheic dermatitis, acne, epifolliculitis, and pustules. In addition, metallic dusts may damage cornea. Asphalt dusts are the possible cause of photodermatitis.

(6) Acute toxicity

Occupational poisoning may occur just because toxic materials such as lead, arsenic and manganese are dissolved in the respiratory system.

(7) Carcinogenicity

Some dusts such as asbestos, free crystalline silica, nickel, chromium, and arsenic compounds are confirmed as Group 1 carcinogens by IARC. Radioactive dusts could induce respiratory tumors.

14.3.1.4 Prevention and control measures

In the past decades, national action program to control pneumoconiosis has been promoted by many developing and developed countries including China. According to primary, secondary and tertiary prevention principles, there are a number of means accomplished to protect workers from productive dusts exposure.

(1) Legislation and regulations

Since the 50s' of the 20th century, a variety of laws and regulations have been issued in China (Table 14-1). One of the most important laws is Prevention and Control Laws of Occupational Diseases issued on May. 1st, 2002, and revised in 2011 and 2016, respectively. Besides, eight-hour time-weight permissible concentrations and excursion limits which represent short-time exposure to 47 productive dusts are listed as the national hygienic standards as follows.

Table 14-1　Laws, regulations and standards of pneumoconiosis control issued in China

Issued year	Laws, regulations and standards
1956	Decision of prevent silica dust hazards in industrial enterprises
1987	Prevention and control regulations of pneumoconiosis
	Health care and treatment program of workers exposed to productive dusts
2002	Prevention and control laws of occupational diseases
2007	Permissible exposure limits of occupational hazards in the workplace Part I: chemical hazards (GBZ 2.1-2007)

(2) Technical measures

The best way to prevent pneumoconiosis is to identify workplace activities that produce dusts and then to eliminate, replace or control the dusts. The engineering controls are the most common methods including substitution of materials such as replacing natural asbestos with artificial asbestos, improvement of process and equipment such as remote control, water spray, air filtering, isolation of the source or workers, enclosed process, local exhaust ventilation, general ventilation system, enclosed cabs and air supply system.

(3) Personal protective measures

To control the dust levels at workplace, personal protective measures may be the final protective measures. The plants are requested to provide personal protective equipment such as mask and goggles against dusts. The workers exposed to dusts need to be trained and educated on work practice such as good housekeeping and maintenance. Besides, good living habit, regular dietary habit and physical fitness are very important to workers exposed to dusts.

(4) Surveillance of worker health and workplace

According to national standards, concentrations of dusts at workplace need to be detected periodically and health risk for workers exposed to dusts need to be evaluated. Meanwhile, periodic health examination such as chest radiography or experimental detection such as biomarkers need to examine to find early damage including pre-job, on-the-job, after leaving stages.

14.3.2　Silicosis

14.3.2.1　Definition

Silicosis is a massive silicotic fibrosis of lung due to dust containing silicon dioxide which was inhaled by the workers and retention in the respiratory system for a long term.

14.3.2.2　Epidemiology

Silicosis is the most common occupational pulmonary disease worldwide. In China, silicosis is one of the most serious pneumoconiosis, which accounts for -40% of the total pneumoconiosis cases. In China, more than 500,000 silicosis cases were recorded between 1991 and 1995, among them 6,000 were new cases. Approximately 2.3 million workers might expose to respirable crystalline silica in the United States. In general, when the concentration of free silica dusts exceeds 10% of total dusts, it is called as occupational silica dust exposure.

14.3.2.3　Chemical and physical properties

Silicon dioxide, all as known silica, is an oxide of silicon with the chemical formula SiO_2, most commonly found in nature, which comprises about 5% within the 16 km of the earth's crust. In many parts of the world, silica is the major constituent of sand, rock and ores. The notable example is quartz which contains about 99% divided finely crystalline silica. According to chemical structure, the inorganic silica is classified as crystalline, crypto-crystalline and amorphous silica. The crystalline silica shows orderly arranged tetrahedron with silicon-oxygen bond such as quartz, tridymite found widespread in quartzite, granite and other minerals. Compared with the crystalline silica, the agate, flint and quartz glass categorized into the crypto crystalline have the tetrahedron of silicon-oxygen bond of is non-orderly arranged. The amorphous silica includes diatomite, silica gel, opal, fused quartz, fumed silica and aerosol. In nature, quartz has different types of isomers with an identical composition while distinct tetrahedron of silicon-oxygen arrangement with the increasing temperature and pressure. With the temperature increasing, these quartz isomers successively form: α-quartz, tridymite, cristobalite, coesite, stishovite and keatite. Compared with α-quartz which is only stable form under normal conditions, the other quartz has lower densities and indices of refraction. Besides, α-quartz will be transformed into cristobalite and tridymite after high-temperature roasting. This phenomenon may be observed in other procedures of roasting silicate minerals such as diatomite.

（1）Potentially occupational exposure

Occupational exposure to inorganic silica dusts can occur in various settings including mining, tunneling, quarrying, construction, manufacturing, smelting, sandblasting, masonry, foundry operations, glass manufacture, ceramic and pottery production, cement and concrete production, gem cutting and polishing, some work with certain materials containing silica. Especially, the workers in the following occupations are at high risk for developing silicosis: highway and bridge construction and repair, building construction, demolition and repair, abrasive blasting, masonry work, concrete finishing, drywall finishing, rock drilling, mining, sand and gravel screening, rock crush for road base.

（2）Classification

There are three types of silicosis according to the disease's severity, rapidity of progression and onset depending on the concentration of respirable crystalline silica.

1）Acute silicosis: Which develops after exposure to high concentrations of high content of free silica and results in symptoms within 1-2 years after initial exposure. Acute silicosis is typically associated with high exposures such as sandblasting or quartz mining. Based on the pathologic characteristics of acute silicosis, it is referred to as silicoproteinosis without typically lung fibrosis.

2）Chronic silicosis: Also called as delayed silicosis, which develops after exposure to relatively low concentrations of free silica and results in symptoms within 15-20 years after initial exposure.

3）Accelerated silicosis: Which develops 5-10 years after the first exposure. Inflammation, fibrosis, and symptoms progress faster in accelerated silicosis than in chronic silicosis.

Beyond that, the onset of silicosis are correlated with types of silica, dispersion of silica, preventive measures and individual characteristics. While different forms of crystalline quartz have different pathogenicity, the sequence from strong to weak is trydimite, crystobalite, quartz, coesite, and stishovite.

（3）Pathogenesis

Although a large body of published papers describes the health effects of silica, the pathogenesis of silicosis is not clear. Several mechanisms have been proposed to explain the cause of the cellular damage. The occurrence of silicosis is correlated with crystalline silica-induced cytotoxicity. Silica dusts were inhaled and deposited in distal airways. After silica dusts were engulfed by alveolar macrophages who are the scavenger in the lung, crystalline silica could directly or indirectly interrupt membrane stability and permeability of alveolar macrophages. Silica dusts could mechanically damage the cell membrane of macrophages, which could change the membrane permeability and induce the inflow of extracellular calcium ion to impair macrophages. Besides, the active hydroxyl group on the surface of silica could form hydrogen bond with alveolar macrophage membrane. Beyond that, dust cells could release the reactive oxygen species and activate reactive oxygen free radicals of white blood cells, which could lead to membrane lipid peroxidation and change the membrane stability.

To date, a lot of in vitro and animals studies have indicated that the occurrence, progress of silicosis were regulated by complicated cell-cytokines network, cell signaling pathways involving lymphocytes, epithelial cells, macrophages, fibroblasts. Stimulation of the alveolar macrophages to release inflammatory factors (e. g. , interleukin-8, leukotriene B_4, platelet-activating factor, tumor necrosis factor, platelet-derived growth factor) and activate inflammasome NLRP3 which stimulates caspase-1, interleukin-1β and interleukin-18 that recruit polymorphonuclear leukocytes and initiate fibroblast production and collagen synthesis which are concerned with interleukin-1β, tumor necrosis factor, plated-derived growth factor, fibronectin, and alveolar macrophage-derived growth factor. Additionally, Th1-type and Th2-type cells play very important roles in regulating silica-induced early inflammation and fibrosis progression. Moreover, myofibroblasts originated from fibroblast transdifferentiation, epithelial-myofibroblast transition or bone marrow-derived cells would produce an excess of extracellular matrix. In addition, autophage is involving in lung fibrosis which would be promoted by silica-induced autophagosome increase regulated by death receptors, mitochondrial and endoplasmic reticulum signaling pathways.

(4) Pathophysiology

Silica dusts inhaled into the distal airway interact with alveolar macrophages. Activated alveolar macrophages would secrete a series of fibroblast growth factors which stimulate the fibroblasts to produce collagen around the silica particles. Continuous accumulation of collagen produces silicotic nodules, peribronchial and perivascular fibrosis.

1) Silicotic nodule: Silicotic nodule is the characteristic pathological change of lung fibrosis from silica dust inhalation. Macroscopically, one can identify small 1-5 mm size pale or dark nodules located predominantly in the upper lung lobes and beneath pleural. Microscopically, in the early stages, silicotic nodules consist of sparse fibers within dust cells. Continuously, fibrotic nodules with concentric "onion-skinned" arrangement of collagen fibers, central hyalinization, and a cellular peripheral zone, with lightly birefringent particles seen under polarized light microscope. In later stages of the disease, the fibrous nodules enlarge and merge, resulting in large areas of fibrosis. Nodules can present central ischemic necrosis. Some small nodules can be calcified in the center. Occasionally, silicotic nodules can be observed in the lymph node.

2) Diffuse interstitial lung fibrosis: It is resulted from inhalation of relatively low concentrations of silica dusts for a long term. The progress of pathological interstitial fibrosis is slow. Diffuse interstitial tissue hyperplasia surrounding alveolar, interlobular septa, small vessels and respiratory bronchioles are detected by electron microscopy.

3) Silicoproteinosis: Sometimes, it is referred to acute silicosis, resulting from relatively short exposure to high concentrations of silica dust, it could be characterized by the presence of proteinaceous fluid in the air spaces.

4) Progressive massive fibrosis (PMF): Along with disease progression, progressive massive fibrosis can be detected resulting from fused smaller silicotic nodules or diffuse fibrosis showing large conglomerate masses of dense fibrosis (size ≥1 cm), usually located in the lung posterior lobe and lower lobe. Macroscopically, the lesions are radiating strands showing cone, spindle or irregular shape with clear boundaries. Microscopically, silicotic nodules, diffused interstitial fibrosis, collagen hyperplasia and central hyalinization can be observed with central ischemic necrosis, thin-wall hollow and calcified lesions accompanying inflammation and emphysema.

5) Silicotuberculosis: Silicosis patients are particularly susceptible to tuberculosis infection, which shows the characteristic pathological changes called as silicotuberculosis. Microscopically, central caseous necrosis in which the tissue appears like cheese can be detected and layers of collagen and dusts are distributed peripherally. Otherwise, the central silicotic nodules can be surrounded by caseous necrosis and tuberculous granuloma tissues.

Most patients with silicosis present mixed dust pneumoconiosis resulting from chronic inhalation of mixed dust with silicotic nodules and diffuse interstitial fibrosis. Some severe silicosis patients have above three types of pathological characteristics including nodules, diffuse interstitial fibrosis and progressive massive fibrosis.

(5) Symptoms and Signs

Symptoms and signs of patients with chronic silicosis may not appear at the early stage. In fact, chronic silicosis could go undetected for 15–20 years after exposure. With silicosis progresses or complications, non-specific symptoms may include chest tightness, shortness of breath, cough (often persistent and sometimes severe), chest pain and coughing up phlegm. These symptoms can become worse over time. Some symptoms and signs may present, including fever, weight loss and respiratory insufficiency resulting from some infection or complications.

Abnormalities in pulmonary function could be detected at the late stage in patients with silicosis. Pulmonary function tests performed by spirometer measure lung volumes [total lung capacity (TLC), vital capacity (VC), inspiratory capacity (IC), functional residual capacity (FRC)], air flow [expiratory volume in 1 second (FEV_1)], blood exchange, and other aspects of lung function. With the progressing of lung fibrosis, the TLC and VC will decrease. The pulmonary function tests of patients with silicosis present mixed ventilation dysfunction due to lung emphysema and chronic inflammation. If a large of pulmonary alveoli were damaged and capillary wall thickened, the lung function tests would show diffusing capacity dysfunction.

(6) Complications

Complications of silicosis can include tuberculosis, pulmonary chronic bronchitis, compensatory emphysema, spontaneous pneumothorax and pulmonary heart diseases. Once complications appears, the symptoms will be worse and lead to death. The most common and dangerous complication is tuberculosis, known as silicotuberculosis, which could largely increase the risk of death. At the same time, the symptoms of tuberculosis accompanying with silicosis is hard to control and treat. The reason for the increased risk is not clear. The probable reason is that silica damages the alveolar macrophages, which are unable to kill the infectious organism Mycobacteria.

Crystalline silica dust was classified as "carcinogenic to humans" by IARC (International Agency for Research on Cancer) in 1997. The crystalline silica was considered a potential occupational carcinogen which increases the risk of incidence of lung cancer based on a lot of studies and meta-analysis.

(7) Diagnosis

The diagnosis of silicosis need to collect the following evidences: the patient history reveal that the sufferer has been exposed to crystalline silica dust in the workplace, chest imaging (usually chest X-ray or digital chest radiography) that shows the imaging changes concurred with pathological progressing, occupational exposure information including shifts, epidemiological data, personal protective equipment from occupational health investigation, clinical manifestation, and pulmonary function test excluding other alternative plausible lung diseases for the findings such as acute or subacute hematogenous disseminated pulmonary tuberculosis, invasive lung tuberculosis, pulmonary hemosiderosis, lung cancer, idiopathic pulmonary fibrosis, allergic pulmonary alveolitis, fungal lung infection, and pulmonary alveolar microlithiasis. Depending on X-ray imaging standard of silicosis, the patients can be diagnosed and by stage at diagnosis.

Most of cases of silicosis don't need a biopsy of the lungs. A few cases exposed to silica dust without diagnosis need autopsy unless last wish or application from family members after one's death. Furthermore, the diagnosis can be done according to pathological diagnostic criteria of pneumoconiosis (GBZ 25–2014, China).

(8) Imaging

Chest radiography is the primary method of diagnosis of silicosis. Generally speaking, the x-ray findings could show the pathological progression. Different sizes and shapes opacities of X-ray imaging may represent silicotic nodules, diffuse interstitial fibrosis, and progressive massive fibrosis. The ILO (International Labor Organization) Classification system of pneumoconiosis provides guidelines and sets of standard radiographs. The doctors compare the patient postero−anterior chest X−ray with those of the standard set. The standard films show different types (shape and size) and severity (profusion) of abnormalities images in the patients with pneumoconiosis (Table 14−2). Besides, hilar shadow, pulmonary emphysema, bronchovascular shadow and pleura shadow can be referred to silicosis diagnosis, which need to be marked using 29 specific symbols issued by ILO (Table 14−3).

Table 14−2   ILO classification system of pneumoconiosis

Small opacities (<10 mm)	
Four−point major scale for profusion *	
0	0/−,0/0,0/1
1	1/0,1/1,1/2
2	2/1,2/2,2/3
3	3/2,3/3,3/+
Round shape and size	
P	≤1.5 mm
Q	1.5−3 mm
R	3−10 mm
Irregular shape and size	
S	≤1.5 mm
T	1.5−3 mm
U	3−10 mm
Large opacities (> 10 mm)	
A	≤5 cm
B	5 cm to the size of the right upper zone
C	Bigger than the right upper zone

* Small opacities are classified into a four−point major category scale with each major category divided into three profusion. Category 0 refers to the absence of small opacity and category 3 refers to the most profusion. The major category (first number) represents the major profusion and diagnosis and the minor category (second number) means the profusion considered as an alternative.

Table 14−3   Abnormality of pneumoconiosis representing as 29 symbols

Symbols	Abnormality	Symbols	Abnormality
at	Significant apical pleural thickening	ca	cancer
bu	Bullae	cn	Calcification of small opacities
cg	Calcified granuloma or lymph node	cp	Cor pulmonale
co	Abnormal cardiac shape or size	di	Marked distortion of an intrathoracic structure
cv	Cavity	em	emphysema
ef	Pleural effusion	fr	Rib fractures
es	Eggshell calcification	ho	honeycombing
hi	Enlargement of non−calcified hilar nodes	ih	Ⅲ−defined heart border
aa	Atherosclerotic aorta	ax	Coalescence of small opacities
id	Ⅲ−defined diaphragm border	me	Mesothelioma (pleural)
kl	Septal (Kerley) lines	pb	Parenchymal bands
pa	Plate atelectasis	px	pneumothorax
pi	Pleural thickening of an interlobar fissure	rp	Rheumatoid pneumoconiosis
ra	Rounded atelectasis	od	Other disease or significant abnormality
tb	Tuberculosis		

* Twenty−nine symbols are additional features related to dust exposure issued by ILO.

1) Round opacities: For simple silicosis, chest x – ray image usually shows small round opacities (<10 mm), often symmetrically distributed in the upper lung zones. The size of small round opacities can be classified into three types according to ILO Classification system: p–type (φ<1.5 mm), q–type (1.5–3.0 mm), r–type (3.0–10 mm). The different sizes of round opacities can interpret pathological changes of silicotic nodules with disease progression from immature nodules to mature and overlapped nodules.

2) Irregular parenchymal opacities: For some patients with silicosis exposed to low concentrations of free silica dust, the chest radiography shows the irregular parenchymal opacities interpreting the diffuse interstitial fibrosis distributed in the lower and middle zones. According to ILO Classification system, small irregular parenchymal opacities have three types: s (φ<1.5 mm), t (1.5–3.0 mm), and u (3.0–10 mm). The image appears like messy web in the base zones.

3) Large opacities: In progressive massive fibrosis, the small opacities become confluent and form large opacities (>10 mm), usually symmetrically located in the upper zones. With the retraction of the lung tissue, there is often compensatory emphysema surrounding large opacities.

4) Pleural abnormabilities: In some severe patients with silicosis, fibrosis occurs in the pleural zones in the base of lung and leads to costophrenic angle obtuse or disappears in the early stage. Over time, the awning–shape shadow appears resulting from pleural tissue retraction and adhesion.

5) Pulmonary emphysema: With the retraction of the lung tissue, there is often compensatory emphysema showing diffuse, limited emphysema around the lesions, and bullae.

6) Pulmonary hilum and markings: For chronic and accelerated silicosis, pulmonary hilum shows enlargement with increasing pulmonary markings resulting from inflammation and fibrosis. Sometimes, the silicotic nodules may be calcified circumferentially, which called as "eggshell" calcification. In the late stage, pulmonary hilum can move up and outside with lung markings disappearing. The X–ray findings of silicoproteniosis show diffuse small featheriness shadows with air bronchogram.

(9) Diagnostic criteria

The silicosis can be diagnosed according to Diagnostic Criteria of Occupational Pneumoconiosis of China (GBZ 70–2015) revised in 2015.

Stage Ⅰ: one of the following radiographic abnormalities:

● Silica exposure: small opacity, total profusion = 1, distribution area >= 4 lung zones.

● Asbestos exposure: small opacity, total profusion = 1, distribution area = 1 lung zones, with pleural plague.

● Asbestos exposure: small opacity, total profusion = 0, while profusion = 0/1 distribution area >= 2 lung zones, with pleural plague.

Stage Ⅱ: one of the following radiographic abnormalities:

● Silica exposure: small opacity, total profusion = 2, distribution area >= 4 lung zones.

● Silica exposure: small opacity, total profusion = 3, distribution area = 4 lung zones.

● Asbestos exposure: small opacity, total profusion = 1, distribution area >4 lung zones, with pleural plague and ill–defined diaphragm or heart border.

● Asbestos exposure: small opacity, total profusion = 2, distribution area = 4 lung zones, with pleural plague and ill–defined diaphragm or heart border.

Stage Ⅲ: one of the following radiographic abnormalities:

● Silica exposure: large opacity, length of diameter >= 20 mm, short radius > 10 mm.

● Silica exposure: small opacity, total profusion = 3, distribution area >4 lung zones with coalescence of small opacities.

● Silica exposure: small opacity, total profusion = 3, distribution area >4 lung zones with large opacities.

● Asbestos exposure: small opacity, total profusion = 3, distribution area >4 lung zones, with pleural plague and ill-defined diaphragm or heart border, with the sum of the length of pleural plagues distributed one-side or both sides of lung zones larger than half of unilateral chest wall or ill-defined diaphragm or shaggy heart.

(10) Treatment

Unfortunately, there is no specific therapy for silicosis to cure or alter the course of the disease. However, there is a variety of treatments available to help manage symptoms and prevent complications associated with the diseases. Though many experimental researches focus on developing medicines to inhibit lung fibrosis, the clinical trial still needs to be evaluated. For acute silicosis, large bronchoalveolar lavage may alleviate symptoms, but does not decrease the overall mortality as well as ensuing the risk of operation complications. Therefore, the comprehensive treatment may be the best options to prevent complications, control tuberculosis, improve life quality including health care and rehabilitation, symptomatic supportive treatment and complications therapy.

1) Health care and rehabilitation: The patients need to stop being exposed to silica dusts. Furthermore, review and follow-up examination need to be done regularly. The doctor would advise patients with silicosis stopping smoke and having good habits such as regular diets and physical training.

2) Symptomatic supportive treatment: The antitussive and expectorant drugs would be administered to expelling phlegm and arrest coughing. Oxygen therapy may improve pulmonary ventilation.

3) Therapy for complications: Antibiotics would be administered to control bacterial lung infection including Mycobacteria which is the most common complications to patients with silicosis. Cardiac stimulants, urinative and vasodilators may be administered to control chronic pulmonary heart diseases, if present. Comprehensive therapies may control respiratory failure such as oxygen administration, correction of electrolytes and acid-base disturbances, anti-inflammation and keeping fluency of respiratory tract.

(11) Identification of pneumoconiosis disability

Based on the results of X-ray imaging diagnosis, pulmonary function testing and respiratory conditions, the disability of patients with silicosis would be evaluated according to the identification of working ability: occupational injury and levels of disability related to occupational diseases (GB/T 16180-2014). There are 7 levels from mild to severe (Table 14-4). If identified, the patients with silicosis should be out of work exposed to silica dusts. The disabilities identified into level 6 and 7 may work at non-dust exposure place. The ones of level 4 may do some moderate workload jobs with rehabilitation. The ones of level 2 and 3 just do some rehabilitation under the guidance of doctors.

Table 14-4 Occupational injury and levels of disability related to occupational diseases

Levels	Identification Criteria
Level 1	Stage III, severe pulmonary function abnormalities, severe hypoxemia [PO_2 <53 kPa (40 mmHg)]
Level 2	Stage III, medium pulmonary function abnormalities, medium hypoxemia or Stage II, severe pulmonary function abnormalities, severe hypoxemia [PO_2 <53 kPa (40 mmHg)] or Stage III, active tuberculosis.
Level 3	Stage III, or Stage II, medium pulmonary function abnormalities, medium hypoxemia or Stage II, active tuberculosis.
Level 4	Stage II, or Stage I, medium pulmonary function abnormalities, medium hypoxemia or Stage I, active tuberculosis.

Continue to Table 14-4

Levels	Identification Criteria
Level 5	/
Level 6	Stage Ⅰ, mild pulmonary function abnormalities, mild hypoxemia.
Level 7	Stage Ⅰ, normal pulmonary function.

14.3.3   Silicatosis

14.3.3.1   Definition

Silicatosis is a type of diffuse interstitial pulmonary fibrosis diseases resulting from long-term inhalation of silicates dust. The histopathological detection of lung tissues from silicatosis shows diffuse interstitial lung fibrosis with ferruginous bodies, microscopically. In Chest X-ray radiograph appears primarily irregular small opacities consistent with pathological changes. Other than silicosis, the sufferers with silicatosis manifest obvious symptoms and signs with pulmonary function abnormalities with obstructive airways and decreased vital capacity in the early stage. With disease progressing, the characteristic pulmonary function finding in silicatosis is restrictive ventilation with air exchange dysfunction.

14.3.3.2   Silicate dust

Silicate is a series of inorganic compounds made up of silicate groups, which contain different ratios of silicon and oxygen with metallic oxide and crystalline water. Natural silicate minerals are widespread in the earth which form about 90% of the Earth's crust such as asbestos, talc and mica. Artificial silicates are made of quartz and base materials by roasting such as glass fiber and cement. According to shapes, silicates dusts are classified into fibrous dusts with a high length/width ratio of silicate dusts (more than 3 : 1) and non-fibrous dusts. The fibrous silicate dusts with diameter<3 μm and length≥5 μm are defined as respirable fibers that can be intercepted in the deep airways and trigger inflammation and fibrosis, whereas, non-respirable fibers with diameter ≥3 μm and length ≥5 μm.

14.3.4   Asbestosis

14.3.4.1   Definition

Asbestosis is a diffused interstitial pulmonary disease resulting from long-term inhalation of asbestos dusts at the workplace which pathological characteristics are diffuse fibrosis distributed all lung zones, not fibrous nodules. Asbestosis is one of the most common and serious silicatosis. Asbestos is widely used in varies of industrials including asbestos mineral mining, processing and application. Asbestos can be found in the roofs, ceilings, walls and floors. Manufacturers also use chrysotile asbestos in automobile brake linings, gaskets and boiler seals, and insulation for pipes, ducts and appliances.

14.3.4.2   Classification of asbestos dusts

Asbestos is a kind of natural fibrous silicate minerals, which are categorized into serpentine and amphibole. As one kind of serpentine, chrysotile or white asbestos, accounting for approximately 95% of asbestos, are widespread applied in many fields and produced primarily in Canada, Russia and China. It is a white, soft, flexible, and fluffy fibrous silicates. Compared with chrysotile, amphibole including crocidolite, amosite, anthophyllite, tremolite, and actinolite shows the features of hard and crisp, of which crocidolite and amosite contribute to the major yields from South Africa, Australia and Finland.

14.3.4.3 Features of asbestos

Asbestos presents considerable tensile strength, resistant to heat, acid, strong bases, and decay. The diameters of asbestos from larger to smaller are in the order: anthophyllite > amosite > chrysotile > crocidolite. Smaller fibers can be inhaled into the deeper airways, more deposition and penetration in the alveoli, therefore, crocidolite, also known as blue asbestos, has the strongest capacity to stimulate fibrosis and carcinogenicity, earlier onset and more asbestos bodies found in the lung tissues among all of asbestos minerals. Chrysotile containing more magnesium oxide is easy to dissolve in the lung and more easily cleared outside of airways than crocidolite and amosite.

Respirable asbestos fibers can be inhaled into the respiratory system and engulfed by alveolar macrophages into dust cells, subsequently, most of which are expelled outside and upside by mucociliary escalator, or by lymphatic circulation, or intercepted in the base of lung. In addition, a portion of dusts with hard and straight fibers can penetrate lung tissue into pleura. The onset and processing of asbestos induced disease are determined by types of asbestos, length of fibers, concentration of respirable dusts, exposure time, and personal susceptibility related to living habits such as tobacco smoking.

14.3.4.4 Pathogenesis and pathophysiology

The pathogenesis of asbestosis is not fully clear, which is probably correlated with physical features of asbestos fibers, cytotoxicity of metal components of asbestos, fiber-induced free radical damage. The pathological features of asbestosis are described as diffuse interstitial pulmonary fibrosis with asbestos bodies forming, visceral pleura thickening, and parietal pleural plaque forming. Gross feature shows both of pleura lightly thickening. With progressing, lung tissues manifest typical diffuse fibrous "basket-webs" gray black appearance. In the late stage, lung volumes become small and stiffening with honeycombing lung.

Microscopically, asbestos is primarily deposited in the respiratory bronchioles and adjacent lung zone, further triggering respiratory bronchioles alveolitis with neutrophilic exudating, serous cellulose secreting, basement membrane swelling, and epithelial necrosis. Over time, granuloma is formed by gathered macrophages and fibroblasts and the web fibers and collagens further break respiratory bronchioles alveolar structure. With progressing, fibrosis is developed from lobules into the base of lung area and fused into webs, representing as fibrosis thickening around lobular septum, pleura, blood vessel and air tract. In the late stage, massive fibrosis with severe honeycombing is a primary manifestation. The remarkable features of progress massive fibrosis in asbestosis tissue section are mostly diffuse fibrosis, alveolar islands and concentrated wide blood vessels and tracts, other than one of silicosis with fused silicotic nodules.

Pleural plaque: It is defined as a continuous confined pleural thickening more than 5 mm in width. The plaque is ivory or grey white, often thickest at the margins, with smooth surface and clear boundary. The most commonly pleural plaque is distributed on the parietal pleura, which lines the inside of the rib cage, but found on the visceral pleura, which lines the lungs. Additionally, pleural plaques can grow on the diaphragm. Microscopically, pleural plaque is composed of bundles of dense hyalinised collagen fibers and relatively acellular, can be calcified over time. Pleural plaque is benign, which can be considered as a pathological and radiographic biomarker of asbestos exposure, which can be found in the populations exposed to asbestos without asbestosis.

Asbestos bodies: Also known as ferruginous bodies. Asbestos fibers are engulfed by macrophage and coated with a layer of iron-rich protein and acid mucopolysaccharide. Microscopically, asbestos bodies are 10-300 μm long, 1-5 μm wide, golden, dumbbell-shape, drumstick-shape or beads-shape. The amounts of asbestos bodies may be not consistent with the degree of lung fibrosis. It can be suggested as an exposure biomarker but not diagnostic evidence.

14.3.4.5   Symptoms and signs

In the early stage, asbestosis can cause shortness of breath, persistent dry cough due to scan tissue to limit air exchange. If having persistent chest pain, lung cancer or mesothelioma should be considered. The stiffening of the lungs can cause crackling sound when patients with asbestosis breath, with progression, the distribution of crackling sound develops from the lower to upper lung zones. Meanwhile, the scar lung tissues result in less oxygen exchange producing insufficient oxygen delivered to blood, which could induce clubbed fingers and toes described that the tips of fingers and toes appears wider and rounder than normal. In addition, the formation of scar can constrict arteries and make it harder to pump blood out of the heart and into the lungs, which means lungs need to work harder and have risk of pulmonary hypertension and heart diseases.

(1)Pulmonary function

Compared with silicosis, the pulmonary function of asbestosis patients is damaged seriously due to diffuse interstitial fibrosis which constrict lung and limit oxygen exchange and deliver into blood. In the early stage, stiffening scar lung tissues lead to lung compliance reducing and vital capacity gradually decreasing. Diffusing capacity, which is a sensitive index to evaluate both of restrictive and obstructive lung diseases, is decreasing earlier than vital capacity. If having emphysema, total lung capacity and residual volume may be normal or slightly high. With progression, most of patients suffer from asbestosis show decrease of vital capacity, forced vital capacity, and total lung capacity without changing of forced expiratory volume in one second/forced vital capacity, which indicate progressive fibrosis showing restrictive lung disease.

(2)Radiographic features

Chest X-ray radiographs usually show irregular opacities and pleural abnormalities. Irregular small opacities along with diffuse interstitial fibrosis are the diagnostic evidence of asbestosis, which distributed on the lower lung zones. With progression, small opacities emerge into basket-web and developed into middle and upper lung zones.

Pleural lesions show pleural plaque, pleural thickening and pleural calcification. The pleural plaque is a diagnostic marker of asbestosis, which is distributed most commonly on the both of lower parietal pleura between the 6th and 10th lib, not developing into lung tip and costodiaphragmatic angle, without tissue adhesion. The shadow of peripheral plaque is overlapped with one of the libs with dense stick or irregular opacities. Diffuse pleural thickening is irregular shadow, distributed in the middle or lower lung zones, often with dense pleural calcification image. On the late stage of asbestosis, shaggy heart is a descriptive term referring to the obscured cardiac silhouette on a chest radiograph, which usually implies pleural fibrosis developing on the mediastinal interface. If happened, it can be documented as an important diagnostic evidence for stage Ⅲ of asbestosis.

14.3.4.6   Complications

Compared with silicosis, asbestosis can more commonly cause respiratory inflammation and severe pulmonary heart disease, but rarely tuberculosis. Lately, repeated infection can lead to heart failure. The most serious complications exposed to asbestos are lung cancer and mesothelioma.

(1)Lung cancer

Asbestos is confirmed as Group 1 carcinogens by IARC. Asbestos exposure or asbestosis can increase the risk of incidence of lung cancer which can be influenced by exposure dose, fiber type, job type, the degree of lung fibrosis and personal behavior such as smoking. Asbestos induced lung cancer usually has a 15-20 years latent. Generally, crocidolite shows the strongest carcinogenesis than chrysotile and amosite.

Histologically, asbestos usually induce peripheral lung adenocarcinoma. The carcinogenesis of asbestos are attributed in special physical features of asbestos fibers, polycyclic aromatic hydrocarbon adsorbed in the suspended asbestosis fibers, radioactive components mixed with asbestos and synergistic effect of tobacco smoking.

(2) Mesothelioma

Mesothelioma is a rare tumor classified into benign and malignant ones. Asbestos exposure is one the most common cause of malignant mesothelioma. Based on the location, mesothelioma is categorized into four types including pleural, peritoneal, pericardial and testicular. As the most common type of asbestos-related cancer, malignant mesothelioma occurs 15-40 years after asbestos exposure. The type of asbestos is one of the important impactors induces malignant mesothelioma. Generally speaking, the initiations of mesothelioma are depending on the physical features of asbestos, especially, the size of fibers. Crocidolite with long and thin fibers is more potent carcinogen than chrysotile with soft and curve fibers. Beyond that, asbestos fibers are easy to be divided into small particles and deposited more in the pleura and hard to be degraded, which can increase the risk of carcinogensis.

14.3.4.7 Diagnosis

According to Diagnostic Criteria of Occupational Pneumoconiosis in China (GBZ 70-2015), the general diagnostic criteria for asbestosis include: evidence of pathological features consistent with asbestosis as documented by imaging or histology, evidence of asbestos exposure as documented by the occupational and environmental history, biomarkers of exposure, exclusion of other diseases.

14.3.5 Coal workers' pneumoconiosis

14.3.5.1 Definition

Coal is one of the primary combustible and chemical materials, which can be classified into lignite, bitumite, and anthracite based on the content of volatiles. Coal mining and the use of coal produce large amounts of coal dust, if inhaled, which can cause adverse health impact on workers and death. The most common diseases induced by inhalation of coal dust is coal workers' pneumoconiosis (CWP), also known as black lung, which is a kind of fibrosis lung disease resulting from long-term exposure to coal dusts at the workplace, especially at coal mining. The prevalence of coal workers' pneumoconiosis is more than 50% of occupational pneumoconiosis in China.

14.3.5.2 Coal mine dust and occupational exposure

All rock and mineral particles produced in the process of coal mining are called coal mine dust, which mainly contains rock dusts and coal dust. However, since the geological structure is complicated and changeable, in which coal bed and rock stratum are co-existing, there are huge amounts of coal and rock dust mixture in coal mining.

(1) Sources of coal mine dust

During underground mining of coal, workers involving in rock drilling, blasting, loading, guniting, transporting, pit propping and underground ventilation can produce dust, mainly containing silica, coal and concrete dust. In the process of rock tunnel boring, drilling operation with pneumatic drills, mechanical coal cutting and blasting have increased greatly the respiratory exposure. Without protective measures, the concentration of coal dust can reach over 1,000 mg/m^3 in the air. Drilling with electric drills and loading of coal onto train cars also have a higher risk of dusts exposure. Opencast working can cause a large quantity of dust while stripping rock stratum and excavating coal beds. Other duties facing higher coal dust exposure are crushing, sizing, washing, and blending of coal at preparation plants.

(2) Physicochemical properties of coal mine dusts

The chemical components of coal mine dust are closely related to sedimentary layer. Coal mine dust is a mixture containing carbon, clay minerals and quartz. Different types of rock have a distinctive constitutes and components. The main chemical components of coal mine dust are: silicon dioxide, aluminium oxide, calcium oxide, magnesium oxide, sodium oxide, potassium oxide, sulfur dioxide, ferrum oxide, etc. The free crystalline silicon dioxide content of coal is usually below 10%.

The physical characteristics of coal mine dust are similar to silicious dust. Higher dispersion and larger specific surface area are more susceptible to produce surface chemical reaction, spontaneous combustion or explosion. Coal mine dust can absorb radon and its daughters, leading to lung cancer or enhancing possibility of pulmonary fibrosis induced by dusts. Newly released dust from the excavation working faces is more likely to get charged than those from return airways. The explosiveness of coal dust is related to the extent of coal's carbonization and volatility. Therefore, bituminous coal with higher volatility (over 20%) is higher explosiveness than meagre coal (10%–20%) and anthracite (less than 10%). The regular coal's lower explosive limit is 30–50 g/m^3.

14.3.5.3 Classification of CWP

The classification of CWP is based on radiographic findings which include classic CWP, silicosis, mixed dust pneumoconiosis called as anthracisilicosis.

CWP is defined as inhalation of simple coal mine dust with the content of silicon dioxide lower than 5% for a long term, usually over 20–30 years, and the typical pathological change is anthracosis such as coal-face workers. The progression of classic CWP is slow, and the hazard is slight.

Silicosis is found primarily in hard-rock tunnel boring workers who are exposed to rock dust usually over 10–15 years, in which the content of free crystalline silicon dioxide is above 10%. This type shows progressive fibrosis similar with silicosis. It accounts for 20–30% of the total CWP patients.

Anthracisilicosis is the most common type of CWP in China. It happens within the patients who work at rock tunnel usually exposed to both rock and coal dusts for 15–20 years. The progression of fibrosis is quite fast and clinical symptoms and signs are severe.

14.3.5.4 Pathophysiology

CWP's pathological features are depending on the ratio of inhaled silicious dust to coal dust. The mixed dust pneumoconiosis is the most common presenting diffuse interstitial fibrosis and nodular pattern. The main pathological changes include:

Coal macula is the most common typical lesion and the basic indicator of pathological diagnosis in CWP patients. On appearance, it is focal, soft, round or irregular shaped, black reticulations or stripes without clear margin. Mostly it is distributed in the crossing corner of interlobular septa and pleura. Microscopically, it is a combination of the coal dust cell focus and the coal dust fibrosis focus. The coal dust cell focus is made of coal dust and macrophages phagocytized coal dust accumulating around pulmonary alveoli, alveolar wall, bronchioles and blood vessels. The most regular spot is secondary respiratory bronchioles wall and the surrounding alveoli. Over time, reticular fibers exist in the cell focus at the beginning, and then, tiny amounts of collagenous fibers form, which turn the coal dust cell focus into the coal dust fibrosis focus.

Perifocal emphysem is another pathological characteristic of CWP. There are two types of emphysema that are common in CWP. One is the localized emphysema, which is dispersed in the expanding air cavity by the coal macula. The other is lobule central emphysema, which is an expanding aerated chamber in the center lobules around the coal or coal dust focus. The formation of lobule central emphysema is attributed in accumulation of coal dust and dust cells around the secondary respiratory bronchioles, which damages smooth muscle of vessel wall and lead to the perifocal emphysema. If the entire acinus distal to the respiratory bronchioles is destructed, it becomes the panlobular emphysema.

Coal silicotic nodule is marked by the 2－5 mm or larger round or irregular shape nodule, which is black, solid, slightly raised to the surface in the lung slice. Microscopically, the typical coal silicotic nodule's center is composed with collagen fibers arranged in swirl surrounding deposited coal dusts, coal dust cells, fibroblast, reticular fibers and radiated collagen fibers. The atypical coal silicotic nodule shows bundles of irregular and loose collagen fibers without core. If high contents of free crystalline silica are inhaled, the typical "onion–skinned" silicotic nodules can be found histologically.

Diffuse interstitial fibrosis in scarring tissues can be found around the alveolar interval, interlobular septa, small blood vessels, bronchi, and under the pleura.

Large scale fibrosis is also known as progressive massive fibrosis (PMF), which is a signal of late stage CWP, but not the inevitable result of terminal CWP. Black mass lesions of 2 cm×2 cm×1 cm with consistent haphazardly arranged dense tissue are distributed mostly in the upper and posterior lungs, preferred to right lung, which is called as fusion shadow radiographically. Microscopically, the pathological type of PMF is classified into diffuse fibrosis with large pieces of scarring tissues around coal dust and coal dust cells without nodules, and predominant interstitial fibrosis with coal silicotic nodules. The massive fibrosis in CWP is different from that of silicosis, with more nodules and less interstitial fibrosis. Sometimes, there are cavities and compensatory emphysema around lesions, and marginal emphysema at the edge of the lung.

Pleural Change is mild－to－moderate incrassating. Beneath the visceral pleura, there are certain amounts of coal dust, coal patches, and coal silicotic nodules.

Ferruginous body can be found in the postmortem lung tissues of coal miners, and the case detection rate can be 83. 8%. The number of ferruginous bodies increase as the degree of the lesion deteriorated. The ferruginous body, also known as coal body, mainly consists of Al, Si, K, S, Ca, and Fe.

14.3.5.5　Clinical manifestations

The patients at the early stage generally are asymptomatic. With progressing, especially developing to progressive massive fibrosis or comorbidity of bronchus and lung infection, respiratory symptoms and signs may appear. For example, after engaging in manual labor or climbing a hill, shortness of breath can be aggravated. Based on pulmonary function testing, CWP patients can only suffer from hypofunction and dysfunction of ventilation, dispersion and gas exchange when extensive pulmonary fibrosis, airway stenosis, and especially alveolar mass destruction caused by compensatory emphysema.

(1) Imaging

1) Small opacities: Chest X–ray radiograph shows the small opacities with p and q type depending on the work duties and the type of dusts. The tunneling workers, who mainly are exposed to mixed dusts containing large amounts of free crystalline silica, show the typical silicosis performance–small round opacities. Coal mining workers, who are exposed to coal dust mixed with a small amount of rock dust, show atypical opacities with star–shape and low–density, which distributed in the middle area of the right lung firstly, followed by the middle of the left one and down area of the right one.

2) Irregular opacities: Irregular opacities are less common. Many of them are reticular. Some intensive ones are honeycombed, and the density is not high. The pathologic bases are coal dust, diffuse interstitial fibrosis, bronchiectasis and pulmonary lobular emphysema.

3) Large opacities: With progression, small opacities can coalesce to form large opacities (larger than 10 mm). Usually, the perifocal emphysema can be found around large opacities located in the middle area

of both sides of two lungs.

In addition, diffuse, localized and bubble emphysema can be observed in the image of CWP. Vesicular emphysema can be seen as a pile of small bubble shadows with a diameter of 1–5 mm, known as "white circle black dot", which can be seen in the late stage of the lung. Sometimes, it can be seen "eggshell" calcification or the mulberry calcification in the lymph node. Pleural thickening and its calcification are rare to be seen, but the costophrenic angle interlocking and adhesion are quite common.

(2) Diagnosis

Coal worker's pneumoconiosis is diagnosed and categorized according to Diagnosis of occupational pneumoconiosis (GBZ 70–2015) consistent with silicosis.

14.3.5.6   Rheumatoid pneumoconiosis (Caplan's Syndrome)

Rheumatoid pneumoconiosis refers to the patients who have rheumatoid arthritis combined with coal pneumoconiosis. The typical chest X–ray image is high density, well–defined uniform round opacities with clear edge. It is one of the complications of the coal worker's pneumoconiosis. In 1953, Dr. Caplan in the United Kingdom firstly described the specific lung shadow found in the lung of coal miners with pneumoconiosis, which is called Caplan's syndrome afterwards. It has been reported that rheumatoid pneumoconiosis patients account for 3.76% of coal worker's pneumoconiosis in China, whereas it accounts for 2.3% –6.2% in other countries. The etiology is not fully clear, but there is a tight relationship with rheumatoid arthritis. The pathological feature of Caplan's syndrome is rheumatoid pneumoconiosis nodules appearing in the setting of pre–existing mild pneumoconiosis. At its early stage, there can be collagen fiber hyperplasia. Over time, the lesions turn into particular necrosis very soon, and inflammatory reaction happens around the necrotic core in fibroblasts and rheumatoid granuloma formation. Large nodules are usually composed of several small nodules. The nodules' diameters are between 3–20 mm, and nodules can fuse to 50 mm. The light–colored area is more active inflammation, while the dark one is the necrotic zone, and the darker area is the coal dust accumulation zone. Immunological examination shows 65% of cases with positive rheumatoid factor. The serum albumin is decreased, while α_2-, $\gamma-$, and $\beta-$globulin are increased with the development of the disease. There are few clinical symptoms and signs in the patients, and only a few cases of pulmonary function have different degrees of damage. Chest X–ray radiograph can present characterized shadow. The lesions may be single or multiple, as round or oval dense shadow, and the boundary is clear, often in the middle and lower lung field. Multiple lesions are similar to metastatic tumors, but the central necrosis is surrounded by a thin wall, usually free of fluid, and a few can be calcified. The patients need to be differentially identified with tuberculosis, metastatic lung cancer, and third–stage pneumoconiosis. Patients may have complication of dyspnea, chest pain, pulmonary hypertension, right ventricular hypertrophy, and right heart failure. It is important to prevent rheumatic pneumoconiosis by making good personal protection, strengthening physical fitness, improving the immune function. Also timely and effectively controlling the infection is also a significant method. There is no radical cure for the disease. The principle of treatment is to exercise the function of joints to prevent joint deformity and muscle contraction under the circumstances of pain–controlling by drugs.

14.3.6   Other pneumoconiosis

A variety of inorganic powder and metal powder can result in pneumoconiosis. Besides pneumoconiosis mentioned before, there are other pneumoconiosis included in occupational disease lists in China such as graphite pneumoconiosis, carbon black pneumoconiosis, aluminosis, welder's pneumoconiosis, founder pneumoconiosis, pottery worker's pneumoconiosis. Of which, the definition, exposure chances, pathological features and clinical manifestations are summarized below (Table 14-5).

Table 14-5 The other pneumoconiosis listed in the occupational diseases in China

	Definition/Classification	Exposure chances	Pathological features	Clinic manifestation	Exposure limits
Graphite Pneumoconiosis	A systemic disease resulting from long-term (15-30 years) inhalation of high concentrations of productive graphite dust, which primarily trigger diffuse pulmonary 1) Graphite pneumoconiosis ($SiO_2 < 5\%$) 2) Graphite silicosis ($SiO_2 > 5\%$)	1) mining, crushing, flotation, drying, sieving and packing of the graphite ore 2) producing graphite-bearing products 3) using graphite as ingot coating, mold coating, reducing agent for atomic reactor 4) producing synthetic graphite, especially in packaging process	Gross Feature: dense, gray black or black, grainy nodules with the size of 2-3 mm; Lymph nodes at the hilum are black and enlarged Microscopically: graphite dust and dust cells are gathering around the bronchioles, alveoli, and small peripheral pulmonary bronchial, leading to the formation of graphite dust cell foci and focal emphysema, which is resemble to black lung	Early stage: mild symptoms, little signs and slow progression. oral cavity, naso-pharyngeal desiccation with cough; coughing up dark sputum but not much shortness of breath after labor Late stage: obstructive ventilation dysfunction Complications: Chronic bronchitis, bronchiectasis, pulmonary tuberculosis, emphysema, severe cardiopulmonary dysfunction Small opacities: p-type, less q-type, rare r-type	PC-TWA(total dusts): 4 mg/m³ PC-TWA (respirable dusts): 2 mg/m³
Carbon Black Pneumoconiosis	A systemic disease resulting from long-term (15-25 years) inhalation of high concentrations of carbon black dust	Carbon black dust is small and light with the size of 0.04-1.04 μm 1) producing carbon black, especially in sieving, package process 2) using carbon black as a pigment and reinforcing agent in making rubber tires and electrodes	Gross feature: Black dust nodules of 0.5-1 mm with ambiguous realm Microscopically: Diffuse interstitial fibrosis with carbon black dust foci containing piles of phagocytic cells, carbon-black dust and collagen fiber Focal emphysema is shown around respiratory bronchioles	No typical symptoms and signs. cough, expectoration, shortness of breath, centrilobular emphysema Obstructive ventilation dysfunction Small opacities: p-type, less s-type	PC-TWA(total dusts): 4 mg/m³

Continue to Table 14-5

	Definition/Classification	Exposure chances	Pathological features	Clinic manifestation	Exposure limits
Aluminosis	A systemic disease resulting from long-term (10-32 years) inhalation of high concentrations of aluminum dust or alumina dust	1) using aluminum powder in producing explosive, fuse primer 2) using alumina powder in producing cryolite, aluminum fluoride	Gross feature: Lung size is slightly reduced, the surface of which is gray black and hard. Pleural thickening, and gray fiber block, fiber strips, black macula and dust foci with unclear boundaries scattered on the section Microscopically: diffuse interstitial fibrosis & severe emphysema	Early stage: mild cough, shortness of breath, chest tightness, general fatigue, pulmonary infection, bronchopneumonia, fever, expectoration, and dry or wet rales Late Stage: limit or hybrid ventilation dysfunction Small opacities p-type	PC-TWA(aluminum): 3 mg/m^3 PC-TWA(alumina): 4 mg/m^3
Welder's Pneumoconiosis	A systemic disease resulting from long-term (15-20 years) inhalation of high concentrations of welding fume	Welding used in the settings including construction, mechanical processing, shipbuilding, national defense and other industries Higher concentration of dust presents in an airtight container such as boiler, oil tank or hull equipment	Gross feature: Increased lung volume and reduced elasticity. Irregular or star shaped dust focuses with diameter > 1 mm. Localized pleural thickening and emphysema Microscopically: 1-3 mm black dust spot or-2 mm nodules scattering in both of lungs, and often accompanied by the perifocal emphysema Iron staining positive, with iron oxide	Early stage: slight chest congestion, chest pain, cough, carbon sputum and shortness of breath Late stage: pulmonary emphysema, Obstructive ventilation dysfunction Small opacities: p-type	PC-TWA(total dusts): 4 mg/m^3
Founder Pneumoconiosis	The workers involving founder in casting and modelling inhale complex dusts with lower content of free SiO_2 for a long time (>20 years), which cause nodular type or dust macular type pulmonary damage accompanied by pulmonary interstitial fibrosis	Exposed to mixed dusts including clay, kaolinite, graphite, coal dust, lime-stone, talc dust with lower contents of free crystalline SiO_2	Similar with carbon pneumoconiosis and silicosis Gross feature: colored or black macula Microscopically: Dust macula around lobular centricity emphysema, typical or atypical silicon nodules	Early stage: no typical symptoms Late Stage: chest tightness, mild chest pain, cough, expectoration and shortness of breath Chronic bronchitis and emphysema Pulmonary function is rare damaged Small opacities: t-type, less s-type, p-type (lower lung zone)	

Continue to Table 14-5

	Definition/Classification	Exposure chances	Pathological features	Clinic manifestation	Exposure limits
Pottery Worker's Pneumoconiosis	A systemic disease resulting from long-term (> 25 years) inhalation of high concentrations of pottery dust free $SiO_2 < 8.7\% - 65\%$ particles<5 μm 70% –90%	Exposed to mixed dust containing quartz and silicates in producing pottery products	Gross feature: lung volume reduced and soft, gray brown dust macula of 1 – 4 mm scattering on the surface and section Microscopically: stellate or plastic dust macula and mixed dust nodules located around the respiratory bronchioles, peripheral and lobular central emphysema, Pleural thickening	Early stage: mild cough, little expectoration, chest tightness and shortness of breath after physical laboring or climbing, marked dyspnea in patients with obstructive emphysema Late Stage: Obvious dyspnea, cyanosis, palpitation Complications: Silicosis, tuberculosis Small opacities: s-, t-type	

14.3.7 Occupational disease-induced by organic dust

14.3.7.1 Introduction

Organic dusts refer to organic particles suspended in the air resulting from plants, animals and microorganisms. With the development of industry and agriculture, the organic dust exposure in industrial and agricultural production environment becomes more complicated, especially the appearance of large-scale intensive management and specialized production of modern agriculture, such as large-scale intensive cultivation instead of a small-scale dispersive cultivation, various agricultural products management instead of a single grain production, greenhouse planting of multiple seasons instead of single field production. There is a wide range of organic dust from plants and animals and diverse in components, usually mixed with microbial pathogenic substances, animal protein and waste, inorganic substances. Though organic dust induced diseases, with lower specificity, are common in population, once attacked, it would do harm to people' health to varying degrees. Organic dust mainly results in respiratory diseases, including acute or chronic respiratory system inflammation, chronic obstructive pulmonary disease (COPD), bronchial asthma, hypersensitivity pneumonitis, organic dust toxic syndrome (ODTS), byssinosis, as well as mixed pneumoconiosis, such as fur-induced mixed pneumoconiosis, wood dust induced nasal and vice nasal cancer.

(1) Sources of organic dust

Organic dust is mainly generated from the industrial and agricultural production, waste management, involving grain, crops, and straw reaping and processing, agricultural production transportation and storage, greenhouse cultivation, production and processing of tea, tobacco, dairy, wood cutting and cotton, linen and silk spinning or woolen or feather processing, pulp and paper manufacture, fur processing, animals slaughter and processing, food condiments production, sugar refining.

(2) Classification of organic dust

Organic dust is mainly divided into plant dust, animal dust and synthetic organic dust.

Plant dust refers to dust broken from plant in the process of industrial and agricultural processing, containing grain dust, plant fiber, wood dust, tea dust, bagasse dust, tobacco dust, etc.

Animal organic dust refers to dust generated in the process of animal feeding and slaughter, such as processing of animal fur, wool, feathers, bone, and silk, etc. It can be mainly divided into fur dust, silk dust, dust with animal protein and serum protein, other animal dust.

Artificial organic dusts have been widely used in many settings of industrial and agricultural production, national defense, and military production. As a consequence, the occupational hazards of synthetic organic dust has been attached much more importance on common people. Synthetic organic dust is primarily divided into synthetic fibrous dust and synthetic resinous dust.

14.3.7.2 Occupational diseases induced by organic dust

(1) Byssinosis

Byssinosis, also as "brown lung disease" or "Monday Fever", due to long-term exposure to vegetable dust like cotton and linen in the inadequately ventilated working environments, is belonging to airway obstructive diseases and characterized by distinctive chest tightness, with or without chest congestion and shortness of breath, accompanied by acute pulmonary ventilation function disorder. Besides, prolonged and recurrent attacks probably result in chronic pulmonary ventilation function damage.

1) Pathogenesis: The etiology and pathogenesis of byssinosis are not fully understood currently. The cotton, flax and hemp dust exposure can all lead to byssinosis. Besides cotton fibers, the cotton stipule, plant debris and microorganism like gram negative bacteria, to great extent affect the occurrence of byssinosis. The pathogenesis of byssinosis is mainly explained in the following three ways. ①Histamine release: Cotton dust inhaled is capable of causing excessive histamine release of lung tissue, leading to the typical symptom of bronchospasm, which can explain the acute symptoms of byssinosis to some extent, nonetheless hard to account for the symptoms of progression and chronic phase. ②Endotoxin: Endotoxin induced inflammation has been identified as important determinants of byssinosis, i. e., patients are infected by gram negative bacteria grow on the cotton and endotoxin, which can activate macrophages to produce bioactive substances, giving rise to neutrophil aggregation and a series of biological reactions, ultimately resulting in acute and chronic inflammation of lung tissue. ③Cell reactions: The cell reaction mainly explains that the lixivium of cotton dust is capable of activating macrophages, which secrete a variety of media to cause bronchospasm symptom.

2) Clinical Manifestation: Depending on the severity and prolonged nature of the exposure, any symptoms may be obvious on Monday and disappear at the end of the working day or in the more severe cases they will persist permanently. In the early stage, cough and fever can appear when workers are exposed to cotton dusts, especially on Monday or the first day back to work. With progressing, symptoms can last for a few days, even whole workdays, accompanied by cough and expectoration. In the terminal phase of byssinosis, it would develop into chronic airway obstruction symptoms, bronchitis, bronchiectasis, even pulmonary edema. Cotton dust induced pulmonary ventilation dysfunction mainly manifests as obstructive ventilation disorder. At the early stage, there is often a modest decrease in the first second forced expiratory volume (FEV1.0) over the work shift, similarly observed in the cotton workers without visible symptoms. At the late stage, chronic pulmonary function damage with the prolonged decreasing of FEV1.0. Furthermore, smoking may increase the hazard to respiratory function. Nonetheless, the chest X-ray image of byssinosis is lack of distinctive radiographic appearance.

3) Diagnosis: According to Diagnosis of Occupational Byssinosis (GBZ 56-2016), the diagnosis and stage standard of byssinosis are as follows: ① Suspected cases. Occasional chest tightness, with or without distinctive respiratory system symptoms such as chest congestion and shortness of breath; FEV1.0 decreasing observed but less than 10% during work shift. ② Class Ⅰ. Frequent chest tightness, with or without

distinctive respiratory system symptoms such as chest congestion and shortness of breath, on most of first days back at work or other days of the working week; FEV1. 0 decreasing obviously observed and exceeding 10% during work shift. ③ Class Ⅱ. Aggravated respiratory system symptoms, accompanied by chronic ventilation function disorder; FEV1. 0 and FVC (Forced vital capacity) less than 80% of predicted.

Treatment: The treatment to byssinosis mainly focuses on the control of obstructive respiratory symptoms. For suspected cases, regular physical examinations are needed to supervise the disease progression. As to class Ⅰ byssinosis patients, it focuses on timely symptomatic treatment and avoidance from dust environment if necessary. For class Ⅱ byssinosis patients, timely symptomatic treatment and avoidance from dust environment are both needed.

(2)Occupational hypersensitivity pneumonitis

Occupational hypersensitivity pneumonitis is one type of granuloma interstitial pneumonitis defined as inhalation of organic dusts adsorbed fungi, bacterial or animal protein. The typical pathological lesions are characterized as immunoreaction mediated inflammatory cells infiltration and granuloma formation in the lung tissue. The common types of occupational hypersensitivity pneumonitis include bagasosis, mushroom worker's lung, and bird breeder's lung, which are induced by some specific antigen such as thermophilic actinomycetes, aspergillus, micropolyspora faeni, avian proteins, and mushroom spores.

1) Pathology: In the acute phase of hypersensitivity pneumonitis, lymphocytes aggregation with increasing plasma cells and macrophages shows pulmonary alveolitis, interstitial pneumonia. In the subacute phase, non-caseating granuloma forms which need to be differentially diagnosed with sarcoidosis. With progressing, chronic patients present pulmonary interstitial fibrosis.

2) Pathogenesis: The pathogenesis of occupational hypersensitivity pneumonitis is attributed to the combination of type Ⅲ and type Ⅳ hypersensitivity. The collected evidence showed that precipitating IgG antibodies against specific antigen can be detected, antigen-antibody complex can be detected in the lung, positive antigen skin test, delayed antigenic bronchial stimulation test, mononuclear cells infiltration and granuloma formation, and activated macrophages mediated immunoreaction.

3) Clinical Manifestation: In the acute phase, symptoms can occur 4-8 hours after exposure to pathogenic organic dust. The patients usually report chills, fever, headache, shortness of breath, cough, significant chest tightness, which symptoms can relief or disappear 2-3 days after cessation of exposure. It is easy to be misdiagnosed as "flu". The characteristic vesicular sound or crepitus can be heard in the base of lungs. The positive results of serum precipitin test can be thought as a recent exposure biomarker. Considerable cases showed subacute symptoms, such as repeated attack of acute hypersensitivity, aggravated shortness of breath and cough after exposure to allergic antigen 2-3 months. Chest X-ray radiograph shows diffuse web shadow and small opacities. When developing to chronic stage, the patients show progressive dyspnea and reducing body weight. After years exposure and repeated attack, irreversible pulmonary fibrosis appears, accompanied by honeycombing lung, restrictive ventilation disorder and diffusion dysfunction.

4) Diagnosis: According to Diagnostic Criteria of Occupational Hypersensitivity Pneumonitis (GBZ 60-2014), the diagnosis and stage are as follows: ① Contact Reaction. after inhalation of provoking allergic agents for 4-8 hours, symptoms show chills, fever, cough, chest tightness, shortness of breath without pathological changes in the chest X-ray film. The symptoms can disappear after cessation of exposure for one week. ② Acute hypersensitivity pneumonitis. after inhalation of biological organic dusts or specific chemicals for a short time, the symptoms show dry cough, chest tightness, dyspnea, accompanied with high fever, chills, sweat, ache and pain, anorexia, headache and muscle pain. Inspiratory crackles can be heard with inflammatory cells infiltration at the both of lungs in the chest X-ray image. ③Chronic hypersensitivity pneu-

monitis. the patients have previous acute hypersensitivity pneumonitis history, or repeated inhalation of biological organic dusts or specific chemicals without detectable symptoms, show progressive dyspnea, cough, expectoration and body weight losing accompanied with fixed inspiratory crackles at both of lungs and interstitial pulmonary fibrosis in the image.

5) Treatment: The best treatment is to avoid exposure to the pathogenic allergic antigens. Corticosteroids may help to control symptoms.

(3) Organic Dust Toxic Syndrome

Organic dust toxic syndrome (ODTS) is defined as non-infectious respiratory inflammation induced by inhalation of high concentrations of organic dusts adsorbed gram-negative bacteria and its endotoxin for a short time. ODTS is a kind of self-healing disease and classified into hay fever, grain fever and mill fever. The occurrence of ODTS is aroused by activated macrophages and epithelial cells to secret inflammatory mediators such as IL-1, which can recruit neurophils aggregation and infiltration and lead to acute pneumonitis, furthermore, which can activate complement to induce macrophages secreting non-specific hydrolyase leading to alveolar edema and diffuse function disorder. Usually, the symptoms arise 4-6 hours after once exposure of high concentration of organic dust workplace. The main symptoms show "flu-like" syndromes including fever, chill, dry cough, headache, and joint pain, lasting for 1-2 days. The result of serum precipitin antibodies is mostly negative with positive respiratory tract stimulation test and reducing pulmonary ventilation function. ODTS is generally self-healing. The best preventive measure is to control exposure to organic dusts.

14.3.8   Other respiratory diseases

Besides occupational pneumoconiosis, occupational asthma, chronic obstructive pulmonary disease induced by chemical irritants, thesaurosis of metal dust, and hard metal lung disease are also listed as the occupational diseases in China.

14.3.8.1   Occupational asthma

Occupational asthma is defined as chronic respiratory tract inflammation resulting from inhalation of allergic agents suspended in the workplace environment, showing intermittent attack of wheezing, shortness of breath, chest tightness or cough. If stopping exposure, the symptoms are generally self-limiting or relieved after treatment.

(1) Exposure

Statistically, there are nearly 300 occupational allergens, which mean asthma provoking allergens suspended in the working environment, widely applied in the settings including chemical industry, artificial fibers, rubber, electronics, pharmacy, textile, farming, etc. There are eight occupational allergens listed in the Diagnostic Criteria of Occupational Asthma in China (GBZ 57-2008), including isocyanate, anhydride, polyamine, β-lactam antibiotics, persulphate salts, formaldehyde, platinum compound salts, and sisal hemp. The common occupational allergens include macromolecular antigen and small one. The macromolecular antigens originated from plant, animal, microbial protein, polysaccharide, glycoprotein and polypeptide can induce allergic asthma directly mediated by IgE antibodies. The small antigens primarily made of hapten or irritants can provoke allergic asthma or stimulatory asthma.

(2) Pathogenesis

The pathogenesis of occupational asthma is complicated, mainly involving hypersensitivity, pharmacological mechanism and neurogenic inflammation.

(3) Clinical Manifestation

The typical symptoms of occupational asthma closely related to working environment show cough, wheezing, chest tightness or nasitis, conjunctivitis, all of which worsen at work and improve during the time away from work, especially induced by macromolecular allergens. The small allergens inducing occupational asthma shows delayed respiratory symptoms after work and be easy to misdiagnose.

(4) Diagnosis

According to Diagnostic Criteria of Occupational Asthma in China (GBZ 57—2008), occupational asthma can be diagnosed.

(5) Treatment

The patients suffered from occupational asthma should leave immediately primary workplace containing occupational allergens, which is the best preventive measure to control symptoms. The prognosis is dependent on the severity and therapeutic sensitivity. Acute asthma patients may be treated using β_2-receptor stimulant, glucocorticoid, anticholinergic drugs, and aminophylline to relieve bronchospasm and control hypoxemia. To chronic asthma, anti-inflammation and comprehensive anti-asthma medication is needed.

14.3.8.2 Chronic obstructive pulmonary disease induced by chemical irritants

Chemicals irritants are toxic substances that may cause injuries to the skin, the eyes or the airways after exposure in lower concentrations. The injuries show that prickling nose or throat, cough, lacrimation, and red eyes, over time or after repeated exposure, developing into chronic respiratory inflammation. In the late stage, irreversible obstructive pulmonary function disorder is the typical signs, which can be defined as chronic obstructive pulmonary disease induced by occupational chemical irritants in the workplace for a long term.

Cause and Pathogenesis: The risk factors of COPD induced by occupational chemical irritants mainly include chloride, sulfur dioxide, nitrogen oxides, amine, formaldehyde, carbonyl chloride, monomethylamine, and phosphorus pentoxide. Smoking behavior can aggravate the pre-exist symptoms. The pathogenesis of this type of COPD is related with inflammatory respiratory tract reaction, imbalance between oxidizing and anti-oxidizing, imbalance between proteinase and anti-proteinase, and airway mucus hypersecretion.

Clinical Manifestation: The main symptoms of COPD exist as progressive cough, expectoration, and dyspnea after exercise. The early signs are atypical, but, in the late stage, cyanosis, barrel chest, prolonged breath-sound, rhonchi, and moist rale. Besides, COPD can arouse other adverse effect on health such as skeletal muscle atrophy.

Diagnosis: According to Diagnostic Criteria of COPD induced by Occupational Chemical Irritants in China (GBZ/T 237-2011), diagnosis can be made based on main evidences from irreversible obstructive ventilation dysfunction, which can be classified into four levels from mild to extreme severe calculated in FEV1% predict value with FEV1/FVC<70%. Meanwhile, the course of the COPD stages can be divided into acute exacerbation phase and stable phase according to severity of respiratory system symptoms.

Treatment: The patients diagnosed as COPD induced by occupational chemical irritants should leave the exposure working environment and get anti-inflammation.

14.3.8.3 Thesaurosis of metal dust

Thesaurosis induced by metal dusts is used to describe the inhalation accumulation of metal and its compounds (tin, iron, antimony and barium) dusts in the lungs in the settings of occupational exposure and classified as non-fibrous pneumoconiosis. Generally, deposited metal dusts may not induce typical lung lesions, occasionally accompanied with mild connective tissues hyperplasia, or pulmonary function abnormality. Once cessation of exposure, the symptoms can disappear or relieve. The main types of thesaurosis of metal dust are stannosis, antimony pneumoconiosis, siderosis and baritosis. The common radiographic characteristics of thesaurosis of metal dust show high dense, discrete small round opacities with clear boundaries in the chest X-ray image due to high radiopacity of metal, without obvious fibrosis, after cessation of exposure, the pathological shadows can disappear automatically. Meanwhile, the patients have no typical symptoms and signs. Presumably, the possible pathogenesis is that deposited metal dusts mainly produce foreign body reaction other than pulmonary fibrosis, which means metal dust and its compounds inhaled and engulfed by macrophages induce macrophagocytitis distributed in the terminal bronchiole and nearby alveolar cavities.

The four types of thesaurosis of metal dust are summarized as follows (Table 14-6).

Table 14-6   The four types of thesaurosis of metal dust

	Cause	Exposure	Clinical Manifestation	Imaging
Stannosis	Tin dust stannic oxides dust	Mining or melting Exposure time: 6-10 years	Early Stage: atypical symptoms and signs Late Stage: Cough, expectoration, fatigue and chest pain Mild emphysema Complications: Lung caner inflammation	Early Stage: Discrete, dense, small round opacities with clear boundaries, p-type, petal-shaped without small opacities fusion Late stage or severe: Irregular dense shadow discretely distributed along bronchus, "casting-like" fused shadows Irregular strip dense shadow discretely distributed along trachea annular cartilage, "coagulate-frost-like" fused shadows Horizontal line shadow (Kerley B line) with the length of 1-3 cm, and the width of 1-2 mm, distributed in the both of lower lateral lungs and costophrenic angle without hilum change
Antimony Pneumoconiosis	Antimony dust antimony compounds	Mining or melting Exposure time: 1-41 years	Pneumonia, bronchiolitis, bronchitis, laryngopharyngitis, perforation of nasal septum	Discrete, dense, small round opacities (0.5-2 mm) with dense web-like lung marking due to radiopacity of antimony
Siderosis	Iron dust Iron oxides dust	Mining or melting Exposure time: 10-20 years	Slowly progressing Cough, expectoration, chest tightness, dyspnea, wheezing, and chest pain Partly, pulmonary emphysema	Discrete, dense, small round or less irregular opacities without fusion shadow. Lung markings disappear partly or mostly. Dense hilum lymph nodules without enlargement. Partly, showing transverse line above diaphragm
Baritosis	Barium dust Barium sulfate dust	Mining or melting	atypical symptoms and signs occasionally, cough, expectoration, without shortness of breath and dyspnea	Short-term exposure: Extremely dense discrete dotted shadows/nodules sizing 1-3 mm, uniformly distribution Clear Kerley B line, dense hilum lymph nodules Shadow disappear or loose after cessation of exposure Long-term exposure: Large and hard shadow resemble to fusion shadow Shadow disappear or loose after cessation of exposure

14.3.8.4   Hard metal lung disease

Hard metal lung disease (HMLD) is defined as pulmonary interstitial disease induced by inhalation of hard metal or its alloy dusts including tungsten, titanium, and cobalt for a long term in the settings of working environment.

(1) Cause

The dusts of tungsten carbide alloys and cobalt alloy, which are the common hard metal alloys, can be created in the settings of processing and molding. The workers engaging in rare metal dusts have higher risk for interstitial lung diseases.

(2) Pathogenesis

The pathogenesis of HMLD is not fully clear. Presumably, hard metal dusts inhaled can activate macrophages, induce macrophages aggregation and form multinuclear giant cells, which can provoke inflammation and lead to pulmonary alveolitis. Furthermore, hard metal dusts can induce lung fibrosis.

(3) Clinic manifestation

Clinic features of HMLD are diversity. The typical symptoms show occupational asthma, partly, some patients show slowly progressive pulmonary interstitial disease. In the early stage, the main symptoms show allergic alveolitis such as cough, rhinitis, chest tightness, progressive dyspnea, fatigue, anorexia, and decreased body weight. Once leaving from exposure workplace, the symptoms and signs can disappear. If repeated exposure, it will develop into irreversible pulmonary interstitial fibrosis. Pulmonary function tests present restrictive ventilation disorder and diffuse disorder. Chest X-ray radiograph shows diffuse small nodules, small opacities. In the late stage, wide web or saclike shadow with tractive bronchiectasis exist in the X-ray film.

▶▶ *Summary*

Pneumoconiosis and other work-related pulmonary fibrosis are induced by occupational dusts exposure. The symptoms vary according to types and features of dusts, exposure intensity, and duration of exposure. The critically important factor of diagnosis to pneumoconiosis and other respiratory diseases is the exposure of industrial dusts in the workplace. What's more, the auxiliary clinical detection such as high-resolution X-ray and spirometer are necessary. In that, pneumoconiosis and other dusts-related pulmonary diseases could be hard to be cured, diseases prevention should be emphasized.

Practice questions:

(1) What is the pneumoconiosis?

(2) What are silicotic nodule and coal speckle?

(3) Please describe the diagnostic criteria of silicosis.

(4) What are the classic X-ray images of silicotic nodule and diffuse interstitial lung fibrosis?

(5) What is byssinosis? Please describe the classic clinical manifestation of byssinosis.

(6) How to prevent pneumoconiosis?

Zhang Qin

14.4   Occupational diseases induced by physical hazards

14.4.1   Heat stress

Body temperature is affected by five fundamental physical processes:

(1)Metabolism—Heat is generated by the biochemical reactions of metabolism.

(2)Evaporation—Heat is lost by evaporation of moisture from the skin and respiratory passages.

(3)Conduction—Heat is transferred to or from matter with which the body is in contact.

(4)Convection—Heat transfer by conduction is greatly facilitated when the body is immersed in a fluid medium (gas or liquid) because of the ability of substance to flow over body surfaces. Conduction in this context is called convection.

(5)Thermal radiation—Heat may be gained or lost due to thermal radiation. The body radiates heat into cold surroundings or gains heat from objects that radiate infrared and other wavelengths of electromagnetic radiation (for example, the sun or a heater). The process is independent of the temperature of matter in contact with the body.

14.4.1.1   Cause

Heat stress may result from alteration of any of the five physical processes involved in determining body temperature. In the occupational setting, heat is most often generated by hard work. Heat transfer is most often impaired by hot and humid air and thus the combination of hard work in a hot and humid environment is the most common scenario resulting in heat stress. Heat transfer can also be impaired by heavy clothing and, in particular, by chemical protective clothing regardless of environmental conditions. Environmental conditions can also be a source of heat. The most common source is the sun, but other common sources are other hot objects, such as engines, furnaces, and molten metal, transferring heat by infrared radiation. Radiant heat is transferred from the hotter to the cooler object, is attenuated by the inverse square of the distance between them, and can be blocked by any object impervious to infrared radiation.

14.4.1.2   Pathophysiology

The body must maintain a relatively constant body temperature in the approximate range from 35 ℃ to 38 ℃. Substantial deviations from normal core body temperatures cause adverse effects ranging from minor annoyance to life-threatening illness. The principal source of body heat is metabolism and as metabolism increases, such as during physical labor, more heat is generated. The acute physiological response to heat stress includes perspiration and dilation of the peripheral blood vessels. Perspiration increases cutaneous moisture, allowing greater evaporative cooling. Peripheral vasodilation reroutes blood flow toward the extremities and body surfaces, thereby enhancing transmission of heat from the body's core to peripheral body parts, from which it can be more readily lost. With continuing exposure to heat stress, a process of physiological adaptation takes place. Although maximal adaptation may take weeks, significant acclimatization occurs within a few days of the first exposure.

14.4.1.3   Clinical classification of heat stress

Heat stress occurs when core body temperature is elevated. Effects can be grouped into three major types, which differ in symptoms, prognosis, and treatment: heat stroke, heat cramps, and heat syncope.

(1) Heat stroke

The most serious illness caused by elevated temperature is heat stroke. Heat stroke, or hyperthermia, is a life-threatening disorder that results from a failure of the core body temperature-regulating system which may cause core temperature exceed to 40 ℃. Heat stroke is usually accompanied by hot and dry skin, mental confusion, convulsions, and unconsciousness. Classically, sweating is said to be absent or diminished, but many victims of clear-cut heatstroke perspire profusely. Death or irreversible organ damage frequently results; the fatality rate for heat stroke may be as high as 50%. A core body temperature above 42 ℃ for more than a few hours is usually fatal, depending on the person's health status. Early recognition and treatment of heat stroke will decrease the risk of death or damage to brain, liver, kidneys, or other organs. Heat stroke is an emergency and medical assistance should be obtained immediately. An approved first aid method for lowing body temperature is to remove the person to a cool and protected environment, remove the outer clothing, wet the skin with water, and fan vigorously. This treatment will maximize body cooling by evaporation and will prevent further body temperature increase while the patient is being transported to a hospital.

(2) Heat Cramps

Heat cramps are muscle cramps, particularly in the legs, arm, or abdominal muscles that occur during or shortly after exercise in a hot environment. They occur when individuals lost excessive amount of salt while sweating during high physical labor and high heat loads. Heat cramps decrease in frequency with athletic training and acclimatization to hot weather. Persons not acclimatized to heat may require additional salt. Increasing salt intake may be helpful.

(3) Heat Syncope

Heat syncope is a transient fall in blood pressure with an associated loss of consciousness. Heat syncope is alarming to the person, but is the least serious of the heat-induced disorders. Heat syncope is characterized by dizziness and/or fainting when immobile, usually standing in the heat for extended period. The condition occurs primarily in individuals who are not acclimatized to the heat, and it results from the pooling of blood in the dilated vessels of the skin and lower extremities with a resulting decrease in blood flow to the brain. Treatment consists of removal of the individual to a cooler area, if possible, and recumbent rest. Recovery is usually prompt and complete.

14.4.1.4 Epidemiology of heat-related illness

Prolonged spells of unusually hot weather can cause dramatic increases in mortality, particularly in the urban areas of temperate regions. Accurate measurement of the occurrence of nonfatal heat stress is unknown. The proportions of heat-related illness in all reported occupational diseases were 0.2%–0.6% from 2010 to 2017 in China. There is average of 32.6 occupational heat-related fatalities each year in the United State from 2000 to 2010; rates are highest in agriculture and construction industry (Table 14-7). In construction, those trades that require substantial manual labor and exposure to hot environment, such as roofers and construction laborers, experience highest rate of fatal injuries. Similarly agricultural workers who are required to perform substantial manual labor with exposure to hot environments experience an elevated rate of heat stress fatalities.

Table 14-7　Occupational heat-related fatality rates in the U. S. ,2000-2010,by Industry

Industry	NAICS code[a]	Average Yearly workers	Average yearly HRI deaths	Average rate per million workers/year	Rate ratio (95% CI)	Percent of all industry sector HRI deaths[b]
Agriculture, Forestry, Fishing, and Hunting	11	2,232,000	6.8	3.06	35. 2 （26. 3 – 47.0）	21.0%
Construction	23	10,503,000	12.0	1.13	13. 0 （10. 1 – 16.7）	36.8%
Support, Waste, and Remediation Services	56	5,846,000	3.3	0.56	6. 4 (4.4 9.4)	10.0%
All other industries	—	121,775,000	10.5	0.09	1.0 (referent)	32.3%

CI-Confidential Interval；HRI-Heat-related illness

[a] North American Industrial Classification System

[b] Numbers may not sum to 100% due to rounding

Source：Diane M. Gubernot, G. Brooke Anderson, and Katherine L. Hunting. Characterizing Occupational Heat–Related Mortality in the United States,2000-2010：An Analysis Using the Census of Fatal Occupational Injuries Database. Am J Ind Med. 2015,58(2)：203-211.

Retrospective reviews of death certificates and clinical records have shown that increases in cardiovascular,cerebrovascular,and respiratory diseases largely account for the heat-related increase. Some studies suggest that heat stress induces some degree of blood hypercoagulability. Thus,external heat may favor the development of thrombi and emboli and may cause an increase in fatal strokes and myocardial infarctions.

14. 4. 1. 5　Prevention of heat stress

Preventing heat stress requires a threefold strategy：Reducing the generation of heat by reducing the work load,reducing heat absorbed from the environment,and promoting heat transfer to the environment.

（1）Reduce the generation of heat

Since the principal source of heat in the occupational setting is metabolic heat,the principal means of reducing the generation of heat is by reducing the physical workload. standards recommended by NIOSH and ACGIH both rely on this method as the principal means for preventing occupational heat stress.

（2）Reduce heat absorbed from the environment

The most common environmental heat sources are hot objects that radiate heat and hot air that transfer heat by conduction and convection. Absorption of radiant heat can be controlled by shielding from the source and increasing the distance from the source. Absorption of heat from hot air （>36 ℃） can be prevented by isolating the work from environment,if it is possible.

（3）Promote heat transfer

Since the principal pathway for heat transfer is by sweat evaporation,it is important to promote evaporation and make sure this pathway is not obstructed. To do so,workers must have ample supplies of portable water to replace that loss by sweat. Strenuous work （>400 kCal/hr） may require a liter of water per hour to maintain body temperature. High humidity （more precisely,the partial pressure of water vapor） is a principal obstruction to sweat evaporation. Reducing humidity is an efficient means of promoting sweat evaporation,but doing so is feasible only in controlled environments,such as inside building,vehicles,booths,or a chemical protective suit. Workers who must don chemical protective ensemble （protective clothing,respirator, gloves, and boots) may be especially vulnerable to heat stress, regardless of environmental conditions. The ensemble that prevents penetration of toxic chemicals also prevents sweat evaporation. Hard work in such an ensemble can quickly elevate the risk of heat. In addition to the usual strategies, adjusted for chemical protective clothing, some form of artificial cooling device may be needed.

14.4.2　Hearing loss

Noise is hazardous to health mainly because it can damage the ear, but it may also influence other bodily functions. A temporary or permanent decrease in hearing acuity, such as that from noise exposure (noise induced hearing loss, NIHL), may impair speech communication. Noise can also mask speech and warning signals and thus poses a risk to safety and to the general health of workers.

14.4.2.1　Cause

Occasionally, a single traumatic exposure to noise typically having intensity in excess of 130 – 140 dB SPL (Sound Pressure Level) may cause hearing loss. More often, however, hearing loss is caused by repeated exposure to noise above 85 dB (A) over long periods, frequently as a mixture of impulsive and continuous–type noise. The amount of NIHL that is acquired is related to the intensity and durations of the noise exposure and the character of the noise (spectrum and time pattern). The character of the noise—whether it is continuous or transient and its spectrum—also play a role and different types of noise pose different degrees of risk to hearing, even though the overall intensity of the noises is the same; impulsive sounds such as that from gunshots generally pose a greater risk than continuous noise. Low–frequency sounds are considered to be less damaging than high–frequency sounds of the same physical intensity. Therefore, when noise intensity is measured with a sound–level meter for predicting its effect on hearing, a frequency weighting is used. The commonly used weighting (A–weighting) gives energy at low frequencies less weight than energy at high frequencies.

14.4.2.2　Pathophysiology

The first effect is noticed when an ear is exposed to sounds above certain intensity and for a certain time is a reduction in the ear's sensitivity (elevated hearing threshold). This reduction in hearing is greatest immediately after the exposure and decreases gradually after the exposure has ended. If the noise has not been too loud or the exposure not too long, hearing will gradually return to its original level. This kind of hearing loss is known as temporary threshold shift (TTS). TTS may be experienced after single exposures to high intensity sounds such as from explosions and from gunfire. If the noise is more intense than a certain value and/or the exposure time longer than a certain time, the hearing threshold never returns to its original value and a permanent threshold shift (PTS) would occurred.

While TTS probably results from temporary impairment of the function of the sensory cells in the cochlea (which is a part of the inner ear), PTS has been associated with irreversible damage to these cells. The usual mechanism of noise–induced hearing loss is gradual destruction of outer hair cells within the Organ of Corti (the sensory organ located within the cochlea). Exposure to loud noise as well as exposure to ototoxic chemicals elicits metabolic/biochemical activity within these hair cells. Metabolites known as reactive oxygen species (ROS) are generated as a byproduct of this activity. These metabolites are known to damage cell membranes, mitochondria, and DNA. With increased noise exposure, there is a corresponding increase in the production of ROS. Eventually, hair cells are unable to counter the damaging effects of the ROS. When this happens, programmed cell death occurs through a process called apoptosis. Sometimes acute traumatic exposure produces hearing loss in a single, sudden blast. In this case, the high sound pressure levels are thought to cause direct, mechanical damage to the hair cells, also leading to cell death.

14.4.2.3 Epidemiology of hearing loss

It has been estimated that there are at least 10 million workers exposed to noise levels greater than 85 dB (A) in China. The proportions of hearing loss in all reported occupational diseases were 1.2% - 4.0% from 2005 to 2017. It has been estimated that there are at least 5 million, and perhaps as many as 30 million, Americans occupationally exposed to noise levels greater than 85 dB (A). Approximately 50% of all occupational noise exposures occur to manufacturing and utilities workers; 20% to transportation workers; and the remainder to workers in agriculture, construction, mining, and the military. Given at least 10 years of noise exposure at 85 dB (A), 8% of workers will develop a material hearing impairment (per the NOISH definition) by age 65. The figure rises to 22%, 38%, and 44% with exposures of 90, 95, and 100 dB (A), respectively. According to the NIH, approximately one-third of all hearing losses can be attributed at least in part to noise exposure, and the most common source of excessive noise exposure is work. The impact of hearing impairment on occupational safety and health was underscored by a recent finding that sensory impairment-particularly hearing loss—is associated with a substantially increased risk of occupational injury.

Although hearing normally declines with age, the average, healthy, non-noise-exposed person will have essentially normal hearing at least up to age 60. According to the American National Standards Institute (ANSI), the median hearing level averaged across 1,000, 2,000, 3,000, and 4,000 Hz for non-exposed 60-year-old males is 17 dB HL (Hearing Level) and females, 12 dB HL. Thus, aging alone should not prevent the average person from enjoying normal hearing throughout to be additive. Because of this and because older workers tend to have greater lifetime noise exposures, the prevalence of occupational hearing loss increases with age.

Individuals vary in their susceptibility to hearing loss. The prevalence of hearing impairment is greater among whites than blacks and higher among males than females. However, there is currently no reliable way to identify particular individuals who may be most susceptible to noise-induced hearing loss.

14.4.2.4 Prevention of hearing loss

Because permanent noise-induced hearing loss is irreversible, prevention is the only way of reducing the burden of this occupational disease.

In the United States, legislation that covers noise includes the Federal Aviation Act of 1958, the 1969 Amendment of the Walsh-Healy Public Contracts Act, the Occupational Safety and Health Act of 1970, the Noise Control Act of 1972, and the Mine Safety and Health Act of 1978. These acts require certain agencies to regulate noise. In Europe, legislation in various countries regarding the limitations on industrial noise has largely been guided by recommendations made by the International Organization for Standardization (ISO). The maximal noise level and duration accepted in most industrial countries is either 85 or 90 dB (A), for 8 hours a day, 5 days a week. In Europe the 85 dB (A) level is more common. In the United States 90 dB (A) is the accepted level stated by the Occupational Safety and Health Administration (OSHA), although certain measures have to be taken if workers are exposed to noise levels above 85 dB (A). The National Institute for Occupational Safety and Health (NIOSH) has recently issued a recommendation that has 85 dB (A) as the limit of accepted exposure level.

Noise measurement is necessary to identify overexposed workers, and should be repeated biennially or sooner if there is a change in equipment or work practices. If hazardous exposure levels are noted, the best strategy is to use engineering controls to reduce noise at the source or shield the worker from the noise. There are many ways to apply engineering controls. Typical approaches involve reducing noise at the source, interrupting the noise path, reducing reverberation, and reducing structure-borne vibration. Nevertheless, implement administrative controls are helpful, such as by scheduling activities at times or locations chosen to minimize workers' exposures, and implementing "buy quiet" policies. When engineering and administrative controls fail to reduce noise to safe levels, exposures must be reduced through hearing protective devices (HPDs), such as earplugs, earmuffs, and canal caps.

Audiometric testing is necessary to monitor workers' hearing. A baseline hearing test should be obtained at the beginning of employment, and monitoring audiograms should be obtained at least annually to identify any change in hearing that might indicate under protection from the noise. Monitoring audiograms are best obtained towards the end of the work shift in order to identify temporary threshold shifts before they become permanent. The annual hearing test is also an excellent opportunity to provide individual worker training and education.

14.4.3 Hand-arm vibration syndrome

Hand-arm vibration syndrome (HAVS) is also known as vibration-induced white finger, traumatic vasospastic disease, or secondary Raynaud's phenomenon of occupational origin. It is a disorder of the blood vessels and nerves in the fingers that is caused by vibration transmitted directly to the hands ("segmental vibration") by tools, parts, or work surfaces. Reduced handgrip strength and hearing loss have also been noted in some groups of exposed workers.

14.4.3.1 Cause

The cause of this syndrome is the direct physical transmission of vibration from a mechanical object to the hand and arm. This occurs through the use of vibrating hand tools or through other hand or arm exposure to segmental vibration, such as that transmitted through a truck or bus steering wheel or a part held to a grinding wheel. Depending on vibration intensity (acceleration), exposure for as little as 1 month is sufficient to initiate the disease process. Latency from first exposure to onset of blanching can range from 1 to 30 years, depending on the daily duration, frequency, and intensity of vibration and on work practices. Therefore, the shorter the latency period until onset, the more severe the expected syndrome if exposure continues. Chronic exposure to cold temperatures or damp conditions, especially during exposure to vibration, exacerbates its effects.

14.4.3.2 Pathophysiology

Circulatory and neurological effects result both from exposure of the hand to vibration, although the exact physiological mechanism is not known. Vibration appears to cause direct injury to peripheral nerves, resulting in the numbness of fingers. Decreased sensation in the hands may be secondary to constriction of the blood vessels, causing ischemia of peripheral nerves. Other physiological and chemical blood vessel changes have been documented, but their causal role is not clear.

An additional mechanism, the tonic vibration reflex (TVR), appears to contribute to soft-tissue damage by affecting tendon function. Vibration interferes with the sensitivity of nerve endings that enable one to sense the force exerted by a tendon. When the hand holds a vibrating object and this sensory feedback is disrupted, muscles are signaled to exert more force than is necessary to grip the object, increasing the strain on the tendons. The tighter grip also increases the amount of vibration transmitted to the hand, resulting in more nerve and blood vessel damage. Tendon nerve endings then lose even more sensitivity and the control reflex is even further disrupted.

14.4.3.3 Epidemiology of hand-arm vibration syndrome

The industries with the highest numbers of workers probably exposed to sources of segmental vibration are construction, farming, and truck and automobile manufacturing. Any worker using a powered hand tool, such as a chain saw, pneumatic drill, chipping hammer, jack hammer, grinder, buffer, or polisher, should be considered at risk.

According to NIOSH estimates, approximately 1.5 million workers in the United States were potentially exposed to vibrating hand tools or other sources of segmental vibration in 1989 and therefore at risk of developing HAVS. A study in 2000 found that 14% of the working population in Great Britain affected by HAVS, 32% in men and 4% in women. Other prevalence estimated range from 20% to 100% among workers exposed to segmental vibration for at least 1 year; however, the intermittent nature of symptoms in the early stages leads to substantial underreporting.

14.4.3.4 Prevention of hand—arm vibration syndrome

Primary prevention consists of measures to reduce exposure to sources of vibration. Redesign of production processes and work methods can help minimize use of vibrating hand tools or equipment. For example, improved quality of metal casings could reduce the need for later grinding and polishing. Where vibration cannot be eliminated from the workplace, engineering controls, work practices, and administrative controls should be considered to reduce the intensity and duration of exposure.

Secondary preventive measures include encouraging workers to report symptoms to their physicians or to the workplace medical service. All workers who use vibrating hand tools should be examined for signs and symptoms of HAVS; work histories should specifically include questions about previous exposure to segmental vibration. Workers with preexisting signs or symptoms should not be assigned to work with vibrating tools. Exposed workers and their supervisors should be informed of the symptoms of HAVS. If tingling, numbness, or blanching occurs, the worker should seek medical attention promptly and should be reassigned to work with little or no exposure to vibration. The jobs of affected workers should be evaluated for implementation of engineering controls. Health care providers should be trained in interview and clinical examination procedures necessary to identify occupational HAVS.

Tertiary measures include calcium channel antagonists to produce peripheral vasodilation. Carpal tunnel syndrome and HAVS sensorineural symptoms are frequently confused. However, carpal tunnel syndrome surgery has shown poor results for cases of neuropathy induced through vibrating hand tools. Reduced grip strength following this surgery may be particularly burdensome for such workers attempting to return to employment.

14.4.4 Diseases induced by non—ionizing radiation

The term non—ionizing radiation refers to several forms of electromagnetic radiation of wavelengths longer than those of ionizing radiation. As wavelength lengthens, the energy value of electromagnetic radiation decreases, and all non—ionizing forms of radiation have less energy than cosmic, gamma, and X—radiation. In order of increasing wavelength, non—ionizing radiation includes ultraviolet (UV) radiation, visible light, infrared radiation, microwave radiation, and radiofrequency radiation. The latter two are often treated as a single category. Laser is an artificial form of non—ionizing radiation with special properties of monochromatic light and low divergence.

14.4.4.1 Ultraviolet Radiation (UVR)

The sun is the major source of UV exposure for most workers. Artificial sources include welding arcs, fluorescent lights, plasma jets, and ultraviolet lights ("black lights"). The amount of UVR reaching the earth varies greatly as a function of time of day, season, atmospheric condition, and geographical position. Window glass and light clothing efficiently filter out ultraviolet radiation.

(1) Cause

UVR is the portion of the electromagnetic spectrum that falls between x-rays and visible light, with wavelengths between 160 and 400 nanometers. The ultraviolet spectrum is further subdivided into UV-A (320-400 nm), UV-B (280-320 nm), and UV-C (160-280 nm). UV-C radiation with the lowest wavelength, and thus the highest energy within the UVR spectrum, actually has sufficient energy to ionize target molecules. Except for the sunlight, there is a wide range of potential occupational exposures to ultraviolet radiation in both outdoor work and industrial settings, such as aircraft workers, glass blowers, metal casting inspectors, and food irradiators.

(2) Pathophysiology

The most common acute effects from UVR exposure are to cause the skin and eyes injury. Eye injury is most common, which is the result of thermal injury, increasing with proximity to source and strength. Skin injury is predominantly photochemical, with injury caused by the products of photochemical reaction with the cell, and potentiated by photosensitizing agents. Sunburn is caused by a resultant vasodilation of exposed skin tissues with a subsequent increase in blood flow. The chronic skin effects of UVR are a result of repeated injury leading to collagen destruction and loss of elasticity. With chronic exposure, the skin atrophies and many abnormal disorderly patterned cells are evident histologically. There areas may be considered "premalignant," at high risk for skin cancer development. Most UVR-associated skin cancers are epithelial in nature, though some studies have shown links between malignant melanomas and UVR. Research also suggests that UVR exposure depresses immune system function.

(3) Epidemiology of disease induced by UVR

More than 90% of skin cancers occur on parts of the body exposed to sunlight. Approximately 40% of all cancers in the United States are skin cancers, and in general they are the most common malignancy in light-skinned populations. Rates for skin cancer vary from less than 2 cases per 100,000 in dark-skinned populations to more than 100 per 100,000 in South African whites and Australians. The incidence of skin cancer on a worldwide bases correlates with decreasing latitude. Great excesses of skin cancer occur among persons with outdoor occupations such as agricultural, forestry, and marine activity.

(4) Prevention

Artificial UV sources should be shielded to the greatest extent possible with materials appropriate for the source. Interlocking access panels are advisable with high-UV-producing sources. Workers operating near these sources must wear clothing with appropriate UV protection factors (UPFs) and goggles with protective qualities matches to the spectral distribution and intensity of the source. Overexposure to natural UVR should be avoided by wearing protective clothing and sunglasses. Most commercial sunscreens offer protection in the UV-B range, though sunscreens provide limited protection from benzophenone and anthranilate in the UV-A range. Opaque sunblock, such as zinc oxide and titanium dioxide, offer the most complete protection, reflecting up to 99% of the radiation in the UVR and visible spectrums, and may be essential if photosensitization.

14.4.4.2　Infrared Radiation (IRR)

Infrared radiation, of longer wavelength than visible light, ranges in wavelength from 700 nm to 1 mm. All objects above absolute zero radiate some infrared radiation. Objects of higher temperature radiate to objects of lower temperature; the sensation of a hot stove results from this. Infrared radiation is the most important part of the spectrum for the production of heat.

(1) Cause

IRR injury is caused by excess absorbed energy from electromagnetic radiation in the IRR region. Wavelengths less than 2,000 nm are responsible for most of the injurious effects of IRR. Occupational exposures to infrared radiation include bakers, foundry workers, chemists, solderers, steel mill workers, and welders.

(2) Pathophysiology

Like UVR, IRR causes damage primarily to the skin and eye. IRR with wavelengths less than 2,000 nm cause molecular excitation and vibration, which is converted to thermal energy in tissue, with subsequent localized injury. In the natural environment, IRR exposure is typically accompanied by a large amount visible light, which triggers the eyes' innate protective mechanisms. Conversely, occupational sources of IRR are often relatively void of visible light, which, coupled with the poor heat sensation and dissipation mechanism of the eye, increase the risk of injury.

(3) Epidemiology of diseases induced by IRR

Significant IRR exposure is nearly always associated with the occupational or laboratory setting, either directly through lamp sources or indirectly through heat sources. Occupations at highest risk for cataract formation are glassblowers and furnace workers. Workers who work with molten metal, drying or dehydrating processes, or thermal conditioning of surfaces are also at significant risk. The proportion of adverse effects that are occupationally related is not known.

(4) Prevention

Engineering controls are the mainstay of IRR protection, with source shielding an effective control. The IRR source should be properly shielded, and eyes should be protected with IRR filters.

14.4.4.3　Radiofrequency Radiation/Microwave (RFR/MW)

Radiofrequency radiation and microwave (RFR/MW) radiation covers the 100 – 300 GHz frequency band of the electromagnetic spectrum. The ambient intensity of the radiation is measured in milliwatts per square centimeter (mW/cm^2) or watts per square meter (W/m^2). Specific absorption rates (SARs) are used to quantify energy delivered to tissues and measured in watts per kilogram (W/kg).

(1) Cause

MW/RFR exposure is prevalent in many occupational settings, especially telecommunications, industries that utilize sealing and heating equipment, RF welding, surgical cautery, and medical diathermy applications. Currently, the most common sources of public exposure to RFR/MW radiation are mobile phones and their associated towers. Television and radio stations use more powerful signals to broadcast their programs. Other high-power sources include radars and satellite uplinks.

(2) Pathophysiology

RFR/MW causes tissue injury, at sufficient power intensity, through thermal effects. The thermal effects caused by RFR/MW exposure can cause cataract formation, testicular degeneration (and decreased sperm counts), focal tissue burns (including keratitis). Tissue injuries through non-thermal mechanisms, below the RFR/MW thermal injury threshold are a much controversial topic. Animal studies have shown that chronic exposure to RFR/MW at intensity levels insufficient to cause thermal injury has been associated with alterations in neurological function (including acute behavior changes), immune cell dysfunction, and possibly cancer. Human studies regarding the health effects of chronic low-intensity RFR/MW have shown mixed results and are difficult to interpret. Associations between RFR/MW exposure and human behavior, immune system dysfunction, reproductive dysfunction, blood-tissue dysfunction, headache, depression, fatigue, endocrine dysfunction, and cardiovascular-system dysfunction have been shown in some studies. The significance of these associations is a subject of investigation and debate.

Whether or not there are any deleterious effects of long-term exposure to microwave radiation remains an open question. The most important public health issue related to nonionizing electromagnetic radiation is the widespread use of mobile (cellular) phones. While much of the concern over mobile phones has been focused on cancer and acoustic neuromas, a number of other effects have also been reported. These include: DNA breaks, increasing the permeability of the blood−brain barrier, changes in brain activity and sleep patterns, activation of stress proteins and changes in reaction times.

(3) Epidemiology of disease induced by RFR/MW

Although RFR/MW exposure is prevalent in many occupational settings, there are far fewer high−quality epidemiological studies of RF/MW−exposed populations. Stanislaw Szmigielski of the Center for Radiobiology and Radiation Safety in Warsaw is the only researcher to ever run a major epidemiological study of military personnel occupationally exposed to RFR/MW radiation. Overall, he found that exposed soldiers had twice the expected rate of cancer, a statistically significant finding. For leukemia and lymphoma, the incidence was six times that of the controls, with even higher rates for younger (20−50−year−old) servicemen.

(4) Prevention

RFR/MW sources must be regularly monitored to detect and control "leakage" of the radiation. Screening should be done to appropriately counsel those with medical devices, which may be affected by RFR/MW. Appropriate shielding and engineering controls should be employed to reduce exposure at the RFR/MW source. Personal protective equipment (PPE) in the form of protective clothing and eyewear is not recommended as a strategy to reduce RFR/MW, as reflection can cause increased risk to others and open circuits on the wearer may actually increase risk. OSHA has established PELs (29 CFR 1910.97), which are based on the thermal power density threshold.

14.4.4.4 Laser radiation

Laser is an acronym of Light Amplification by the Stimulated Emission of Radiation, an artificially generated nonionizing radiation. Laser radiation is a focused beam of monochromatic (single−wavelength) photons, from the ultraviolet, visible, or infrared portion of the electromagnetic spectrum that have a high energy density. Laser radiation exhibits a low level of divergence, which allows energy transfer over great distances.

(1) Cause

Laser radiation is unique among forms of radiant energy in its low divergence and highly directional nature. Laser radiation is able to cause tissue injury over great distances when the beam path is crossed. Non−beam hazards are created when the laser creates a potential health hazard through interaction of the beam with another medium. These can range from metal fumes, toxic gases/vapors, electricity, plasma radiation, fires, and explosions.

(2) Pathophysiology

Thermal injury from laser exposure is caused by the direct absorption of the radiant energy creating movement of molecules within eye or skin tissue, which is dissipated as heat to the exposed tissue. Photochemical injury is also caused by visible light lasers up to 550 nm (blue through green). The products of light−induced chemical reactions within the tissues are responsible for the photochemical injury. Ocular damage can also occur indirectly from exposure to diffuse reflections from high−power lasers. Lasers producing nonvisible radiation can be particularly hazardous, given that exposure may not be readily apparent.

(3) Epidemiology of disease induced by laser

The use of lasers has increased dramatically in recent years, particularly in such areas as construction, industry, medicine, communications, entertainment, education, and the military. In the United States, all products containing lasers must be certified under the Federal Laser Product Performance Standard. Part of this standard requires that all laser products be classified from Class 1 to Class 4 in increasing order of power output, and thus injury risk. Any laser greater than Class 1 can cause eye injury by direct exposure; Class

4 lasers are high-power devices, which can also cause ocular injury through different reflection of the laser beam. The proportion of adverse effects that are occupationally related is not known.

(4) Prevention

Laser installations should be well marked and isolated, and should utilize attenuating or terminating interlocks when possible. Laser beams must be terminated by a nonreflective, fireproof material. Goggles can help only if they afford protection specific to the wavelength of the laser being used, and must not be utilized as a substitute for engineering controls. Proper worker education and surveillance eye exams are important components of the safety program.

14.4.5   Ionizing radiation and adverse effect

Ionizing radiations differ from other forms of radiant energy in being able to disrupt atoms and molecules on which they impinge, giving rise to ions and free radicals in the process. Ionizing radiation consists of short-wavelength, high-frequency electromagnetic radiations (X-rays and gamma rays) as well as various particulate radiations (electrons, protons, neutron, alpha particles, and other atomic particles).

14.4.5.1   Types of adverse health effects

Ionizing radiation can cause many types of adverse health effects, depending on the dose of radiation that is absorbed, the rate at which it is absorbed, the quality (linear energy transfer) of the radiation, and the conditions of exposure. Most of the adverse health effects of ionizing radiation, including various types of tissue injury, such as erythema of the skin, cataract of the lens, impairment of fertility, and depression of hematopoiesis, are produced only when the relevant threshold dose are exceeded. However, mutagenic and carcinogenic effects are assumed to have no threshold.

(1) Effects on genes and chromosomes

The frequency of mutations and chromosome aberrations appears to increase linearly with the dose of radiation in the low-to-intermediate dose range. Such changes are not pathognomonic of radiation exposure, however, since they can result from other causes. Furthermore, heritable effects of radiation have yet to be demonstrated in humans, and the dose required to double their frequency in human germ cells is estimated to be at least 1 Sievert.

(2) Effects on tissues

Mitotic inhibition and other cytological abnormalities are detectable almost immediately after exposure to a large dose of ionizing radiation. A dose that is large enough to kill a major percentage of progenitor cells in the marrow or intestinal mucosa, such as >2 Sieverts absorbed in a single brief exposure, will cause the acute radiation syndrome. The typical prodromal symptoms of this syndrome include anorexia, nausea, and vomiting during the first a few hours after exposure, followed by a symptom-free interval until the main phase of the illness. The main phase of the intestinal form of the illness typically begins 2-3 days after exposure, with abdominal pain, fever, and increasingly severe diarrhea, dehydration, toxemia, and shock, leading to death within 7-14 days. In the hematopoietic form, the main phase typically begins in the second or third week after exposure, with a reduction in white blood cells and platelets; if damage to the bone marrow has been severe enough, death from septicemia or exsanguination may occur between the fourth and sixth week after irradiation.

(3) Effects on the growth and development of the embryo

Embryonal and fetal tissues are unusually radiosensitive. Thus, intensive exposure in utero can cause prenatal death, various malformations, or other disturbances in growth and development, including mental retardation.

(4) Effects on the incidence of cancer

The incidence of many types of cancer may be increased by exposure to ionizing radiation. The induced cancers include leukemia and cancers of the thyroid, lung, breast, digestive tract, and bone. Such cancers don't appear until years or decades after exposure. They have no distinguishing features caused by radiation. For the most part, moreover, they could be detected only after relatively large doses (0.5-2.0 Sieverts) exposure. Therefore, the carcinogenic risks from low doses can be estimated only by interpolation or extrapolation from higher doses, based on assumptions about the dose-response relationship.

14.4.5.2 Epidemiology of diseases induced by ionizing radiation

Because of the relatively large doses that are required to elicit acute tissue reactions, the occurrence of such reactions is limited primarily to radiotherapy patients and heavily exposed radiation accident victims. Smaller doses, however, have been observed to increase the risks of lung cancer in underground hard-rock miners, leukemia in early radiologists, and cancers of additional types in various other exposed populations. The weight of existing evidence implies, moreover, that although less than 3% of all cancers in the United States can be attributed to natural background irradiation, up to 10% of lung cancers in the U.S. may result from exposure to radon in indoor air.

14.4.5.3 Prevention

The guiding principle in radiation protection holds that the dose should be kept as low as reasonably achievable. In addition, absolute limits have been set on the permissible doses to radiation workers and other members of the population. The doses equivalent (DE) limit that has been recommended to prevent the impairment of organ function has been set at 0.50 Sv (50 rem) per year for all organs other than thelens of the eye, for which the recommended annual DE limit has been set at 0.15 Sv (15 rem). To restrict the risks of mutagenic and carcinogenic effects to levels that are acceptably low, additional DE limits have been recommended for the various organs of the body, as well as for the body as a whole—which is 50 mSv (5 rem) in any one year, but no more than 20 mSv per year, on average.

In order to restrict radiation exposure to acceptable levels, radiation sources, facilities where they are produced or used, and work procedures must be designed accordingly. This requires thorough training and supervision of involved personnel, implementation of a well-conceived radiation protection program, and systematic health physics oversight and monitoring. Also needed is careful provisions for dealing with radiation accidents, emergencies, and other contingencies; systematic recording and updating of each worker's exposures; thorough labeling of all radiation sources and exposure fields; appropriate monitoring of facilities and interlocks to guard against inadvertent irradiation; and various other precautionary measures.

▶▶ *Summary*

The preventive measures taken against various kinds physical hazards are different. The general principle is to control physical hazards in the appropriate range of parameter.

Practice questions:

(1) State the fundamental physical processes affected body temperature.

(2) Describe the clinical classification of heat stress.

(3) Describe the pathophysiology of hearing loss induced by noise.

(4) Describe the principle of prevention of hand-arm vibration syndrome.

(5) Define the following terms: UVR, IRR, RFR/MW and laser radiation.

(6) Describe types of adverse health effects induced by ionizing radiation.

Yang Jin

14.5 Occupational cancers

14.5.1 Introduction

Occupational cancers are the cancers caused by occupational hazards in the workplace. Approximately 5%–10% of all human cancers are thought to be caused by occupational exposure to carcinogens. The risks within an occupationally exposed population may be much higher. Several cancers have been directly associated to occupational hazards, including chimney sweeps' carcinoma, lung cancer, mesothelioma, leukemia, and others. The first report of workplace exposures associated with human cancers, scrotum cancer among London chimney sweeps, was published by Percival Pott in 1775. The occupational carcinogens have not been identified at that time. However, the identification of occupational carcinogens is important at least in part because most occupational cancers are completely preventable with appropriate personnel practices and strict protective legislation.

Carcinogens are any substances, radionuclide or radiation that promotes carcinogenesis, the formation of cancer in mammals, including humans. The International Agency for Research on Cancer (IARC) has developed the most used classification system for carcinogens, in which carcinogens is divided into five groups. Group 1 carcinogens definitely cause cancer in humans. Group 2A is probably carcinogenic to humans, Group 2B is possibly carcinogenic, the carcinogenicity of Group 3 in humans is unclassifiable, and Group 4 is probably not carcinogenic to humans. Only a little more than 100 are classified as Group 1 cancer-causing substances, including ultraviolet radiation, benzene and nickel compounds, etc. Tables 14–8 and 14–9 list the IARC established and strongly suspected human occupational carcinogens, and examples of occurrence. There are several routes to identify potential human carcinogens, including human epidemiologic studies, evaluations done in animal models, in vitro testing systems, and analysis of structure–activity relationships, in which epidemiologic studies have the highest potential; however, they are difficult and expensive to carry out.

Occupational cancers are usually indistinguishable, histopathologically and symptomatically, from non-occupational cancers. Nevertheless, there are several characteristics for occupational carcinogens. Firstly, they tend to occur earlier than "spontaneous" cancers of the same sites. Secondly, exposure to the putative agent is repeated, but not necessarily continuous. Thirdly, the latent period is 10–40 years. Fourthly, the cancers are often multiple in a given organ. Lastly, the proportion of all cancers caused by occupation is in the range of 3%–8%, however, if one adds in the interaction of occupational exposures with other risk, the range doubles to 5%–15%.

The identification of relationship between occupational exposures and cancer is a challenging problem for several reasons. One issue is the long latency period between exposures to possible carcinogens and subsequent development of cancer. Latency refers to the period of time between the first exposure to a carcinogen and the development of a malignancy. Many human carcinogens are said to follow the "20–year rule", where the onset of an increase in malignancy rates is seen two decades after the onset of exposure. Another issue is the threshold of carcinogens. For many nonmalignant diseases there appears to be a threshold of exposure that be crossed before disease is seen in individuals. However, there is no threshold for carcinogens and the legally allowable workplace levels should not be considered safe. A third issue is that of multiple factor interaction. The multiple exposures to carcinogens can greatly increase the risk for individuals in certain types of developing cancers. The synergistic or multiple-factor interactions have been documented for a variety of carcinogenic substances acting together.

14.5.2 Occupationally associated cancer

14.5.2.1 Lung cancer

According to WHO statistics, 10% of lung cancer deaths worldwide are related to workplace risks. About half of the burden of occupational cancer is from lung cancer. Processes strongly associated with occupational lung cancer: aluminum production, coke production, coal gasification, underground hematite mining (radon), iron and steel founding, nickel refining (nickel oxides and sulfides), painters, and passive smoking. Agents (IARC Group 1) strongly associated with occupational lung cancer: arsenic compounds, hexavalent chromium compounds, asbestos, beryllium, cadmium compounds, ionizing radiation, crystalline silica, soots, and talc containing asbestiform fibers. Bis(chloromethyl)ether and chloromethyl methyl ether (technical grade) are strongly associated with lung (oat cell) cancer. "There is sufficient evidence in humans for the carcinogenicity of coal-tar pitch as encountered in paving and roofing. Coal-tar pitch as encountered in paving and roofing causes cancer of the lung. " Ionizing radiation was strongly associated with lung cancer in studies of Japanese A-bomb survivors, patients treated with radiation for Hodgkin's disease, underground miners, and Mayak workers with heavy exposure to plutonium. However, no associations were found in studies of radiologists, nuclear workers, uranium workers, and populations exposed to background radiation. IARC announced on June 12, 2012 that diesel exhaust had been reclassified as a Group 1 carcinogen and that the evidence was sufficient for lung cancer.

The primary lung cancer often causes cough, hemoptysis, wheezing, dyspnea, or pneumonitis secondary to obstruction. Tumor spread may cause tracheal obstruction or esophageal compression, and superior vena cava syndrome may result from compression of vascular structures. Non-specific symptoms, such as weight loss, anorexia, and fatigue, may be evident. The diagnosis of lung cancer may be made on the basis of sputum cytologic examination and flexible fiberoptic bronchoscopy. The chest radiograph is the most important tool for the diagnosis of lung cancer. The most effective method of reducing the mortality rate for lung cancer is primary prevention, which includes identification of etiologic agents in the workplace, adherence to strict workplace standards, and worker education. Medical monitoring in the workplace has been attempted as a model of secondary prevention to aid in early detection.

14.5.2.2 Bladder cancer

Bladder cancer accounts for approximately 5% of all malignant tumors. Use of tobacco is the leading risk factor for bladder cancer. The increase in cancer of the bladder is also considered secondary to the relationship between bladder and smoking. As with most cancers, the incidence of bladder cancer increases with age, with a peak incidence in the seventh decade. Suspected bladder carcinogens include benzidine-based dyes, O-toluidine, 4-chloro-O-toluidine, and MBOCA. Other occupational exposures associated with bladder cancer include PAHs (aluminum production, coal gasification, coal-tar pitches, benzo[a]pyrene, and diesel exhaust), and hair dyes (hairdresser or barber). Diesel exhaust had a positive association with bladder cancer in many case-control studies, but was negative in cohort studies of transportation workers. "An open question is whether occupational exposures in industries identified in the past as high risk can still be linked to an excess risk of bladder cancer. " Occupational carcinogens with strong evidence include 4-aminobiphenyl, benzidine, and 2-naphthylamine, aluminum production, coal gasification, magenta manufacture, and the rubber industry. Ingestion of arsenic contaminated drinking water is linked to bladder cancer. Previously classified as 2A, MBOCA was reclassified by IARC as Group 1 in 2012. "There is sufficient evidence in humans for the carcinogenicity of ortho – toluidine. ortho – Toluidine causes cancer of the urinary bladder. "

The most common presenting symptom of bladder cancer is hematuria and usually is painless, gross, and intermittent. Other symptoms include vesical irritability with increased frequency, dysuria, urgency, and nocturia. The diagnosis of bladder cancer bases on urinary cytologic examination. Prevention of exposure to known carcinogens is the most effective means of preventing occupational urinary tract cancer. The recommended means of control are by engineering methods aimed at zero exposure levels. The other means are by personal protective equipment. In addition, the appealing means of control is screening.

14.5.2.3 Skin cancer

The major risk for outdoor workers is exposure to ultraviolet light. Other agents carcinogenic to the skin include: PAHs (coal tar, shale oil, or mineral oils); arsenic (pesticide manufacturing; sheep dip; copper, lead or zinc smelting); and ionizing radiation (radiologists); arsenic exposure is associated with an increased risk of basal cell cancer after a long latency. Sun exposure increases risk for basal cell cancer, squamous cell cancer, and melanoma. Chronic arsenic poisoning causes keratoses of palms and soles, patchy hyperpigmentation, and skin cancer (squamous and basal cell). The evidence is strong for associations between the following agents or processes and occupational skin cancer: arsenic and compounds; coal tars and pitches; coal gasification; coke production; dibenz[a, h] anthracene; mineral oils, untreated and mildly treated; shale oils or shale−derived lubricants; solar radiation; and soots. Studies of ionizing radiation and skin cancer have found "meaningful associations" for Japanese A−bomb survivors, tinea capitis patients treated with radiation, and radiologists working in earlier decades.

Basal cell epithelioma frequently presents as a nodular or nodular−ulcerative lesion on the skin of the head and neck. The lesion generally is smooth, shiny, and translucent, with telangiectatic vessels just beneath the surface. It is usually not painful or tender. Basal cell carcinoma rarely metastasizes. Squamous cell carcinoma presents first in a premalignant stage characterized by actinic karatosis, a rough, reddened plaque on sun−exposed skin. Metastases are more common than from basal cell cancer. The most important step in prevention of occupation related skin cancers is avoidance of UV light. Protective clothing is the most effective barrier to UV radiation exposure in outdoor workers. Effective sunscreens should be used daily. Periodic examinations are recommended to detect the presence of malignant and premalignant skin lesions.

14.5.2.4 Other cancers

Leukemias represent 3% of all malignant neoplasms. Ionizing radiation, benzene, and cytotoxic drugs are known causes of acute leukemia. In atomic bomb survivors, the incidence of acute leukemias peaked at 2−5 years and declined after 10 years. After chemotherapy, the incidence peaks at 5 – 8 years. There is strong evidence for associations between the following and occupational leukemia: boot and shoe manufacture and repair, benzene, ionizing radiation, and ethylene oxide. In studies of ionizing radiation and leukemia, strong associations were found for Japanese A−bomb survivors, radiation treatments for spondylitis, and use of Thorotrast as a contrastagent. Meaningful associations were found for radiologists working in past decades and Mayak workers. Ionizing radiation increases risks for acute lymphocytic and acute myeloid leukemias and chronic myeloid leukemia, but not for chronic lymphocytic leukemia. "There is sufficient evidence in humans for a causal association of formaldehyde with leukemia". "Studies from the styrene−butadiene industry show an excess of leukaemia, and a dose−response relationship with cumulative exposure to butadiene, while studies from the monomer industry show an excess of haematolymphatic malignancies in general, attributable both to leukaemia and malignant lymphoma".

Agents associated with sino−nasal cancer include cigarette smoking, wood and leather dust, nickel refining, chromates, mustard gas manufacturing, isopropanol manufacturing (sulfuric acid mists), and possibly formaldehyde and welding. Softwood dust is associated with squamous cell carcinoma, and hardwood dust is associated with adenocarcinoma of the nasal cavity. An increased risk exists for sawmill workers, furniture workers, wood products workers, and carpenters. Sino-nasal cancer is associated with occupational exposure to nickel (refining), wood dusts (furniture making), boot and shoe dusts (manufacturing), hexavalent chromium (pigment manufacturing), and radium (dial painting). Strong evidence: Boot and shoe manufacture and repair; furniture and cabinet making; isopropanol manufacture, strong acid process (sulfuric acid); nickel refining (nickel oxides and sulfides); and wood dust. Suggestive evidence: chromium compounds, hexavalent; formaldehyde; and mineral oils, untreated and mildly treated.

Increased risk of angiosarcoma of the liver (ASL) was found in workers exposed to vinyl chloride while cleaning reactor vessels for the production of polyvinyl chloride. There is suggestive evidence that German vineyard workers exposed to arsenic in the 1930s and 1940s had increased incidence of angiosarcoma of the liver. This cancer occurs most commonly in middle-aged men, and the mean age at presentation is 53 years.

Bone cancer is an uncommon form of cancer that originates in the bone. Studies have identified increased death rates from bone cancer among former employees of nuclear facilities. Documented causes of radiation-induced bone cancer in humans include 226, 228-radium, 224-radium, plutonium, Thorotrast (thorium oxide), and radiotherapy. "Radiation-induced bone cancer appears, it seems, only at very high doses, and it is rarely reported at doses under 5 Gy." There was strong evidence of work-related bone cancer in radium dial painters and a "meaningful association" in Mayak workers who had very high exposure to plutonium.

14.5.3　Prevention of occupational cancer

Occupational cancers have been and continue to be a serious problem in workplace. Occupational exposures to carcinogenic substances are highly preventable. It is imperative that workers could be protected by reducing or eliminating exposure. In addition, workers should be educated about potential carcinogenic risks at their workplace. The best principles of occupational medicine, such as getting a good history of exposure, monitoring workplaces, undertaking appropriate medical surveillance, and educating workers, are all extremely important when dealing with potential carcinogens. According to the National Occupational Research Agenda Team, "Focus on occupational cancer research methods is important both because occupational factors play a significant role in a number of cancers, resulting in significant morbidity and mortality, and also because occupational cohorts often provide unique opportunities to evaluate health effects of occupational toxicants and understand the carcinogenic process in humans. Progress in occupational cancer will require interdisciplinary research involving epidemiologists, industrial hygienists, toxicologists, and molecular biologists".

▶▶ *Summary*

Occupational cancers are the cancers caused by occupational hazards in the workplace. Occupational cancers are usually indistinguishable, histopathologically and symptomatically, from non-occupational cancers. Nevertheless, there are several common characteristics for occupational carcinogens. Occupational cancers may include lung cancer, bladder cancer, and skin cancer, among others. Occupational exposures to carcinogenic substances are highly preventable.

Practice questions:

(1) Define the following terms: occupational cancers, carcinogenesis, and occupational carcinogens.

(2) State the characteristics for occupational carcinogens.

(3) Which occupational exposures are believed to increase the risk of cancer? Give five examples of such exposures.

(4) Describe three cancer diagnoses that have been linked to the work environment and discuss methods of their prevention.

(5) Describe work-related exposures associated with lung cancer.

Table 14-8   Established human occupational carcinogens (IARC group 1)

Industrial processes	
Aluminum production	
Auramine manufacturing	
Boot and shoe manufacturing and repair	
Coal gasification	
Coke production	
Furniture and cabinetmaking	
Iron and steel founding	
Isopropyl alcohol manufacturing (strong acid process)	
Magenta manufacturing	
Painting	
Rubber industry	
Underground hematite mining with radon exposure	
Chemicals and mixtures	Exposures examples of occurrence
Aflatoxins	Grains, peanuts
4-Aminoobiphenyl	Rubber industry
Arsenic and arsenic compounds	Insecticides
Asbestos	Insulation
Benzene	Chemical industry
Benzidine	Rubber and dye industries
Bis(chloromethyl) ether and chloromethyl methyl ether	Chemical industry
Chromium(VI) compounds	Metal plating, pigments
Coal tar pitches	Coal distillation
Coal tars	Coal distillation
Erionite	Environmental (Turkey)
Mineral oils	Machining, jute processing
Mustard gas	Production, war gas
β-Naphthylamine	Rubber and dye industries
Nickel compounds	Nickel refining and smelting
Radon and its decay products	Indoor environmentals, mining
Shale oils	Energy production
Soots	Chimneys, furnaces
Talc containing asbestiform fibers	Talc mining, pottery and manufacturing

Table 14-9   Strongly suspected human occupational carcinogens (IARC group 2A)

Industrial processes	
Vinyl chloride	Plastics industry
Petroleum refining(certain exposures)	
Insecticide application(nonarsenicals)	
Chemicals and mixtures	
Exposures examples of occurrence	
Acrylonitrile	Plastics industry
Benz[a]anthracene	Coal distillation
Benzidine-based dyes	Dye industry
Benzo[a]pyrene	Coal and petroleum-derived products
Beryllium and Be compounds	Be extraction, electronics
Cadmium and cadmium compounds	Battery and alloy manufacturing
Creosotes	Wood preservatives
Dibenz[a,h]anthracene	Coal distillation
Diesel engine exhaust	Motor vehicles
Diethyl sulfate	Petrochemical industry
Dimethylcarbamoyl chloride	Dimethylcarbamoyl chloride manufacturing
Dimethyl sulfate	Chemical industry
Epichlorhydrin	Resin manufacturing
Ethylene dibromide	Fumigant, gasoline additive
Ethylene oxide	Sterilizing agent
Formaldehyde	Building materials
4,4'-methylene bis(2-chloroaniline) (MBOCA)	Resin manufacturing
N-nitrosodiethylamine	Solvent
N-nitrosodimethylamine	Solvent
Polychlorinated biphenyls	Electrical equipment
Propylene oxide	Chemical industry
Silica, crystalline	Glass and porcelain manufacturing
Styrene oxide	Chemical industry
Vinyl bromide	Plastics industry

Meng Xiaojing

14.6 Job stress related disorders

14.6.1 Introduction

Psychosocial risks are a particular form of workplace hazard. According to the European Agency for Safety and Health at Work, psychosocial risk may result in work-related stress, burnout and depression.

14.6.2 Job stress and job stress-related diseases

An increasingly accepted definition of job stress is described as "a psychological state which is part of and reflects a wider process of interaction between the person and their work environment". In another word, occupational stress is a pattern of physiological, emotional cognitive, and behavioral responses that occur when workers are presented with work demands not matched to their knowledge, skills, or abilities and which challenge their ability to cope.

Workplace and occupational stress is an area that has drawn a great deal of attention. Stress within the working environment is not avoidable and therefore labelling stressful events as being the sole reason why an individual might be negatively affected in terms of their health would be inaccurate. It has long been recognized that certain forms of "positive stress" or "eustress", can result in increased mindful focus on the task in hand, and can be a rewarding experience. An example might be where a veterinary staff member regularly finds themselves "under pressure", but also regularly achieves positive, appreciated outcomes.

On the other hand, when an employee is repeatedly exposed to stress within their working environment and lacks the ability to adaptively cope with it, there is an increasing risk of damage to their psychological wellbeing or "distress". Long hours, tight deadlines, and ever-increasing demands can leave the employee feeling worried, drained, and overwhelmed. And when stress exceeds his ability to cope, it stops being helpful and starts causing damage to his mind and body—as well as to his job satisfaction. Excessive stress can interfere with his productivity and performance, impact his physical and emotional health, and affect his relationships and home life. It can even mean the difference between success and failure on the job.

Job stress exerts the effect through job strain. Job strain refers to the physical and psychological hardships that go along with a job when a worker has inadequate power to respond to the demands and expectations imposed upon him or her. It is characterized by a combination of high demands and low levels of control regarding one's job. A meta-analysis published in 2012 found a positive association between job strain and coronary heart disease risk. Another meta-analysis published in 2015 found a similar association between job strain and stroke; the association was especially strong for women. Job strain has also been found to increase the risk of higher blood pressure but not obesity.

Job strain has two primary consequences, acute stress response, including physiological, psychological and behavioral changes, and job stress-related illness, including depression, headaches, migraines, sleep disturbance, insomnia, backache, heart problem, stomach ulcers, chronic fatigue syndrome, fertility and menstrual problems.

14.6.2.1 Depression caused by stress

Stress can either cause depression or exacerbate it in those already suffering from the illness. Poor sleep brought on by stress can also trigger depression in some people.

14.6.2.2 Stress related headaches and migraines

When we are stressed, our body naturally tenses up; a bodily response to increased levels of hormones such as cortisol which control our fight or flight instinct. It is thought that tension is responsible for many of the headaches suffered, maybe as many as 80% and perhaps an even higher percentage for migraine headaches.

14.6.2.3 Stress-induced sleep disturbances and insomnia

Sleep deprivation has been used as a form of torture which perhaps illustrates the serious implications of lack of sleep. Lack of quality sleep alone will make us ill. The body repairs and rejuvenates itself while we sleep and if there isn't enough sleep, then the implications are obvious.

Poor sleeping patterns are a very common sign of stress. When we are anxious or over stimulated, we find it difficult to sleep.

14.6.2.4 Backache caused by stress

Most body aches including backaches are a form of stress induced illness. This is the most common result of constantly tense muscles which can lead to poor posture and body alignment. In addition, tense muscles are prone to injury and tear which will lead to soreness and general aches and pains.

14.6.2.5 Heart problems

The raised risk of cardiovascular problems from prolonged stress has been much in the news for several years now. Although the exact links are not known, it is accepted that they are there none the less.

14.6.2.6 Stress and high blood pressure

Continuously stress-induced high blood pressure increases the risk of stroke and coronary disease.

14.6.2.7 Colds and other infectious llnesses

It is known that there is a link between high stress levels and lowered immunity which may mean picking up every bug that's going. Although in most cases this isn't serious, it is believed that in the most ominous of cases the risk of cancer becomes higher. At present, research has being done on this to prove or disprove this theory.

14.6.2.8 Stomach ulcers caused by stress

Stress can lead to the secretion of excess acid which can harm the stomach wall and cause ulcers.

14.6.2.9 Stress related digestive disorders

It is thought that the muscle tension that leads to conditions such as backache and migraines can also affect the body internally. Digestive system muscle contractions can lead to stomach cramps, digestive disorders and Irritable Bowel Syndrome (IBS).

14.6.2.10 Chronic fatigue syndrome (CFS)

General fatigue and lethargy can arise from prolonged stress and in more severe cases will result in a chronic condition that has a serious knock on effect and other ill health implications.

14.6.2.11 Fertility problems and menstrual cycle disorders

Severe stress can have the effect of temporarily suspending the menstrual cycle so it stands to reason for affecting fertility.

14.6.3 Burnout

Burnout is a state of emotional, mental, and physical exhaustion caused by excessive and prolonged stress. It occurs when you feel overwhelmed, emotionally drained, and unable to meet constant demands. As the stress continues, you begin to lose the interest and motivation that led you to take on a certain role in the first place. Burnout reduces productivity and saps your energy, leaving you feeling increasingly helpless, hopeless, cynical, and resentful. Eventually, you may feel like you have nothing more to give.

14.6.3.1　Causes of burnout

Burnout often stems from your job. But anyone who feels overworked and undervalued is at risk for burnout—from the hardworking office worker who hasn't had a vacation in years, to the frazzled stay—at—home mom struggling to care for kids, housework, and an aging parent.

Your lifestyle and personality traits can also contribute to burnout. What you do in your downtime and how you look at the world can play just as big of a role in causing burnout as work or home demands.

(1) Work—related causes of burnout
- Feeling like you have little or no control over your work.
- Lack of recognition or reward for good work.
- Unclear or overly demanding job expectations.
- Doing work that's monotonous or unchallenging.
- Working in a chaotic or high—pressure environment.

(2) Lifestyle causes of burnout
- Working too much, without enough time for socializing or relaxing.
- Lack of close, supportive relationships.
- Taking on too many responsibilities, without enough help from others.
- Not getting enough sleep.

(3) Personality traits can contribute to burnout
- Perfectionistic tendencies; nothing is ever good enough.
- Pessimistic view of yourself and the world.
- The need to be in control; reluctance to delegate to others.
- High—achieving, type A personality.

14.6.3.2　Signs and symptoms of burnout

Most of us have days when we feel helpless, overloaded, or unappreciated—when dragging ourselves out of bed requires the determination of Hercules. If you feel like this most of the time, however, you may have burnout.

Burnout is a gradual process. The signs and symptoms are subtle at first, but they get worse as time goes on. Think of the early symptoms as red flags that something is wrong that needs to be addressed. If you pay attention and act to reduce your stress, you can prevent a major breakdown. If you ignore them, you'll eventually burn out.

(1) Physical signs and symptoms of burnout
- Feeling tired and drained most of the time.
- Lowered immunity, getting sick a lot.
- Frequent headaches or muscle pain.
- Change in appetite or sleep habits.

(2) Emotional signs and symptoms of burnout
- Sense of failure and self—doubt.
- Feeling helpless, trapped, and defeated.
- Detachment, feeling alone in the world.

- Loss of motivation.
- Increasingly cynical and negative outlook.
- Decreased satisfaction and sense of accomplishment.

(3) Behavioral signs and symptoms of burnout

- Withdrawing from responsibilities.
- Isolating yourself from others.
- Procrastinating, taking longer to get things done.
- Using food, drugs, or alcohol to cope.
- Taking out your frustrations on others.
- Skipping work or coming in late and leaving early.

14.6.4   Prevention of job stress

Stress is something which affects all of us at times and where it is temporary or manageable then will do little or no harm. However, where the stress is prolonged, it is clearly indicated that steps must be taken to address the issue before serious medical conditions arise.

Interventions against job stress can be divided into primary prevention, secondary prevention and tertiary prevention. Primary prevention is primarily about the prevention of stress factors and is directed towards workers (e. g. , stress control training), workplaces (job redesign, Occupational Safety and health strategies) or workers interacting with the workplace (e. g. , selection processes). Secondary prevention is primarily individual and prevents further stress reactions (such as employee assistance programming, treatment or counselling). Level 3 prevention is the treatment, recovery and return to work of stress-related diseases.

Ensuring adequate and restful sleep is one positive step to take. Meditation, relaxation techniques, yoga and massage can all help to manage stress levels. Regular exercise and a healthy diet will also contribute positively. Just simply taking time out and spending time doing things you enjoy are crucial to managing stress.

As stress related ailments are so often serious, it is advisable to seek medical advice in cases of severe or prolonged stress.

▶▶ *Summary*

Job stress is a new type of occupational hazard, which can induce occupational staff appear physiological, psychological, behavioral changes and burnout, jobstress-related diseases. Intervention job stress must follow tertiary prevention principle.

Practice questions:

(1) Please state the conception of job stress, job strain and burnout.

(2) How many kinds of outcome the job stress can cause?

(3) Please describe the symptoms and signs of burnout.

(4) what means tertiary prevention principle of job stress?

14.7   Work-related musculo skeletal disorders

14.7.1   Introduction

Work-related musculoskeletal disorders (WMSDs) are a group of painful disorders of muscles, tendons, and nerves. Carpal tunnel syndrome, tendonitis, thoracic outlet syndrome, and tension neck syndrome are examples.

For the purpose of developing injury prevention strategies, many health and safety agencies include only disorders that develop gradually and are caused by the overuse of the above constituents of the musculoskeletal system. The traumatic injuries of the muscles, tendons and nerves due to accidents are not considered to be WMSDs or are considered separately. However, there are organizations, such as the European Agency for Safety and Health at Work, that include acute traumas and fractures within in the WMSD group.

Here will discuss those injuries resulting from overuse and those that develop over time. Work activities which are frequent and repetitive, or activities with awkward postures cause these disorders which may be painful during work or at rest.

Almost all work requires the use of the arms and hands. Therefore, most WMSD affect the hands, wrists, elbows, neck, and shoulders. Work using the legs can lead to WMSD of the legs, hips, ankles, and feet. Some back problems also result from repetitive activities.

14.7.1.1   Mechanism of WMSD

(1) Tendon injury

Tendons consist of numerous bundles of fibres that attach muscles to bones. Tendon disorders related to repetitive or frequent work activities and awkward postures occur in two major categories—tendons with sheaths (Figure 14-1), found mainly in the hand and wrist; and tendons without sheaths (Figure 14-2), generally found around the shoulder, elbow, and forearm.

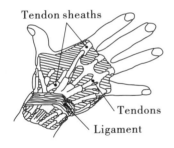

Figure 14-1   Finger tendons and their sheaths

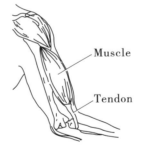

Figure 14-2   Tendon, muscle, bone unit

The inner walls of the sheaths contain cells that produce a slippery fluid to lubricate the tendon. With repetitive or excessive movement of the hand, the lubrication system may malfunction. It may not produce enough fluid, or it may produce a fluid with poor lubricating qualities. Failure of the lubricating system creates friction between the tendon and its sheath, causing inflammation and swelling of the tendon area. Repeated episodes of inflammation cause fibrous tissue to form. The fibrous tissue thickens the tendon sheath, and hinders tendon movement. Inflammation of the tendon sheath is known as tenosynovitis. When inflamed, a tendon sheath may swell up with lubricating fluid and cause a bump under the skin. This is referred to as a ganglion cyst.

Tendons without sheaths are vulnerable to repetitive motions and awkward postures. In fact, when a tendon is repeatedly tensed, some of its fibres can tear apart. The tendon becomes thickened and bumpy, causing tendonitis. In some cases, such as in the shoulder, tendons pass through a narrow space between bones. A sac called the bursa filled with lubricating fluid is inserted between the tendons and the bones as an anti-friction device. As the tendons become increasingly thickened and bumpy, the bursa is subject to a lot of friction and becomes inflamed. Inflammation of the bursa is known as bursitis.

(2) Nerve injury

Nerves carry signals from the brain to control activities of muscles. They also carry information about temperature, pain and touch from the body to the brain, and control bodily functions such as sweating and salivation. Nerves are surrounded by muscles, tendons, and ligaments. With repetitive motions and awkward postures, the tissues surrounding nerves become swollen, and squeeze or compress nerves (Figure 14-3 and Figure 14-4).

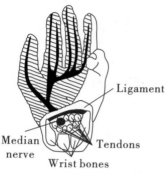

Figure 14-3　Wrist in natural

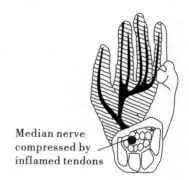

Figure 14-4　Wrist showing symptoms of carpal tunnel symptoms

Compression of a nerve causes muscle weakness, sensations of "pins and needles" and numbness. Dryness of skin, and poor circulation to the extremities, may also occur.

14.7.1.2　Symptoms of WMSDs

Pain is the most common symptom associated with WMSDs. In some cases, there may be joint stiffness, muscle tightness, redness and swelling of the affected area. Some workers may also experience sensations of "pins and needles", numbness, skin colour changes, and decreased sweating of the hands (Table 14-10).

WMSDs may progress in stages from mild to severe.

Table 14-10　Stage and symptoms of WMSDs

Stage	Symptoms
Early stage	Aching and tiredness of the affected limb occur during the work shift but disappear at night and during days off work. No reduction of work performance
Intermediate stage	Aching and tiredness occur early in the work shift and persist at night. Reduced capacity for repetitive work
Late stage	Aching, fatigue, and weakness persist at rest. Inability to sleep and to perform light duties

Not everyone goes through these stages in the same way. In fact, it may be difficult to say exactly when one stage ends and the next begins. The first pain is a signal that the muscles and tendons should rest and recover. Otherwise, an injury can become longstanding, and sometimes, irreversible. The earlier people recognize symptoms, the quicker they should respond to them (Table 14-11).

The table below outlines occupational risk factors and symptoms of the most common disorders of the upper body associated with WMSDs.

Table 14-11   Identified disorders, occupational risk factors and symptoms

Disorders	Occupational risk factors	Symptoms
Tendonitis/tenosynovitis	Repetitive wrist motions Repetitive shoulder motions Sustained hyper extension of arms Prolonged load on shoulders	Pain, weakness, swelling, burning sensation or dull ache over affected area
Epicondylitis (elbow tendonitis)	Repeated or forceful rotation of the forearm and bending of the wrist at the same time	Same symptoms as tendonitis
Carpal tunnel syndrome	Repetitive wrist motions	Pain, numbness, tingling, burning sensations, wasting of muscles at base of thumb, dry palm
DeQuervain's disease	Repetitive hand twisting and forceful gripping	Pain at the base of thumb
Thoracic outlet syndrome	Prolonged shoulder flexion Extending arms above shoulder height Carrying loads on the shoulder	Pain, numbness, swelling of the hands
Tension neck syndrome	Prolonged restricted posture	Pain

14.7.1.3   Recognition of WMSDs

The evaluation of WMSDs includes identifying workplace risks. Evaluation begins with a discussion of the person's employment and requires a detailed description of all the processes involved in a typical workday. Consideration is given to the frequency, intensity, duration, and regularity of each task performed at work.

Diagnosis of WMSDs is confirmed by performing laboratory and electronic tests that determine nerve or muscle damage. One such test, electroneuromyography (ENMG), encompasses two areas: electromyography (EMG) and nerve conduction velocity (NCV). Magnetic resonance imaging (MRI), an alternative to X-rays, provides images of tendons, ligaments, and muscles and improves the quality of the diagnostic information.

14.7.1.4   WMSDs treatment

(1) Restriction of movement

The first approach to treatment of WMSDs is to avoid the activities causing the injury. This often requires work restrictions. In some cases, transfer to a different job should be considered. A splint can also be used to restrict movements or to immobilize the injured joint. However, the use of splints in occupational situations requires extreme caution. If used inappropriately, splints can cause more damage than good. Splints are usually used for two reasons: to mechanically support a joint where an excessive load on the joint is anticipated, or to restrict the movement of the injured joint.

In the occupational context, splints should not be used as a mechanical support for the joint. Instead, the job should be redesigned to avoid the extreme load on the worker's joint in the first place. To be effective, the use of splints to immobilize an affected joint also requires that the work activity that caused the injury be stopped or changed. If injurious work continues, then the worker is exposed to risk of injury to other joints that have to compensate for the one that is splinted.

(2) Application of heat or cold

Applying heat or cold seems to relieve pain and may accelerate the repair process. Cold reduces pain and swelling and is recommended for injuries and inflammations (tissues that are swollen, red, hot and inflamed). The use of ice is not recommended in case of muscle pain (spasm) because cold temperature will contract the muscle even more. Application of ice on painful muscle is recommended only immediately after an injury occurred, and only for few days.

Heat is recommended for muscle pain relief. Heat increases the flow of blood which facilitates the elimination of lactic acid build up. It is not recommended for injuries with significant inflammation and swelling.

(3) Exercise

Stretching is beneficial because it promotes circulation and reduces muscle tension. However, people suffering from WMSDs should consult a physical therapist before exercising. Stretching or exercise programs can aggravate the existing condition if not properly designed.

(4) Medication and surgery

Anti-inflammatory drugs can reduce pain and inflammation. The doctor may try more elaborate treatments or even surgery if all other approaches fail.

14.7.1.5 WMSDs prevention

Hazards are best eliminated at the source; this is a fundamental principle of occupational health and safety. In the case of WMSDs, the prime source of hazard is the repetitiveness of work. Other components of work such as the applied force, fixed body positions, and the pace of work are also contributing factors. Therefore the main effort to protect workers from WMSDs should focus on avoiding repetitive patterns of work through job design which may include mechanization, job rotation, job enlargement and enrichment or teamwork. Where elimination of the repetitive patterns of work is not possible or practical, prevention strategies involving workplace layout, tool and equipment design, and work practices should be considered.

(1) Job design

1) Mechanization: One way to eliminate repetitive tasks is to mechanize the job. Where mechanization is not feasible or appropriate, other alternatives are available.

2) Job rotation: Job rotation is one possible approach. It requires workers to move between different tasks, at fixed or irregular periods of time. But it must be a rotation where workers do something completely different. Different tasks must engage different muscle groups in order to allow recovery for those already strained. However, job rotation alone will not be effective in reducing WMSDs if not combined with the proper design of workstations. And it will not be effective while the high pace of work persists.

3) Job enlargement and enrichment: Another approach is job enlargement. This increases the variety of tasks built into the job. It breaks the monotony of the job and avoids overloading one part of the body. Job enrichment involves more autonomy and control for the worker.

4) Team work: Team work can provide greater variety and more evenly distributed muscular work. The whole team is involved in the planning and allocation of the work. Each team member carries out a set of operations to complete the whole product, allowing the worker to alternate between tasks, hence, reducing the risk of WMSDs.

(2) Workplace design

The guiding principle in workplace design is to fit the workplace to the worker. Evaluation of the workplace can identify the source or sources of WMSD. Proper design of the workstation decreases the effort required of the worker to maintain a working position. Ideally, the workstation should be fully adjustable, providing a worker with the options to work in standing, sitting or sitting-standing positions, as well as fitting the worker's body size and shape. Detailed information about proper workplace design can be found in the OSH Answers documents Working in a Standing Position and Working in a Sitting Position.

（3）Tools and equipment design

Proper design of tools and equipment significantly decreases the force needed to complete the task.

Providing the worker with the proper jigs or fixtures for tasks that require holding elements saves a lot of muscular effort in awkward positions.

Good tools, maintained carefully and where necessary frequently changed, can also save a lot of muscle strain. More information about hand tools and preventing WMSD resulting from their use can be found in the OSH Answers document Hand Tool Ergonomics.

（4）Work practices

A well-designed job, supported by a well-designed workplace and proper tools, allows the worker to avoid unnecessary motion of the neck, shoulders and upper limbs. However, the actual performance of the tasks depends on individuals.

Training should be provided for workers who are involved in jobs that include repetitive tasks. Workers need to know how to adjust workstations to fit the tasks and their individual needs. Training should also emphasize the importance of rest periods and teach how to take advantage of short periods of time between tasks to relax the muscles, and how to consciously control muscle tension throughout the whole work shift.

Increased communication and support together with an increased ability of the worker to control his job (where possible) are work practices that improve worker's satisfaction and have a positive impact on reducing the risk of WMSDs.

14.7.2 Lower back pain

14.7.2.1 Introduction

Occupational low back pain has multifactorial etiology and elevated incidence and prevalence. It is characterized by pain of varying intensity and duration and can lead to work incapacity and invalidity. Low back pain causes workers suffering and increases the costs of employers and of social security and healthcare systems.

14.7.2.2 Epidemiology

Second only to headaches in the ranking of painful disorders that affect humans, low back pain is a common cause of morbidity and incapacity and is associated with significant social and economic impact. Epidemiological studies indicate that the prevalence of low back pain in the general population is between 50% and 80%. Low back pain is one of the principal causes of medical consultations, hospitalizations and surgical interventions and commonly affects men over the age of 40 and women between 50 and 60 years of age; in the case of women this is probably the result of the increased prevalence and the consequences of osteoporosis. Occupational low back pain is the largest single health problem related to work and absenteeism at most common cause of incapacity among workers aged less than 45, it primarily affects young adults and is responsible for approximately one quarter of all cases of premature invalidity. Since occupational lower back pain affects the economically active part of the population, is related to work incapacity, causes suffering to patients, involves costs due to lost productivity, days off work, medical and legal expenses and social security and insurance payments for invalidity, it should not only analyze as a medical issue, but also as a social and economic problem.

14.7.2.3 Classifications

Low back pain can be classified as either primary or secondary, with or without neurological involvement; mechanical degenerative; non-mechanical; inflammatory, infectious, metabolic, neoplastic or secondary to the effects of systemic diseases. There is also an important group of non-organic low back pain, which is extremely important in an occupational or compensation context, because of the frequency of secondary rewards related to these situations. Non-organic low back pain includes pain secondary to Munchausen syndrome (uncommon), simulated low back pain in the direct and conscious interest of obvious secondary rewards (usually financial) and psychosomatic low back pain, the consequences of psychological conflicts that are usually unconscious and which may or may not be concomitant with somatic complaints. Secondary rewards may also be related to psychosomatic back pain, although in a more complex manner than simple simulated pain. Low back pain can also be classified from the point of view of tissue damage of muscular or ligament origin: low back pain caused by fatigue of the paravertebral musculature and low back pain caused by muscle or ligament distension; originating in the spinal mobility and stability system: low back pain caused by lumbar spine torsion or unhealthy lumbar pelvic rhythm and low back pain caused by joint instability; originating in the intervertebral discs: low back pain caused by disc protrusion in the nucleus pulposus and low back pain caused by intervertebral disc hernia; or as predominantly psychological: low back pain as a form of psychosomatic conversion or with the objective of gaining secondary rewards.

The World Health Organization's International Classification of Impairments, Disabilities and Handicaps recognizes low back pain as a condition revealing loss or abnormality of the structure of the lumbar spine with psychological, physiological or anatomic etiology or, as a deficiency that causes a disability limiting or preventing full performance of physical activities. Still from the perspective of this classification, low back pain may be evidence of overuse, compressive or postural syndromes, be related to muscle imbalances, muscle weakness, reductions in amplitude or coordination of movements, increased tiredness or trunk instability.

In 1984, Schilling proposed a classification of work-related diseases based on three groups.

(1) Diseases in which is a necessary cause, such as accidents at work.

(2) Diseases in which occupation is one of the contributing factors or a risk factor.

(3) Diseases in which occupation aggravates or provokes a latent or preexisting disorder or a risk factor.

Within the Schilling classification, occupational low back pain may be classed as Schilling II, if work is considered to be one of the factors contributing to onset, or Schilling III, if work is considered to be an aggravating factor in a preexisting disorder or pathology.

Low back pain can also be classified according to the clarity with which an etiologic diagnosis is arrived at; specific, when the cause is well-defined, for example, caused by a case of disc herniation, or non specific, when the diagnosis is ill-defined. Nonspecific low back pain accounts for 80% of all cases recorded in adults and primarily affects people aged 20-55. It can be classified further as either static, when caused by poor posture (static overload), or kinetic, when caused by dynamic overload.

14.7.2.4 Etiology and risk factors

The causal factors most directly related with occupational low back pain are mechanical, postural, traumatic and psychosocial. Age, posture and fatigue at work are considered factors that contribute to the high percentage of low back pain relapses. Working long hours, heavy duties, lifting weights, lack of physical exercise and psychological problems are some of the factors that contribute to low back becoming chronic. Frequent complaints of pain in the lumbar spine are associated with paravertebral muscle tension caused by uncomfortable positions and premature degeneration of intervertebral discs due to excessive physical exertion. It is believed that many cases of low back pain are caused by abnormal pressures on the muscles and ligaments that support the spinal column. The dynamic forces related to displacements, carrying loads and using steps, ladders or stairs, and the static forces related to supporting heavy loads, to uncomfortable positions and to restriction of movement, can contribute to joint injuries and to intervertebral discs. Factors that have been identified as conferring a risk of occupational low back pain include cumulative traumas, dynamic activities related to movements of trunk flexion and rotation, heavy physical work, bending or squatting, macro traumas, lifting or carrying loads, exposure to long work shifts without pauses, whole-body vibrations and static and inadequate postures.

Many different factors have been identified as contributors to painful lumbar syndromes becoming chronic, in particular psychosocial factors, dissatisfaction with work, inactivity, obesity, smoking, performing heavy duties, depressive syndromes, employment lawsuits and tribunals, climatic changes, genetic and anthropological factors, changes in atmospheric pressure and temperature, postural habits and educational level. Risk factors for chronicity and incapacity from nonspecific low back pain include previous history of low back pain, absenteeism during the previous 12 months, pain irradiating to the legs, reduced amplitude leg elevation, signs of neurological involvement, reduced muscle strength and stamina of the trunk, physical unfitness, smoking, signs of depression and psychological stress, low job satisfaction, personal problems related to alcohol abuse, marital problems and financial difficulties.

Other authors emphasize the importance of psychosocial aspects, and conclude that there is a strong psychosocial factor in incapacity related to chronic low back pain that is so strong as to predict which patients with acute low back pain will require early intervention to prevent progression to a chronic state.

One study found that preexisting differences in health status were not associated with differences in the behavior of patients with chronic low back pain or with reported pain scales. Progression of symptoms and reported pain had a statistically significant relationship with secondary social and economic rewards. This finding is of fundamental importance for healthcare professionals involved in assessing these patients, in particular employment compensation doctors. The same study divided patients with chronic low back pain into classes, depending on their degree of social and economic interests (potential rewards); comparing groups of patients with the same degree of "social rewards", but with different secondary economic rewards. In a group with the same level of secondary economic rewards, the greater the secondary social reward was, the greater the number of days off sick, the greater the number of complaints of domestic incapacity and the more frequent depression, revealing that the secondary rewards had an equal influence on these parameters, irrespective of whether they were economic or social. The only differences observed between these groups were related to pain and nonspecific symptoms. Patients with chronic low back pain who were in the group with greater secondary social interests reported greater pain intensity and more nonspecific symptoms, which are common to diseases related to chronic anxiety.

This is a reminder of the undeniable fact that treatments directed exclusively at the physical component (rest, localized exercises, local heat, etc.) may not stimulate the desired therapeutic effects. Freud concluded that secondary rewards are the major problem for psychoanalytic treatment. This Freudian deduction is confirmed by the objective data, with relation to management of chronic low back pain. The intense modifications of behavior and of the clinical course of the disease caused by secondary rewards have also been investigated by other researchers.

There are also risk factors or factors associated with chronic low back pain, which are apparently bizarre, but which is equally necessary for specialists and compensation doctors and other professionals involved to be aware of. Foremost among these is the influence of solicitous spouses (or partners) on the pain reported or felt by the patient. Studies demonstrated that the greater the solicitousness (dedication, gentleness, detailed care) of the partners of patients with chronic low back pain, the greater the intensity of the pain they perceived and the greater the degree of incapacity they reported, irrespective of other factors. It should be pointed out that this factor is actually part of the secondary rewards, bearing in mind that the greater the pain or incapacity reported, the greater the patient's appeal for solicitousness, sympathy and attention from their partners or spouses. Finally, a recent study demonstrated that low back pain with gradual onset was significantly associated with psychological aspects and not with occupational activities.

14.7.2.5 Diagnosis

The elevated incidence of abnormal findings in imaging exams conducted on asymptomatic people mean that it is imperative to correlate these findings with information from patient history and physical examinations. It should also be pointed out that dissimulation maneuvers should generally be employed. A diagnosis of occupational low back pain also demands detailed occupational history taking and careful analysis of the way work is organized and of the environment in which it takes place.

It is not enough to simply wait for the patients to mention their complaints. They should be actively elicited. The physician must avoid adopting a posture of directing questioning exclusively at symptoms located in the lumbar region and expanded to thearsenal of questions in order to detect with greater precision the true origin of low back pain and characterize the non-organic symptoms that are often present, without being led by the appearance of imaging exams.

Sudden "loss of strength" of a muscle or group of muscles (instantaneous refusal at a certain point during a maneuver requiring strength) is behavior that is characteristic of non-organic pain. Diseases that cause muscle weakness manifest during physical examination with a consistent degree of loss of strength. This loss of strength (smooth and constant) is almost impossible to simulate people with non-organic symptoms.

The possibility of allodynia should always be investigated, and attention should be paid to possible histrionic facial expressions, trembling and exaggerated verbalization of pain, which is not to be expected even in painful diseases with organic causes. Some patients may exhibit increased diaphoresis or fainting. In general, fainting conforms to the characteristics of psychogenic syncope or non-epileptic psychogenic convulsions, in which patients' falls never result in head traumas (when observed directly by a physician).

Patients who claim to be unable to work because they are lame, should have signs of uneven shoe sole wear. Symmetrically worn soles (in the absence of heel deviations) may be a sign that the limping or claudication is non-organic. Using questionable or unprescribed ortheses, including walking sticks and kidney belts, is another sign associated with non-organic complaints, especially when there is no corresponding atrophy or cutaneous signs of prolonged use.

Checking for calluses on the hands may verify whether a worker is indeed leaving off physical activities. Lacerated hands and dirt under the nails are also useful signs. An absence of muscle atrophy after a prolonged period of inactivity and maintenance of muscle tone of the trunk and pectoral girdle are indications of non-organic pain.

The World Health Organization (WHO) warns that fibromyalgia should not be ignored as a common cause of chronic low back pain. The WHO publication states that "chronic back pain is a more difficult problem, which often has strong psychological overlay: work dissatisfaction, boredom, and a generous compensation system contribute to it. Among the diagnoses offered for chronic pain is fibromyalgia." It also states that "although disc protrusions detected on X-ray are often blamed, they rarely are responsible for the pain".

Many patients with fibromyalgia only complain of regional pain during consultations, and those with chronic low back pain should also be assessed for the possible presence of this syndrome, bearing in mind that patients with chronic low back pain tend to present with pain in other anatomic sites and nonspecific symptoms, when there are secondary interests.

Another publication, which supports the WHO's warnings, states that the appearance of intervertebral discs is not a predictive factor of greater occupational functional limitations. That study was conducted using a larger and more appropriate cohort than previous studies. It found that there was only a weak statistical association between moderate or severe disc abnormalities and poor prognosis. Not even a provocative discogram is capable of predicting any type of future adverse event related to back pain or to work. The authors concluded that the incapacity of patients with chronic low back pain, even those with significant abnormal intervertebral disc imaging findings, cannot be assessed on the basis of the appearance of their discs on imaging exams. The only factors capable of predicting incapacity related to chronic low back pain, with a significant statistical power, were psychosocial factors.

14.7.2.6   Prognosis

The occupational prognosis of patients with chronic low back pain should not be based on the appearance of images (degeneration of discs or osteophytes) of the lumbar spine of the patient or compensation seeker. Detection of signs suggestive of non-organic pain does not imply poor prognosis—if patients are treated properly. The presence of unfavorable psychosocial factors can predict a greater number of days off work, if the sufferer is not treated correctly. One group of researchers has proven that even patients with apparently refractory chronic low back pain strongly associated with psychosocial factors may exhibit significant improvements, if managed with multidisciplinary rehabilitation that adequately deals with the somatic symptoms and not just the regional physical pains or with supposed anatomic findings that are of little relevance. Another study supported these conclusions that treatment and improvement is possible with patients with chronic low back pain, even in long-term cases.

This raises the need to better publicize these technical concepts and evidence among compensation doctors, given the countless invalidity retirements for chronic low back pain. Systematically ignoring this medical evidence cannot have any other result than to substantially increase public expenditure, reducing the number of economically active people in the employment market and causing irreparable damage to the patients themselves, who would have a chance of being treated, were they not so labeled. In some cases it may be necessary to change employment activities, not retiring because of invalidity, but undergoing professional rehabilitation or simply changing duties.

The true findings have shown that there are solutions for chronic low back pain, which reveal that patients who won financial compensation (e. g., favorable employment tribunal or compensation claim outcomes) reported more intense low back pain than patients who apparently had the same condition but did not receive compensation. The rationale of cause and effect could be questioned, in this case, on a logical basis. It could be postulated that those with chronic low back pain who received financial compensation had more severe spinal injuries, justifying their financial gains. However, patients who received financial compensation did not have more severe injuries than those who did not receive it. Financial compensation does in fact have an influence on reported pain in the context of chronic low back pain.

14.7.2.7   Treatment

Elimination of risk factors, drug treatments, physiotherapy and patient reeducation are the foundations of occupational low back pain treatment.

With regard to physiotherapy, no scientific evidence has yet been found that electrotherapy with local heat or electrical stimulation has any proven relevance for the treatment of chronic low back pain. It is guided physical exercise that is most relevant to treatment. Although the majority of episodes of low back pain are self-limiting, they should be treated promptly and effectively in order to avoid progression to chronicity. Once specific causes have been ruled out, treatment should be centered on symptomatic pain control in order to allow functional recovery as quickly as possible. During the acute phase, rest is effective, but should not be prolonged because of the deleterious effects of inactivity on the locomotor system. Where there are inflammatory processes, treatment should cover, in addition to anti-inflammatory medication, alleviation of overloads and promotion of a working environment that is favorable to the reestablishment of good health. Corticoids can benefit patients with disc herniation and radicular involvement. Muscle relaxants are indicated in cases of acute low back pain with associated muscle contracture. Muscle relaxants combined with other anti-inflammatories and analgesics can provide additional pain relief. Tricyclic antidepressants can have good results in chronic low back pain cases, even when there is no depression present. Epidural infiltration of glucocorticoids, anesthetics or opiates is an option for the relief of acute radicular pain after conservative treatment has failed. Surgical treatment of low back and sciatic pain due to herniated discs is indicated in cases of significant neurological involvement or of absolute failure of clinical treatment.

Multidisciplinary treatment has proven effective for improving the prognosis of patients with chronic low back pain. However, physicians should be cautious about mentioning the influence of psychosocial factors to their patients, because of laypeople's limited understanding of the true origin of their low back pain, so that confronting patients directly (explaining that their symptoms are unrelated to the imaging results and actually have a psychological or socio-cultural origin) is unwise and should be avoided, since such action may result in patients who are unconvinced abandoning treatment or may even cause inappropriate and prejudicial behavior. Explanations should not devalue the symptoms reported by patients.

Since no differences have been detected between flexion or extension for the lumbar spine, it was established that nonspecific exercises should be recommended. One group of authors has concluded that physical rehabilitation for chronic low back pain should emphasize more intense exercise, canceling out the influence of these patients' tendency to limit their own movements (kinesiophobia). Correct physical activity effectively reduces pain, both anticipated pain (fear of pain), and pain induced by movement, and there is no doubt about the positive influence of physical exercise for reducing work incapacity.

14.7.2.8 Prevention

Prevention of occupational low back pain involves physical, organizational and cognitive measures. The physical measures should deal with the biomechanical aspects, posture at work, handling of material and loads, repetitive movements, job descriptions and occupational health and safety. Organizational prevention should focus on communication, resource management, job descriptions, the organization of time at work, teamwork, paradigms of work, cooperative working, organizational culture, organizational networking, teleworking and quality management. The cognitive component involves studying psychological processes, mental workload at work, decision making, specialist performance, man-machine interaction, stress and training. In this way, the psychosocial factors that contribute to the emergence of occupational low back pain can be prevented, including job dissatisfaction, monotonous work and the wear provoked by work overload, by the lack of autonomy and by competition with colleagues.

14.7.3 Carpal tunnel syndrome

Carpal tunnel syndrome (CTS) is a medical condition due to compression of the median nerve as it travels through the wrist at the carpal tunnel. The main symptoms are pain, numbness, and tingling, in the thumb, index finger, middle finger, and the thumb side of the ring fingers. Symptoms typically start gradually and during night. Pain may extend up the arm. Weak grip strength may occur and after a long period of time the muscles at the base of the thumb may waste away. In more than half of cases both sides are affected.

About 5% of people in the United States have carpal tunnel syndrome. It usually begins in adulthood and women are more commonly affected than men. Up to 33% of people may improve without specific treatment over approximately a year. Carpal tunnel syndrome was first fully described after World War Ⅱ.

14.7.3.1   Causes and epidemiology

(1) Causes

Most cases of CTS are of unknown cause. Carpal tunnel syndrome can be associated with any condition that causes pressure on the median nerve at the wrist. Some common conditions that can lead to CTS include obesity, hypothyroidism, arthritis, diabetes, prediabetes, and trauma. Genetics play a role. Other causes of this condition include intrinsic factors that exert pressure within the tunnel, and extrinsic factors (pressure exerted from outside the tunnel), which include benign tumors such as lipomas, ganglion, and vascular malformation.

The international debate regarding the relationship between CTS and repetitive motion in work is ongoing. The Occupational Safety and Health Administration (OSHA) has adopted rules and regulations regarding cumulative trauma disorders. Occupational risk factors of repetitive tasks, force, posture, and vibration have been cited. The relationship between work and CTS is controversial; in many locations, workers diagnosed with carpal tunnel syndrome are entitled to time off and compensation.

Some speculate that carpal tunnel syndrome is provoked by repetitive movement and manipulating activities and that the exposure can be cumulative. It has also been stated that symptoms are commonly exacerbated by forceful and repetitive use of the hand and wrists in industrial occupations, but it is unclear as to whether this refers to pain (which may not be due to carpal tunnel syndrome) or the more typical numbness symptoms.

A review of available scientific data by the National Institute for Occupational Safety and Health (NIOSH) indicated that job tasks that involve highly repetitive manual acts or specific wrist postures were associated with incidents of CTS, but causation was not established, and the distinction from work-related arm pains that are not carpal tunnel syndrome was not clear. It has been proposed that repetitive use of the arm can affect the biomechanics of the upper limb or cause damage to tissues. It has also been proposed that postural and spinal assessment along with ergonomic assessments should be included in the overall determination of the condition. Addressing these factors has been found to improve comfort in some studies. A 2010 survey by NIOSH showed that 2/3 of the 5 million carpal tunnel cases in the US were related to work. Women have more work-related carpal tunnel syndrome than men.

Speculation that CTS is work-related is based on claims such as CTS being found mostly in the working adult population, though evidence is lacking for this. For instance, in one recent representative series of a consecutive experience, most patients were older and not working. Based on the claimed increased incidence in the workplace, arm use is implicated, but the weight of evidence suggests that this is an inherent, genetic, slowly but inevitably progressive idiopathic peripheral mononeuropathy.

(2) Epidemiology

Carpal tunnel syndrome is estimated to affect one out of ten people during their lifetime and is the most common nerve compression syndrome. It accounts for about 90% of all nerve compression syndromes. In the U. S. ,5% of people have the carpal tunnel syndrome. Caucasians have the highest risk of CTS compared with other races such as non-white South Africans. Women suffer more from CTS than men with a ratio of 3 : 1 between the ages of 45-60 years. Only 10% of reported cases of CTS are younger than 30 years. Increasing age is a risk factor. CTS is also common in pregnancy.

As of 2010,8% of U. S. workers reported ever having carpal tunnel syndrome and 4% reported carpal tunnel syndrome in the past 12 months. Prevalence rates for carpal tunnel syndrome in the past 12 months were higher among females than among males; among workers aged 45–64 than among those aged 18–44. Overall,67% of current carpal tunnel syndrome cases among current/recent workers were reportedly attributed to work by health professionals, indicating that the prevalence rate of work–related carpal tunnel syndrome among workers was 2% , and that there were approximately 3. 1 million cases of work–related carpal tunnel syndrome among U. S. workers in 2010. Among current carpal tunnel syndrome cases attributed to specific jobs,24% were attributed to jobs in the manufacturing industry, a proportion 2. 5 times higher than the proportion of current/recent workers employed in the manufacturing industry, suggesting that jobs in this industry are associated with an increased risk of work–related carpal tunnel syndrome.

14.7.3.2　Pathophysiology

The carpal tunnel is an anatomical compartment located at the base of the palm. Nine flexor tendons and the median nerve pass through the carpal tunnel that is surrounded on three sides by the carpal bones that form an arch. The median nerve provides feeling or sensation to the thumb, index finger, long finger, and half of the ring finger. At the level of the wrist, the median nerve supplies the muscles at the base of the thumb that allow it to abduct, move away from the other four fingers, as well as move out of the plane of the palm. The carpal tunnel is located at the middle third of the base of the palm, bounded by the bony prominence of the scaphoid tubercle and trapezium at the base of the thumb, and the hamate hook that can be palpated along the axis of the ring finger. From the anatomical position, the carpal tunnel is bordered on the anterior surface by the transverse carpal ligament, also known as the flexor retinaculum. The flexor retinaculum is a strong, fibrous band that attaches to the pisiform and the hamulus of the hamate. The proximal boundary is the distal wrist skin crease, and the distal boundary is approximated by a line known as Kaplan's cardinal line. This line uses surface landmarks, and is drawn between the apex of the skin fold between the thumb and index finger to the palpated hamate hook. The median nerve can be compressed by a decrease in the size of the canal, an increase in the size of the contents (such as the swelling of lubrication tissue around the flexor tendons) , or both. Since the carpal tunnel is bordered by carpal bones on one side and a ligament on the other, when the pressure builds up inside the tunnel, there is nowhere for it to escape and thus it ends up pressing up against and damaging the median nerve. Simply flexing the wrist to 90 degrees will decrease the size of the canal.

Compression of the median nerve as it runs deep to the transverse carpal ligament (TCL) causes atrophy of the thenar eminence, weakness of the flexor pollicis brevis, opponens pollicis, abductor pollicis brevis, as well as sensory loss in the digits supplied by the median nerve. The superficial sensory branch of the median nerve, which provides sensation to the base of the palm, branches proximal to the TCL and travels superficially to it. Thus, this branch spared in carpal tunnel syndrome, and there is no loss of palmar sensation.

14.7.3.3　Signs and symptoms

People with CTS experience numbness, tingling, or burning sensations in the thumb and fingers, in particular the index and middle fingers and radial half of the ring finger, because these receive their sensory and motor function (muscle control) from the median nerve. Ache and discomfort can possibly be felt more proximally in the forearm or even the upper arm. Less–specific symptoms may include pain in the wrists or hands, loss of grip strength, and loss of manual dexterity.

Some suggest that median nerve symptoms can arise from compression at the level of the thoracic outlet or the area where the median nerve passes between the two heads of the pronator teres in the forearm, although this is debated.

Numbness and paresthesias in the median nerve distribution are the hallmark neuropathic symptoms (NS) of carpal tunnel entrapment syndrome. Weakness andatrophy of the thumb muscles may occur if the condition remains untreated, because the muscles are not receiving sufficient nerve stimulation. Discomfort is usually worse at night and in the morning.

14.7.3.4 Diagnosis

There is no consensus reference standard for the diagnosis of carpal tunnel syndrome. A combination of described symptoms, clinical findings, and electrophysiological testing may be used. CTS work up is the most common referral to the electrodiagnostic lab. Historically, diagnosis has been made with the combination of a thorough history and physical examination in conjunction with the use of electrodiagnostic (EDX) testing for confirmation. Additionally, evolving technology has included the use of ultrasonography in the diagnosis of CTS. However, it is well established that physical exam provocative maneuvers lack both sensitivity and specificity. Furthermore, EDX cannot fully exclude the diagnosis of CTS due to the lack of sensitivity. A Joint report published by the American Association of Neuromuscular and Electrodiagostic Medicine (AA-NEM), the American Academy of Physical Medicine and Rehabilitation (AAPM and R) and the American Academy of Neurology defines practice parameters, standards and guidelines for EDX studies of CTS based on an extensive critical literature review. This joint review concluded median and sensory nerve conduction studies are valid and reproducible in a clinical laboratory setting and a clinical diagnosis of CTS can be made with a sensitivity greater than 85% and specificity greater than 95%. Given the key role of electrodiagnostic testing in the diagnosis of CTS, The American Association of Neuromuscular & Electrodiagnostic Medicine has issued evidence-based practice guidelines for the diagnosis of carpal tunnel syndrome.

Numbness in the distribution of the median nerve, nocturnal symptoms, thenar muscle weakness/atrophy, positive Tinel's sign at the carpal tunnel, and abnormal sensory testing such as two-point discrimination have been standardized as clinical diagnostic criteria by consensus panels of experts. Pain may also be a presenting symptom, although less common than sensory disturbances.

Electrodiagnostic testing (electromyography and nerve conduction velocity) can objectively verify the median nerve dysfunction. Normal nerve conduction studies, however, do not exclude the diagnosis of CTS. Clinical assessment by history taking and physical examination can support a diagnosis of CTS.

14.7.3.5 Treatment

Generally accepted treatments include: physiotherapy, steroids either orally or injected locally, splinting, and surgical release of the transverse carpal ligament. Limited evidence suggests that gabapentin is no more effective than placebo for CTS treatment. There is insufficient evidence for therapeutic ultrasound, yoga, acupuncture, low level laser therapy, vitamin B_6, and exercise. Change in activity may include avoiding activities that worsen symptoms.

The American Academy of Orthopedic Surgeons recommends proceeding conservatively with a course of nonsurgical therapies tried before release surgery is considered. A different treatment should be tried if the current treatment fails to resolve the symptoms within 2–7 weeks. Early surgery with carpal tunnel release is indicated where there is evidence of median nerve denervation or a person elects to proceed directly to surgical treatment. Recommendations may differ when carpal tunnel syndrome is found in association with the following conditions: diabetes mellitus, coexistent cervical radiculopathy, hypothyroidism, polyneuropathy, pregnancy, rheumatoid arthritis, and carpal tunnel syndrome in the workplace.

(1) Splints

The importance of wrist braces and splints in the carpal tunnel syndrome therapy is known, but many people are unwilling to use braces. In 1993, The American Academy of Neurology recommend a non-invasive treatment for the CTS at the beginning (except for sensitive or motor deficit or grave report at EMG/ENG): a therapy using splints was indicated for light and moderate pathology. Current recommendations generally don't suggest immobilizing braces, but instead activity modification and non-steroidal anti-inflammatory drugs as initial therapy, followed by more aggressive options or specialist referral if symptoms don't improve.

Many health professionals suggest that, for the best results, one should wear braces at night and, if possible, during the activity primarily causing stress on the wrists.

(2) Corticosteroids

Corticosteroid injections can be effective for temporary relief from symptoms while a person develops a long-term strategy that fits their lifestyle. This form of treatment is thought to reduce discomfort in those with CTS due to its ability to decrease median nerve swelling. The use of ultrasound while performing the injection is more expensive but leads to faster resolution of CTS symptoms. The injections are done under local anesthesia. This treatment is not appropriate for extended periods, however. In general, local steroid injections are only used until more definitive treatment options can be used. Corticosteroid injections do not appear to be very effective for slowing disease progression.

(3) Surgery

Release of the transverse carpal ligament is known as "carpal tunnel release" surgery. It is recommended when there is static (constant, not just intermittent) numbness, muscle weakness, or atrophy, and when night-splinting or other conservative interventions no longer control intermittent symptoms. The surgery may be done with local or regional anesthesia with or without sedation, or under general anesthesia. In general, milder cases can be controlled for months to years, but severe cases are unrelenting symptomatically and likely to result in surgical treatment.

Surgery is more beneficial in the short term to alleviate symptoms (up to six months) than wearing an orthosis for a minimum of 6 weeks. However, surgery and wearing a brace resulted in similar symptom relief in the long term (12–18 month outcomes).

(4) Physical therapy

A recent evidence based guideline produced by the American Academy of Orthopedic Surgeons assigned various grades of recommendation to physiotherapy (also called physical therapy) and other nonsurgical treatments. One of the primary issues with physiotherapy is that it attempts to reverse (often) years of pathology inside the carpal tunnel. Practitioners caution that any physiotherapy such as myofascial release may take weeks of persistent application to effectively manage carpal tunnel syndrome.

Again, some claim that pro-active ways to reduce stress on the wrists, which alleviates wrist pain and strain, involve adopting a more ergonomic work and life environment. For example, some have claimed that switching from a QWERTY computer keyboard layout to a more optimised ergonomic layout such as Dvorak was commonly cited as beneficial in early CTS studies; however, some meta-analyses of these studies claim that the evidence that they present is limited.

14.7.3.6 Prognosis

Most people relieved of their carpal tunnel symptoms with conservative or surgical management find minimal residual or "nerve damage". Long-term chronic carpal tunnel syndrome (typically seen in the elderly) can result in permanent "nerve damage", i. e., irreversible numbness, muscle wasting, and weakness.

Those that undergo a carpal tunnel release are nearly twice as likely as those not having surgery to develop trigger thumb in the months following the procedure.

While outcomes are generally good, certain factors can contribute to poorer results that have little to do with nerves, anatomy, or surgery type. One study showed that mental status parameters or alcohol use yields much poorer overall results of treatment. Recurrence of carpal tunnel syndrome after successful surgery is rare.

14.7.3.7   Prevention

Suggested healthy habits such as avoiding repetitive stress, work modification through use of ergonomic equipment [mouse pad, taking proper breaks, using keyboard alternatives (digital pen, voice recognition, and dictation)], and have been proposed as methods to help prevent carpal tunnel syndrome. The potential role of B vitamins in preventing or treating carpal tunnel syndrome has not been proven. There is little or no data to support the concept that activity adjustment prevents carpal tunnel syndrome. The evidence for wrist rest is debated.

Stretches and isometric exercises will aid in prevention for persons at risk. Stretching before the activity and during breaks will aid in alleviating tension at the wrist. Place the hand firmly on a flat surface and gently press for a few seconds to stretch the wrist and fingers. An example for an isometric exercise of the wrist is done by clenching the fist tightly, releasing and fanning out fingers. None of these stretches or exercises should cause pain or discomfort.

Biological factors such as genetic predisposition and anthropometric features had significantly stronger causal association with carpal tunnel syndrome than occupational/environmental factors such as repetitive hand use and stressful manual work. This suggests that carpal tunnel syndrome might not be preventable simply by avoiding certain activities or types of work/activities.

14.7.4   Tenosynovitis

Tenosynovitis is the inflammation of the sheath (called the synovium) that surrounds atendon. Tenosynovitis symptoms include pain, swelling and difficulty moving the joint where the inflammation occurs.

The condition occurs most often in the hands, wrists, and elbows, and has specific diagnoses based on location such as trigger digit, de Quervain's disease (tenosynovitis of the thumb extensor and abductor tendons), and medial or lateral epicondylitis.

In its acute stage, infectious tenosynovitis can create pus (purulent exudate), which compromises the space for the tendon even further. Bacterial causes of tenosynovitis include Neisseria gonorrhoeae, Staphylococcus, Streptococcus, Pasteurella multocida (cat bites), Eikenella corrodens (human bites), and Mycobacterium in immunocompromised individuals.

14.7.4.1   Causes

Individuals at risk for tenosynovitis of the upper extremities include carpenters, painters, welders, swimmers, tennis players, and baseball players. Although wrist tenosynovitis usually occurs in individuals who perform repetitive grasping or pinching motions with the thumb, it sometimes develops spontaneously in pregnant women. Runners, who engage in repetitive movements of the lower extremities, are at risk of tenosynovitis of the knee, ankle, and foot, but this type of tenosynovitis is less common. Women are more prone than men to irritative or frictional tenosynovitis.

Most causes of tenosynovitis are unknown. Irritation to the synovial lining can be related to injury, overuse, repetitive strain, trauma, rheumatoid arthritis (RA), or infection, any of which may increase the symptoms of tenosynovitis.

Gonococcal tenosynovitis, a complication of gonorrhea, typically affects teenagers and young adults. Common sites of infection include the top (dorsum) of the hand, wrist, and ankle. Other types of infectious tenosynovitis may result from puncture wounds or lacerations, usually to the hands.

14.7.4.2 Diagnosis

(1) History

A complete medical history should be obtained including recent trauma, history of sexually transmitted diseases (STDs), prior fractures or orthopedic surgery, underlying medical conditions (especially diabetes mellitus, RA, osteoarthritis, gout), medications, allergies, and occupation. A description of repetitive activities is helpful.

Although specific symptoms vary according to the location of the affected tendon sheath, pain, swelling (edema), and restricted motion in the affected area are common complaints with tenosynovitis. Some individuals may notice a crackling or squeaking noise (crepitus) accompanying tendon use.

(2) Physical exam

Findings on examination are specific to the location of tenosynovitis and include pain, swelling and difficulty moving the particular joint where the inflammation occurs. Careful observation and examination of the entire tendon sheath is crucial since infection can easily spread along tissue planes. The affected area may be fixed in slight flexion and the individual may report pain when touched (palpated) in the area over the involved tendon. In some cases, tendon thickening and nodularity can be palpated. There may also be decreased range of motion. In particularly painful cases, the involved joint may exhibit weakness, and the affected area may show redness (erythema), edema, and warmth to the touch. When tenosynovitis is caused by an infection, there may be additional systemic symptoms including rash and fever.

(3) Tests

Laboratory tests are not necessary for diagnosis, but if differential diagnosis includes gout and uric acid levels may be evaluated. Tests for suspected infectious tenosynovitis may include a complete blood count (CBC), erythrocyte sedimentation rate (ESR), and cultures. In some cases, fluid may be withdrawn (aspirated) from a swollen joint for further diagnostic evaluation.

14.7.4.3 Treatment

Treatment usually begins with modification of the activity that is associated with the pain. Individuals are often advised to wear a splint temporarily to avoid recurrence. Nonsurgical (conservative) treatment for tenosynovitis may utilize ultrasound, iontophoresis, and electrical stimulation, along with heat or ice for local pain control and to reduce swelling and inflammation.

Oral nonsteroidal anti-inflammatory drugs (NSAIDs) may be prescribed to control mild to moderate pain. In some cases, injection of lidocaine or a corticosteroid may be helpful. Repeated injections into tendons can weaken the tendon, so injections are limited to 2–3 over a period of several months. Weight-bearing tendons, such as the patellar tendon and Achilles tendon, are at greater risk for rupture from injections.

Surgery to incise part or the entire sheath (release of tendon sheath) may be necessary when conservative measures fail. When tenosynovitis causes swelling in a confined space such as the base of the thumb (de Quervain's disease), the swelling may need to be relieved by surgical incision of the constrictive tendon sheath. Surgery may also be necessary for a painful trigger finger or thumb.

Infectious tenosynovitis may require hospitalization for intravenous antibiotics, drainage if pus is suspected, and/or surgery.

14.7.4.4 Prognosis

Depending on the location and severity of tenosynovitis, symptoms may persist for a few days or for several weeks. Symptoms with activities may persist. Improvement may take several months. If rest and conservative medical management fail to provide relief, surgery to release the tendon sheath usually is effective.

14.7.4.5 Rehabilitation

The rehabilitation of tenosynovitis aims to control pain and swelling and to allow the tendon, muscle, and joint structures involved to regain motion, flexibility, strength, and endurance. The ultimate goal is to return the individual to full function in work and recreational activities with minimal risk of recurrence.

When pain is intense and disabling, application of ice to the injured tendon, muscle, and joint region may reduce pain. Later, heat treatments may reduce inflammation and pain, especially when stretching the involved tendon and muscle.

Once movement is allowed, passive range of motion exercises should begin with the therapist bending and straightening the involved area. As increased motion of the involved joint improving flexibility, the individual begins to perform all the motions independently. The physical therapist also uses joint mobilization techniques to restore joint motion affected by tenosynovitis, as well as to aid in the stretching of surrounding muscles and tendons. Early in the strengthening phase, the therapist will instruct the individual in isometric strengthening exercises. Once both range of motion and isometric exercises are tolerated, the individual progresses to isotonic strengthening involving movement at and around the joint. An occupational therapist may fabricate a splint for the individual to help immobilize and protect the involved area.

Modifications may need to be made by the physical therapist for individuals who have arthritis or other muscle or joint conditions. If the affected tendon requires surgical repair, some restrictions may be placed on range of motion and strengthening exercises, depending on the degree or type of surgery that was performed. If surgery is involved, the physician will guide the rehabilitation.

14.7.4.6 Complications

Complications of tenosynovitis include chronic pain, decreased range of motion, and amputation. Tendon rupture is a possible complication of chronic tenosynovitis. Risk of tendon rupture increases with the use of corticosteroid injections that may weaken the tendon. Untreated, infectious tenosynovitis can develop into septic arthritis or spread into adjacent bone, causing osteomyelitis.

14.7.5 Tension neck syndrome

Tension neck syndrome refers to a condition whereby pain and stiffness occur in the neck. Upon further examination, palpation tenderness in the trapezius muscle is usually discovered. Headache and fatigue are other indications of the presence of the condition. There is normally a trigger point of the condition, from whence the pain and stiffness originates. This condition is common amongst office and factory workers due to the nature of the jobs. Commonly affected are those who work on assembly lines, such as cashiers and packers.

14.7.5.1 Causes

There are many possible causes of this condition, including chronic strain, poor posture and even psychogenic factors such as stress, depression and tension. The condition might also occur due to muscular and mental fatigue as a result of repetitive arm and hand work. One theory points to the load that is put on our bodies as a result of repetitive motions involving any part of the time. Unnatural arm position and increased muscular workload are often factors. Other factors, such as working environment, also played a part in the development of the condition. Constant elevation of the arms is another possible cause of the onset of the condition.

The usage of a computer mouse has been associated with neck and shoulder pain. The connection between the two is possible but not certain. It has been found that the prevalence of the condition amongst those who use a mouse for more than 25 hours per week is higher than normal. Those who use a computer as part of their job are believed to be at a higher risk of developing the condition.

Generally, the condition is believed to be caused by localized muscle fatigue. This fatigue can occur due to repetitive motion or static, sustained contraction. Lack of oxygen supply and the accumulation of metabolic end products are thought to be primary causes of muscle fatigue.

These primary causes can be worsened or developed by other factors, such as the psychological constitution of the sufferer. It is thought that the pain can be enhanced by motivational or social factors. Many findings with regard to this condition are inconsistent, but it is generally believed that the psychological and physical condition of the sufferer both contribute to its development. It has been established, however, that the connection between workload and muscle fatigue does exist.

14.7.5.2 Symptoms

The most obvious symptom of the condition is an aching discomfort that is felt at the back of the neck and the upper back. There might also be headaches, which can occur as a result of tension in the neck muscles. One might also experience muscle spasms in the neck and dull pain in the upper arm, elbow, forearm and hands.

▶▶ *Summary*

Work-related musculoskeletal disorders (WMSDs) are a group of painful disorders of muscles, tendons, and nerves. Carpal tunnel syndrome, tendonitis, and tension neck syndrome are examples. Each WMSD has it own characteristics and causes. The prevention measurements should according to its characteristics and causes.

Practice questions:
(1) What's WMSDs?
(2) How many kinds of WMSDs?
(3) How to prevent WMSDs?

Yao Sanqiao

Chapter 15

Prevention and Control of Occupational Hazards

15.1   Introduction

Work is essential for life, development and personal fulfilment. Unfortunately, indispensable activities such as food production, extraction of raw materials, manufacturing of goods, energy production and services involved processes, operations and materials which can, to a greater or lesser extent, create hazards to the health of workers and those in nearby communities, as well as to the general environment. However, the generation and release of harmful agents in the work environment can be prevented, through adequate hazard control interventions, which not only protect workers' health but also limit the damage to the environment often associated with industrialization. If a harmful chemical is eliminated from a work process, it will neither affect the workers nor go beyond, to pollute the environment.

The profession that aims specifically at the prevention and control of hazards arising from work processes is occupational hygiene. The goals of occupational hygiene include the protection and promotion of workers' health, the protection of the environment and contribution to a safe and sustainable development. The need for occupational hygiene in the protection of workers' health cannot be overemphasized. Even when feasible, the diagnosis and the cure of an occupational disease will not prevent further occurrences, if exposure to the etiological agent does not cease. So long as the unhealthy work environment remains unchanged, it remains potential to impair health. Only the control of health hazards can break the vicious circle. However, preventive action should start much earlier, not only before the manifestation of any health impairment but even before exposure actually occurs. The work environment should be under continuous surveillance so that hazardous agents and factors can be detected and removed, or controlled, before they cause any ill effects; this is the role of occupational hygiene.

Occupational health requires a multidisciplinary approach and involves fundamental disciplines, one of which is occupational hygiene, along with others which include occupational medicine and nursing, ergonomics and work psychology. It is important that decision makers, managers and workers themselves, as well as all occupational health professionals, understand the essential role that occupational hygiene plays in the protection of workers' health and of the environment, as well as the need for specialized professionals in this field. The close link between occupational and environmental health should also be kept in mind, since the prevention of pollution from industrial sources, through the adequate handling and disposal of hazardous effluents and waste, should be started at the workplace level.

To control occupational hazards, first we should recognize the hazars, and then evaluate the impairment on workers' health, third should forecast the risk on peoples' health, and the last, take all kinds of step to control the risk of hazards.

15.1.1　Recognition of hazards

A workplace hazard can be defined as any condition that may adversely affect the well-being or health of exposed persons. Recognition of hazards in any occupational activity involves characterization of the workplace by identifying hazardous agents and groups of workers potentially exposed to these hazards. The hazards might be of chemical, biological or physical origin. Some hazards in the work environment are easy to recognize—for example, irritants, which have an immediate irritating effect after skin exposure or inhalation. Others are not so easy to recognize—for example, chemicals which are accidentally formed and have no warning properties. Some agents like metals (e. g. , lead, mercury, cadmium, manganese) , which may cause injury after several years of exposure, might be easy to identify if you are aware of the risk. A toxic agent may not constitute a hazard at low concentrations or if no one is exposed. Basic to the recognition of hazards are identification of possible agents at the workplace, knowledge about health risks of these agents and awareness of possible exposure situations.

15.1.1.1　Identification and classification of hazards

Before any occupational hygiene investigation is performed, the purpose must be clearly defined. The purpose of an occupational hygiene investigation might be to identify possible hazards, to evaluate existing risks at the workplace, to prove compliance with regulatory requirements, to evaluate control measures or to assess exposure with regard to an epidemiological survey. This article is restricted to programmes aimed at identification and classification of hazards at the workplace. Many models or techniques have been developed to identify and evaluate hazards in the working environment. They differ in complexity, from simple checklists, preliminary industrial hygiene surveys, job—exposure matrices and hazard and operability studies to job exposure profiles and work surveillance programmes. No single technique is a clear choice for everyone, but all techniques have parts which are useful in any investigation. The usefulness of the models also depends on the purpose of the investigation, size of workplace, type of production and activity as well as complexity of operations. Identification and classification of hazards can be divided into three basic elements: workplace characterization, exposure pattern and hazard evaluation.

15.1.1.2　Workplace characterization

A workplace might have from a few employees up to several thousands and have different activities (e. g. , production plants, construction sites, office buildings, hospitals or farms) . At a workplace different activities can be localized to special areas such as departments or sections. In an industrial process, different stages and operations can be identified as production is followed from raw materials to finished products.

Detailed information should be obtained about processes, operations or other activities of interest, to identify agents utilized, including raw materials, materials handled or added in the process, primary products, intermediates, final products, reaction products and by—products. Additives and catalysts in a process might also be of interest to identify. Raw material or added material which has been identified only by trade name must be evaluated by chemical composition. Information or safety data sheets should be available from manufacturer or supplier.

Some stages in a process might take place in a closed system without anyone exposed, except during maintenance work or process failure. These events should be recognized and precautions should be taken to prevent exposure to hazardous agents. Other processes take place in open systems, which are provided with or without local exhaust ventilation. A general ventilation system should be provided, including local exhaust system.

When possible, hazards should be identified in the planning or design of new plants or processes, when changes can be made at an early stage and hazards might be anticipated and avoided. Conditions and procedures that may deviate from the intended design must be identified and evaluated in the process state. Recognition of hazards should also include emissions to the external environment and waste materials. Facility locations, operations, emission sources and agents should be grouped together in a systematic way to form recognizable units in the further analysis of potential exposure. In each unit, operations and agents should be grouped according to health effects of the agents and estimation of emitted amounts to the work environment.

15.1.1.3   Exposure patterns

The main exposure routes for chemical and biological agents are inhalation and dermal uptake or incidentally by ingestion. The exposure pattern depends on frequency of contact with the hazards, intensity of exposure and time of exposure. Working tasks have to be systematically examined. It is important not only to study work manuals but to look at what actually happens at the workplace. Workers might be directly exposed as a result of actually performing tasks, or be indirectly exposed because they are located in the same general area or location as the source of exposure. It might be necessary to start by focusing on working tasks with high potential to cause harm even if the exposure is of short duration. Non-routine and intermittent operations (e. g. ,maintenance, cleaning and changes in production cycles) have to be considered. Working tasks and situations might also vary throughout the year.

Within the same job title exposure or uptake might differ because some workers wear protective equipment and others don't. In large plants, recognition of hazards or a qualitative hazard evaluation is seldom performed for every single worker. Therefore workers with similar working tasks have to be classified in the same exposure group. Differences in working tasks, work techniques and work time will result in considerably different exposure and have to be considered. Persons working outdoors and those working without local exhaust ventilation have been shown to have a larger day-to-day variability than groups working indoors with local exhaust ventilation. Work processes, agents applied for that process/job or different tasks within a job title might be used, instead of the job title, to characterize groups with similar exposure. Within the groups, workers potentially exposed must be identified and classified according to hazardous agents, routes of exposure, health effects of the agents, frequency of contact with the hazards, intensity and time of exposure. Different exposure groups should be ranked according to hazardous agents and estimated exposure in order to determine workers at greatest risk.

15.1.1.4   Chemical agents

Chemicals can be grouped into gases, vapours, liquids and aerosols (dusts, fumes, mists).

(1) Gases

Gases are substances that can be changed to liquid or solid state only by the combined effects of increased pressure and decreased temperature. Handling gas always implies risk of exposure unless they are processed in closed systems. Gases in containers or distribution pipes might accidentally leak. In processes with high temperatures (e. g. ,welding operations and exhaust from engines) gases will be formed.

(2) Vapours

Vapours are the gaseous form of substances that normally are in the liquid or solid state at room temperature and normal pressure. When a liquid evaporates, it changes to a gas and mixes with the surrounding air. A vapour can be regarded as a gas, where the maximal concentration of a vapour depends on the temperature and the saturation pressure of the substance. Any process involving combustion will generate vapours or gases. Degreasing operations might be performed by vapour phase degreasing or soak cleaning with solvents. Work activities like charging and mixing liquids, painting, spraying, cleaning and dry cleaning might generate harmful vapours.

(3) Liquids

Liquids may consist of a pure substance or a solution of two or more substances (e. g. , solvents, acids, alkalis). A liquid stored in an open container will partially evaporate into the gas phase. The concentration in the vapour phase at equilibrium depends on the vapour pressure of the substance, its concentration in the liquid phase, and the temperature. Operations or activities with liquids might give rise to splashes or other skin contact, besides harmful vapours.

(4) Dusts

Dusts consist of inorganic and organic particles, which can be classified as inhalable, thoracic or respirable, depending on particle size. Most organic dusts have a biological origin. Inorganic dusts will be generated in mechanical processes like grinding, sawing, cutting, crushing, screening or sieving. Dusts may be dispersed when dusty material is handled or whirled up by air movements from traffic. Handling dry materials or powder by weighing, filling, charging, transporting and packing will generate dust, as well activities like insulation and cleaning work.

(5) Fumes

Fumes are solid particles vaporized at high temperature and condensed to small particles. The vaporization is often accompanied by a chemical reaction such as oxidation. The single particles that make up a fume are extremely fine, usually less than 0. 1 μm, and often aggregate in larger units. Examples are fumes from welding, plasma cutting and similar operations.

(6) Mists

Mists are suspended liquid droplets generated by condensation from the gaseous state to the liquid state or by breaking up a liquid into a dispersed state by splashing, foaming or atomizing. Examples are oil mists from cutting and grinding operations, acid mists from electroplating, acid or alkali mists from pickling operations or paint spray mists from spraying operations.

15. 2　Evaluation

15. 2. 1　Hazard surveillance and survey methods

Occupational surveillance involves active programmes to anticipate, observe, measure, evaluate and control exposures to potential health hazards in the workplace. Surveillance often involves a team of people that includes an occupational hygienist, occupational physician, occupational health nurse, safety officer, toxicologist and engineer.

Depending upon the occupational environment and problem, three surveillance methods can be employed: medical, environmental and biological. Medical surveillance is used to detect the presence or absence of adverse health effects for an individual from occupational exposure to contaminants, by performing medical examinations and appropriate biological tests. Environmental surveillance is used to document potential exposure to contaminants for a group of employees, by measuring the concentration of contaminants in the air, in bulk samples of materials, and on surfaces. Biological surveillance is used to document the absorption of contaminants into the body and correlate with environmental contaminant levels, by measuring the concentration of hazardous substances or their metabolites in the blood, urine or exhaled breath of workers.

15.2.1.1   Medical surveillance

Medical surveillance is performed because diseases can be caused or exacerbated by exposure to hazardous substances. It requires an active programme with professionals who are knowledgeable about diagnoses and treatment of occupational diseases. Medical surveillance programmes provide steps to protect, educate, monitor and, in some cases, compensate the employee. It can include pre-employment screening programmes, periodic medical examinations, specialized tests to detect early changes and impairment caused by hazardous substances, medical treatment and extensive record keeping. Pre-employment screening involves the evaluation of occupational and medical history questionnaires and results of physical examinations. Questionnaires provide information concerning past illnesses and chronic diseases (especially asthma, skin, lung and heart diseases) and past occupational exposures. There are ethical and legal implications of pre-employment screening programmes if they are used to determine employment eligibility. However, they are fundamentally important when used to provide a record of previous employment and associated exposures, establish a baseline of health for an employee and test for hypersusceptibility. Medical examinations can include audiometric tests for hearing loss, vision tests, tests of organ function, evaluation of fitness for wearing respiratory protection equipment, and baseline urine and blood tests. Periodic medical examinations are essential for evaluating and detecting trends in the onset of adverse health effects and may include biological monitoring for specific contaminants and the use of other biomarkers.

15.2.1.2   Environmental and biological surveillance

Environmental and biological surveillance starts with an occupational hygiene survey of the work environment to identify potential hazards and contaminant sources, and determine the need for monitoring. For chemical agents, monitoring could involve air, bulk, surface and biological sampling. For physical agents, monitoring could include noise, temperature and radiation measurements. If monitoring is indicated, the occupational hygienist must develop a sampling strategy that includes which employees, processes, equipment or areas to sample, the number of samples, how long to sample, how often to sample, and the sampling method. Industrial hygiene surveys vary in complexity and focus depending upon the purpose of the investigation, type and size of establishment, and nature of the problem.

There are no rigid formulas for performing surveys; however, thorough preparation prior to the on-site inspection significantly increases effectiveness and efficiency. Investigations that are motivated by employee complaints and illnesses have an additional focus of identifying the cause of the health problems. Indoor air quality surveys focus on indoor as well as outdoor sources of contamination. Regardless of the occupational hazard, the overall approach to surveying and sampling workplaces is similar; therefore, this chapter will use chemical agents as a model for the methodology.

(1) Survey of the exposure routes

The mere presence of occupational stresses in the workplace does not automatically imply that there is a significant potential for exposure or the agent must reach the worker. For chemicals, the liquid or vapour form of the agent must make contact with and/or be absorbed into the body to induce an adverse health effect. If the agent is isolated in an enclosure or captured by a local exhaust ventilation system, the exposure potential will be low, regardless of the chemical's inherent toxicity.

The route of exposure can impact the type of monitoring performed as well as the hazard potential. For chemical and biological agents, workers are exposed through inhalation, skin contact, ingestion and injection; the most common routes of absorption in the occupational environment are through the respiratory tract and the skin. To assess inhalation, the occupational hygienist observes the potential for chemicals to become airborne as gases, vapours, dusts, fumes or mists.

Skin absorption of chemicals is important primarily when there is direct contact with the skin through splashing, spraying, wetting or immersion with fat—soluble hydrocarbons and other organic solvents. Immersion includes body contact with contaminated clothing, hand contact with contaminated gloves, and hand and arm contact with bulk liquids. For some substances, such as amines and phenols, skin absorption can be as rapid as absorption through the lungs for substances that are inhaled. For some contaminants such as pesticides and benzidine dyes, skin is the primary route of absorption, and inhalation is a secondary route. Such chemicals can readily enter the body through the skin, increase body burden and cause systemic damage. When allergic reactions or repeated washing dries and cracks the skin, there is a dramatic increase in the number and type of chemicals that can be absorbed into the body. Ingestion, an uncommon route of absorption for gases and vapours, can be important for particulates, such as lead. Ingestion can occur from eating contaminated food, eating or smoking with contaminated hands, and coughing and then swallowing previously inhaled particulates.

Injection of materials directly into the bloodstream can occur from hypodermic needles inadvertently puncturing the skin of health care workers in hospitals, and from high—velocity projectiles released from high—pressure sources and directly contacting the skin. Airless paint sprayers and hydraulic systems have pressures high enough to puncture the skin and introduce substances directly into the body.

(2) The walk—through inspection

The purpose of the initial survey, called the walk—through inspection, is to systematically gather information to judge whether a potentially hazardous situation exists and whether monitoring is indicated. An occupational hygienist begins the walk—through survey with an opening meeting that can include representatives of management, employees, supervisors, occupational health nurses and union representatives. The occupational hygienist can powerfully impact the success of the survey and any subsequent monitoring initiatives by creating a team of people who communicate openly and honestly with one another and understand the goals and scope of the inspection. Workers must be involved and informed from the beginning to ensure that cooperation, not fear, dominates the investigation.

During the meeting, requests are made for process flow diagrams, plant layout drawings, past environmental inspection reports, production schedules, equipment maintenance schedules, documentation of personal protection programmes, and statistics concerning the number of employees, shifts and health complaints. All hazardous materials used and produced by an operation are identified and quantified. A chemical inventory of products, by—products, intermediates and impurities is assembled and all associated Material Safety Data Sheets are obtained. Equipment maintenance schedules, age and condition are documented because the use of older equipment may result in higher exposures due to the lack of controls.

After the meeting, the occupational hygienist performs a visual walk—through survey of the workplace, scrutinizing the operations and work practices, with the goal of identifying potential occupational stresses, ranking the potential for exposure, identifying the route of exposure and estimating the duration and frequency of exposure.

The occupational hygienist uses the walk—through inspection to observe the workplace and have questions answered. Questions could address:

- Non—routine tasks and schedules for maintenance and cleaning activities.
- Recent process changes and chemical substitutions.
- Recent physical changes in the work environment.
- Changes in job functions.
- Recent renovations and repairs.

Non—routine tasks can result in significant peak exposures to chemicals that are difficult to predict and measure during a typical workday. Process changes and chemical substitutions may alter the release of substances into the air and affect subsequent exposure. Changes in the physical layout of a work area can alter the effectiveness of an existing ventilation system. Changes in job functions can result in tasks performed by inexperienced workers and increased exposures. Renovations and repairs may introduce new materials and chemicals into the work environment which are off—gas volatile organic chemicals or irritants.

(3) Indoor air quality surveys

Indoor air quality surveys are distinct from traditional occupational hygiene surveys because they are typically encountered in non—industrial workplaces and may involve exposures to mixtures of trace quantities of chemicals, none of which alone appears capable of causing illness. The goal of indoor air quality surveys is similar to occupational hygiene surveys in terms of identifying sources of contamination and determining the need for monitoring. However, indoor air quality surveys are always motivated by employee health complaints. In many cases, the employees have a variety of symptoms including headaches, throat irritation, lethargy, coughing, itching, nausea and non—specific hypersensitivity reactions that disappear when they go home. When health complaints do not disappear after the employees leave work, non—occupational exposures should be considered as well. Non—occupational exposures include hobbies, other jobs, urban air pollution, passive smoking and indoor exposures in the home. Indoor air quality surveys frequently use questionnaires to document employee symptoms and complaints and link them to job location or job function within the building. The areas with the highest incidence of symptoms are then targeted for further inspection.

Sources of indoor air contaminants that have been documented in indoor air quality surveys include: inadequate ventilation (52%), contamination from inside of the building (17%), contamination from outside of the building (11%), microbial contamination (5%), contamination from the building materials (3%), unknown causes (12%). For indoor air quality investigations, the walk—through inspection is essentially a building and environmental inspection to determine potential sources of contamination both inside and outside of the building. Inside building sources include: building construction materials such as insulation, particleboard, adhesives and paints; human occupants that can release chemicals from metabolic activities; human activities such as smoking; equipment such as copy machines; ventilation systems that can be contaminated with micro—organisms.

15.2.2   Sampling and measurement strategies

15.2.2.1   Occupational exposure limits

After the walk—through inspection is completed, the occupational hygienist must determine whether sampling is necessary; sampling should be performed only if the purpose is clear. The occupational hygienist must ask, "What will be made of the sampling results and what questions will the results answer?" It is relatively easy to sample and obtain numbers; it is far more difficult to interpret them.

Air and biological sampling data are usually compared to recommended or mandated occupational exposure limits (OELs). Occupational exposure limits have been developed in many countries for inhalation and biological exposure to chemical and physical agents. To date, out of a universe of over 8 millions commercially used chemicals, approximately 600 have been evaluated by a variety of organizations and countries. The philosophical bases for the limits are determined by the organizations that have developed them. The most widely used limits, called threshold limit values (TLVs), are those issued in the United States by the American Conference of Governmental Industrial Hygienists (ACGIH). Most of the OELs used by the Occupational Safety and Health Administration (OSHA) in the United States are based upon the TLVs. However, the National Institute for Occupational Safety and Health (NIOSH) of the US Department of Health and Human Services has suggested their own limits, called recommended exposure limits (RELs). For airborne exposures, there are three types of TLVs: an eight–hour time–weighted–average exposure, TLV–TWA, to protect against chronic health effects; a fifteen–minute average short–term exposure limit, TLV–STEL, to protect against acute health effects; and an instantaneous ceiling value, TLV–C, to protect against asphyxiants or chemicals that are immediately irritating. Guidelines for biological exposure levels are called biological exposure indices (BEIs). These guidelines represent the concentration of chemicals in the body that would correspond to inhalation exposure of a healthy worker at a specific concentration in air. Outside of the United States as many as 50 countries or groups have established OELs, many of which are identical to the TLVs. In Britain, the limits are called the Health and Safety Executive Occupational Exposure Standards (OES), and in Germany OELs are called Maximum Workplace Concentrations (MAKs). OELs have been set for airborne exposures to gases, vapours and particulates; they do not exist for airborne exposures to biological agents. Therefore, most investigations of bioaerosol exposure compare indoor with outdoor concentrations. If the indoor/outdoor profile and concentration of organisms is different, an exposure problem may exist. There are no OELs for skin and surface sampling, and each case must be evaluated separately. In the case of surface sampling, concentrations are usually compared with acceptable background concentrations that were measured in other studies or are determined in the current study. For skin sampling, acceptable concentrations are calculated based upon toxicity, rate of absorption, amount absorbed and total dose. In addition, biological monitoring of a worker may be used to investigate skin absorption.

15.2.2.2　Sampling strategy

An environmental and biological sampling strategy is an approach to obtaining exposure measurements that fulfils a purpose. A carefully designed and effective strategy should be scientifically defensible, optimize the number of samples obtained, be cost–effective and prioritizes needs. The goal of the sampling strategy guides decisions concerning what to sample (selection of chemical agents), where to sample (personal, area or source sample), whom to sample (which worker or group of workers), sample duration (real–time or integrated), how often to sample (how many days), how many samples, and how to sample (analytical method). Traditionally, sampling performed for regulatory purposes involves brief campaigns (one or two days) that concentrate on worst–case exposures. While this strategy requires a minimum expenditure of resources and time, it often captures the least amount of information and has little applicability to evaluating long–term occupational exposures. To evaluate chronic exposures so that they are useful for occupational physicians and epidemiological studies, sampling strategies must involve repeated sampling overtime for large numbers of workers.

(1) Purpose

The goal of environmental and biological sampling strategies is either to evaluate individual employee exposures or to evaluate contaminant sources. Employee monitoring may be performed to:

- Evaluate individual exposures to chronic or acute toxicants.
- Respond to employee complaints about health and odours.
- Create a baseline of exposures for a long–term monitoring program.

- Determine whether exposures comply with governmental regulations.
- Evaluate the effectiveness of engineering or process controls.
- Evaluate acute exposures for emergency response.
- Evaluate exposures at hazardous waste sites.
- Evaluate the impact of work practices on exposure.
- Evaluate exposures for individual job tasks.
- Investigate chronic illnesses such as lead and mercury poisoning.
- Investigate the relationship between occupational exposure and disease.
- Carry out an epidemiological study.

Source and ambient air monitoring may be performed to:

- Establish a need for engineering controls such as local exhaust ventilation systems and enclosures.
- Evaluate the impact of equipment or process modifications.
- Evaluate the effectiveness of engineering or process controls.
- Evaluate emissions from equipment or processes.
- Evaluate compliance after remediation activities such as asbestos and lead removal.
- Respond to indoor air, community illness and odour complaints.
- Evaluate emissions from hazardous waste sites.
- Investigate an emergency response.
- Carry out an epidemiological study.

When monitoring employees, air sampling provides surrogate measures of dose resulting from inhalation exposure. Biological monitoring can provide the actual dose of a chemical resulting from all absorption routes including inhalation, ingestion, injection and skin. Thus, biological monitoring can more accurately reflect an individual's total body burden and dose than air monitoring. When the relationship between airborne exposure and internal dose is known, biological monitoring can be used to evaluate past and present chronic exposures.

Biological monitoring has its limitations and should be performed only if it accomplishes goals that cannot be accomplished with air monitoring alone. It is invasive, requiring samples to be taken directly from workers. Blood samples generally provide the most useful biological medium to monitor; however, blood is taken only if non-invasive tests such as urine or exhaled breath are not applicable. For most industrial chemicals, data concerning the fate of chemicals absorbed by the body are incomplete or non-existent; therefore, only a limited number of analytical measurement methods are available, and many are not sensitive or specific. Biological monitoring results may be highly variable between individuals exposed to the same airborne concentrations of chemicals; age, health, weight, nutritional status, drugs, smoking, alcohol consumption, medication and pregnancy can impact uptake, absorption, distribution, metabolism and elimination of chemicals.

(2) What to sample

Most occupational environments have exposures to multiple contaminants. Chemical agents are evaluated both individually and as multiple simultaneous assaults on workers. Chemical agents can act independently within the body or interact in a way that increases the toxic effect. The question is of what to measure and how to interpret the results depends upon the biological mechanism of action of the agents when they are within the body. Agents can be evaluated separately if they act independently on altogether different organ systems, such as an eye irritant and a neurotoxin. If they act on the same organ system, such as two respiratory irritants, their combined effect is important. If the toxic effect of the mixture is the sum of the separate effects of the individual components, it is termed additive. If the toxic effect of the mixture is greater than the sum of the effects of the separate agents, their combined effect is termed synergistic. Exposure to cigarette smoking and inhalation of asbestos fibres gives rise to a much greater risk of lung cancer than a simple additive effect.

Sampling all the chemical agents in a workplace would be both expensive and not necessarily defensible. The occupational hygienist must prioritize the laundry list of potential agents by hazard or risk to determine which agents receive the focus.

Factors involved in ranking chemicals include: whether the agents interact independently, additively or synergistically; inherent toxicity of the chemical agent; quantities used and generated; number of people potentially exposed; anticipated duration and concentration of the exposure; confidence in the engineering controls; anticipated changes in the processes or controls; occupational exposure limits and guidelines.

(3) Where to sample

To provide the best estimate of employee exposure, air samples are taken in the breathing zone of the worker (within a 30 cm radius of the head), and are called personal samples. To obtain breathing zone samples, the sampling device is placed directly on the worker for the duration of the sampling. If air samples are taken near the worker, outside of the breathing zone, they are called area samples. Area samples tend to underestimate personal exposures and do not provide good estimates of inhalation exposure. However, area samples are useful for evaluating contaminant sources and measuring ambient levels of contaminants. Area samples can be taken while walking through the workplace with a portable instrument, or with fixed sampling stations. Area sampling is routinely used at asbestos abatement sites for clearance sampling and for indoor air investigations.

(4) Whom to sample

Ideally, to evaluate occupational exposure, each worker would be individually sampled for multiple days over the course of weeks or months. However, unless the workplace is small (<10 employees), it is usually not feasible to sample all the workers. To minimize the sampling burden in terms of equipment and cost, and increase the effectiveness of the sampling program, a subset of employees from the workplace is sampled, and their monitoring results are used to represent exposures for the larger work force.

To select employees who are representative of the larger work force, one approach is to classify employees into groups with similar expected exposures, called homogeneous exposure groups (HEGs). After the HEGs are formed, a subset of workers is randomly selected from each group for sampling. Methods for determining the appropriate sample sizes assume a lognormal distribution of exposures, an estimated mean exposure, and a geometric standard deviation of 2.2 to 2.5. Prior sampling data might allow a smaller geometric standard deviation to be used. To classify employees into distinct HEGs, most occupational hygienists observe workers at their jobs and qualitatively predict exposures.

There are many approaches to forming HEGs; generally, workers may be classified by job task similarity or work area similarity. When both job and work area similarity is used, the method of classification is called zoning. Once airborne, chemical and biological agents can have complex and unpredictable spatial and temporal concentration patterns throughout the work environment. Therefore, proximity of the source relative to the employee may not be the best indicator of exposure similarity. Exposure measurements made on workers initially expected to have similar exposures may show that there is more variation between workers than predicted. In these cases, the exposure groups should be reconstructed into smaller sets of workers, and sampling should continue to verify that workers within each group actually have similar exposures.

Exposures can be estimated for all the employees, regardless of job title or risk, or it can be estimated only for employees who are assumed to have the highest exposures; this is called worst–case sampling. The selection of worst–case sampling employees may be based upon production, proximity to the source, past sampling data, inventory and chemical toxicity. The worst–case method is used for regulatory purposes and does not provide a measure of long–term mean exposure and day–to–day variability. Task–related sampling involves selecting workers with jobs that have similar tasks that occur on a less than daily basis.

There are many factors that enter into exposure and can affect the success of HEG classification, including the following: Employees rarely perform the same work even when they have the same job description, and rarely have the same exposures; employee work practices can significantly alter exposure; workers who are mobile throughout the work area may be unpredictably exposed to several contaminant sources throughout the day; air movement in a workplace can unpredictably increase the exposures of workers who are located a considerable distance from a source; exposures may be determined not by the job tasks but by the work environment.

(5) Sample duration

The concentrations of chemical agents in air samples are either measured directly in the field, obtaining immediate results (real–time or grab), or are collected over time in the field on sampling media or in sampling bags and are measured in a laboratory. The advantage of real–time sampling is that results are obtained quickly onsite, and can capture measurements of short–term acute exposures. However, real–time methods are limited because they are not available for all contaminants of concern and they may not be analytically sensitive or accurate enough to quantify the targeted contaminants. Real–time sampling may not be applicable when the occupational hygienist is interested in chronic exposures and requires time–weighted–average measurements to compare with OELs.

Real–time sampling is used for emergency evaluations, obtaining crude estimates of concentration, leak detection, ambient air and source monitoring, evaluating engineering controls, monitoring short–term exposures that are less than 15 minutes, monitoring episodic exposures, monitoring highly toxic chemicals (carbon monoxide), explosive mixtures and process monitoring. Real–time sampling methods can capture changing concentrations over time and provide immediate qualitative and quantitative information. Integrated air sampling is usually performed for personal monitoring, area sampling and for comparing concentrations to time–weighted–average OELs. The advantages of integrated sampling are that methods are available for a wide variety of contaminants; it can be used to identify unknowns; accuracy and specificity is high and limits of detection are usually very low. Integrated samples that are analysed in a laboratory must contain enough contaminant to meet minimum detectable analytical requirements; therefore, samples are collected over a predetermined time period.

In addition to analytical requirements of a sampling method, sample duration should be matched to the sampling purpose. For source sampling, duration is based upon the process or cycle time, or when there are anticipated peaks of concentrations. For peak sampling, samples should be collected at regular intervals throughout the day to minimize bias and identify unpredictable peaks. The sampling period should be short enough to identify peaks while also providing a reflection of the actual exposure period.

For personal sampling, duration is matched to the occupational exposure limit, task duration or anticipated biological effect. Real–time sampling methods are used for assessing acute exposures to irritants, asphyxiants, sensitizers and allergenic agents. Chlorine, carbon monoxide and hydrogen sulphide are examples of chemicals that can exert their effects quickly and at relatively low concentrations.

Chronic disease agents such as lead and mercury are usually sampled for a full shift (7 hours or more per sample), using integrated sampling methods. To evaluate full shift exposures, the occupational hygienist uses either a single sample or a series of consecutive samples that cover the entire shift. The sampling duration for exposures that occur for less than a full shift are usually associated with particular tasks or processes. Construction workers, indoor maintenance personnel and maintenance road crews are examples of jobs with exposures that are tied to tasks.

(6) How many samples and how often to sample?

Concentrations of contaminants can vary minute to minute, day to day and season to season, and variability can occur between individuals and within an individual. Exposure variability affects both the number of samples and the accuracy of the results. Variations in exposure can arise from different work practices, changes in pollutant emissions, the volume of chemicals used, production quotas, ventilation, temperature changes, worker mobility and task assignments. Most sampling campaigns are performed for a couple of days in a year; therefore, the measurements obtained are not representative of exposure. The period over which samples are collected is very short compared with the unsampled period; the occupational hygienist must extrapolate from the sampled to the unsampled period. For long-term exposure monitoring, each worker selected from a HEG should be sampled multiple times over the course of weeks or months, and exposures should be characterized for all shifts. While the day shift may be the busiest, the night shift may have the least supervision and there may be lapses in work practices.

15.2.2.3 Measurement techniques

(1) Active and passive sampling

Contaminants are collected on sampling media either by actively pulling an air sample through the media, or by passively allowing the air to reach the media. Active sampling uses a battery-powered pump, and passive sampling uses diffusion or gravity to bring the contaminants to the sampling media. Gases, vapours, particulates and bioaerosols are all collected by active sampling methods; gases and vapours can also be collected by passive diffusion sampling.

For gases, vapours and most particulates, once the sample is collected the mass of the contaminant is measured, and concentration is calculated by dividing the mass by the volume of sampled air. For gases and vapours, concentration is expressed as parts per million (ppm) or mg/m^3, and for particulates concentration is expressed as mg/m^3.

In integrated sampling, air sampling pumps are critical components of the sampling system because concentration estimates require knowledge of the volume of sampled air. Pumps are selected based upon desired flowrate, ease of servicing and calibration, size, cost and suitability for hazardous environments. The primary selection criterion is flowrate: low-flow pumps (0.5-500 mL/min) are used for sampling gases and vapours; high-flow pumps (500-4,500 mL/min) are used for sampling particulates, bioaerosols and gases and vapours. To insure accurate sample volumes, pumps must be accurately calibrated. Calibration is performed using primary standards such as manual or electronic soap-bubble meters, which directly measure volume, or secondary methods such as wet test meters, dry gas meters and precision rotameters that are calibrated against primary methods.

(2) Sampling media: gases and vapours

Gases and vapours are collected using porous solid sorbent tubes, impingers, passive monitors and bags. Sorbent tubes are hollow glass tubes that have been filled with a granular solid that enables adsorption of chemicals unchanged on its surface. Solid sorbents are specific for groups of compounds; commonly used sorbents include charcoal, silica gel and Tenax. Charcoal sorbent, an amorphous form of carbon, is electrically nonpolar, and preferentially adsorbs organic gases and vapours. Silica gel, an amorphous form of silica, is used to collect polar organic compounds, amines and some inorganic compounds. Because of its affinity for polar compounds, it will adsorb water vapour; therefore, at elevated humidity, water can displace the less polar chemicals of interest from the silica gel. Tenax, a porous polymer, is used for sampling very low concentrations of nonpolar volatile organic compounds.

The ability to accurately capture the contaminants in air and avoid contaminant loss depends upon the sampling rate, sampling volume, and the volatility and concentration of the airborne contaminant. Collection efficiency of solid sorbents can be adversely affected by increased temperature, humidity, flowrate, concentration, sorbent particle size and number of competing chemicals. As collection efficiency decreases chemicals will be lost during sampling and concentrations will be underestimated. To detect chemical loss, or breakthrough, solid sorbent tubes have two sections of granular material separated by a foam plug. The front section is used for sample collection and the back section is used to determine breakthrough. Breakthrough has occurred when at least 20% -25% of the contaminant is present in the back section of the tube. Analysis of contaminants from solid sorbents requires extraction of the contaminant from the medium using a solvent. For each batch of sorbent tubes and chemicals collected, the laboratory must determine the desorption efficiency, the efficiency of removal of chemicals from the sorbent by the solvent. For charcoal and silica gel, the most commonly used solvent is carbon disulphide. For Tenax, the chemicals are extracted using thermal desorption directly into a gas chromatograph. Impingers are usually glass bottles with an inlet tube that allows air to be drawn into the bottle through a solution that collects the gases and vapours by absorption either unchanged in solution or by a chemical reaction. Impingers are used less and less in workplace monitoring, especially for personal sampling, because they can break, and the liquid media can spill onto the employee. There are a variety of types of impingers, including gas wash bottles, spiral absorbers, glass bead columns, midget impingers and fritted bubblers. All impingers can be used to collect area samples; the most commonly used impinger, the midget impinger can be used for personal sampling as well.

Passive, or diffusion monitors are small, have no moving parts and are available for both organic and inorganic contaminants. Most organic monitors use activated charcoal as the collection medium. In theory, any compound that can be sampled by a charcoal sorbent tube and pump can be sampled using a passive monitor. Each monitor has a uniquely designed geometry to give an effective sampling rate. Sampling starts when the monitor cover is removed and ends when the cover is replaced.

Most diffusion monitors are accurate for eight-hour time-weighted-average exposures and are not appropriate for short-term exposures.

Sampling bags can be used to collect integrated samples of gases and vapours. They have permeability and adsorptive properties that enable storage for a day with minimal loss. Bags are made of Teflon (polytetrafluoroethylene) and Tedlar (polyvinylfluoride).

(3) Sampling media: particulate materials

Occupational sampling for particulate materials, or aerosols, is currently in a state of flux; traditional sampling methods will eventually be replaced by particle size selective (PSS) sampling methods. Traditional sampling methods will be discussed first, followed by PSS methods.

The most commonly used media for collecting aerosols are fibre or membrane filters; aerosol removal from the air stream occurs by collision and attachment of the particles to the surface of the filters. The choice of filter medium depends upon the physical and chemical properties of the aerosols to be sampled, the type of sampler and the type of analysis. When selecting filters, they must be evaluated for collection efficiency, pressure drop, hygroscopicity, background contamination, strength and pore size, which can range from 0.01 to 10 μm. Membrane filters are manufactured in a variety of pore sizes and are usually made from cellulose ester, polyvinylchloride or polytetrafluoroethylene. Particle collection occurs at the surface of the filter; therefore, membrane filters are usually used in applications where microscopy will be performed. Mixed cellulose ester filters can be easily dissolved with acid and are usually used for collection of metals for analysis by atomic absorption. Nucleopore filters (polycarbonate) are very strong and thermally stable, and are used for sampling and analysing asbestos fibres using transmission electron microscopy. Fibre filters are usually made of fibreglass and are used to sample aerosols such as pesticides and lead.

For occupational exposures to aerosols, a known volume of air can be sampled through the filters, the total increase in mass (gravimetric analysis) can be measured (mg/m^3 air), the total number of particles can be counted (fibres/cc) or the aerosols can be identified (chemical analysis). For mass calculations, the total dust that enters the sampler or only the respirable fraction can be measured. For total dust, the increase in mass represents exposure from deposition in all parts of the respiratory tract. Total dust samplers are subject to error due to high winds passing across the sampler and improper orientation of the sampler. Strong winds and filters facing upright can result in collection of extra particles and overestimation of exposure.

For respirable dust sampling, the increase in mass represents exposure from deposition in the gas exchange (alveolar) region of the respiratory tract. To collect only the respirable fraction, a preclassifier called a cyclone is used to alter the distribution of airborne dust presented to the filter. Aerosols are drawn into the cyclone, accelerated and whirled, causing the heavier particles to be thrown out to the edge of the air stream and dropped to a removal section at the bottom of the cyclone. The respirable particles that are less than 10 μm remain in the air stream and are drawn up and collected on the filter for subsequent gravimetric analysis.

Sampling errors encountered when performing total and respirable dust sampling result in measurements that do not accurately reflect exposure or relate to adverse health effects. Therefore, PSS has been proposed to redefine the relationship between particle size, adverse health impact and sampling method. In PSS sampling, the measurement of particles is related to the sizes that are associated with specific health effects. The International Organization for Standardization (ISO) and the ACGIH have proposed three particulate mass fractions: inhalable particulate mass (IPM), thoracic particulate mass (TPM) and respirable particulate mass (RPM). IPM refers to particles that can be expected to enter through the nose and mouth, and would replace the traditional total mass fraction. TPM refers to particles that can penetrate the upper respiratory system past the larynx. RPM refers to particles that are capable of depositing in the gas-exchange region of the lung, and would replace the current respirable mass fraction. The practical adoption of PSS sampling requires the development of new aerosol sampling methods and PSS-specific occupational exposure limits.

(4) Sampling media: biological materials

There are few standardized methods for sampling biological material or bioaerosols. Although sampling methods are similar to those used for other airborne particulates, viability of most bioaerosols must be preserved to ensure laboratory culturability. Therefore, they are more difficult to collect, store and analyse. The strategy for sampling bioaerosols involves collection directly on semisolid nutrient agar or plating after collection in fluids, incubation for several days and identification and quantification of the cells that have grown. The mounds of cells that have multiplied on the agar can be counted as colony-forming units (CFU) for viable bacteria or fungi, and plaque-forming units (PFU) for active viruses. With the exception of spores, filters are not recommended for bioaerosol collection because dehydration causes cell damage.

Viable aerosolized micro-organisms are collected using all-glass impingers (AGI-30), slit samplers and inertial impactors. Impingers collect bioaerosols in liquid and the slit sampler collects bioaerosols on glass slides at high volumes and flowrates. The impactor is used with one to six stages, each containing a Petri dish, to allow for separation of particles by size. Interpretation of sampling results must be done on a case-by-case basis because there are no occupational exposure limits. Evaluation criteria must be determined prior to sampling; for indoor air investigations, in particular, samples taken outside of the building are used as a background reference. A rule of thumb is that concentrations should be ten times background to suspect contamination.

When using culture plating techniques, concentrations are probably underestimated because of losses of viability during sampling and incubation.

(5) Skin and surface sampling

There are no standard methods for evaluating skin exposure to chemicals and predicting dose. Surface sampling is performed primarily to evaluate work practices and identify potential sources of skin absorption and ingestion. Two types of surface sampling methods are used to assess dermal and ingestion potential: direct methods, which involve sampling the skin of a worker, and indirect methods, which involve wipe sampling surfaces.

Direct skin sampling involves placing gauze pads on the skin to absorb chemicals, rinsing the skin with solvents to remove contaminants and using fluorescence to identify skin contamination. Gauze pads are placed on different parts of the body and are either left exposed or are placed under personal protective equipment. At the end of the work day, the pads are removed and are analysed in the laboratory. The distribution of concentrations from different parts of the body are used to identify skin exposure areas. This method is inexpensive and easy to perform, however, the results are limited because gauze pads are not good physical models of the absorption and retention properties of skin, and measured concentrations are not necessarily representative of the entire body.

Skin rinses involve wiping the skin with solvents or placing hands in plastic bags filled with solvents to measure the concentration of chemicals on the surface. This method can underestimate dose because only the unabsorbed fraction of chemicals is collected.

Fluorescence monitoring is used to identify skin exposure for chemicals that naturally fluoresce, such as polynuclear aromatics, and to identify exposures for chemicals in which fluorescent compounds have been intentionally added. The skin is scanned with an ultraviolet light to visualize contamination. This visualization provides workers with evidence of the effect of work practices on exposure. Research is underway to quantify the fluorescence intensity and relate it to dose.

Indirect wipe sampling methods involve the use of gauze, glass fibre filters or cellulose paper filters, to wipe the insides of gloves or respirators, or the tops of surfaces. Solvents may be added to increase collection efficiency. The gauze or filters are then analysed in the laboratory. To standardize the results and enable comparison between samples, a square template is used to sample a $100 \, cm^2$ area.

(6) Biological media

Blood, urine and exhaled air samples are the most suitable specimens for routine biological monitoring, while hair, milk, saliva and nails are less frequently used. Biological monitoring is performed by collecting bulk blood and urine samples in the workplace and analysing them in the laboratory. Exhaled air samples are collected in Tedlar bags, specially designed glass pipettes or sorbent tubes, and are analysed in the field using direct-reading instruments, or in the laboratory. Blood, urine and exhaled air samples are primarily used to measure the unchanged parent compound (same chemical that is sampled in workplace air), its metabolite or a biochemical change (intermediate) that has been induced in the body. For example, the parent compound lead is measured in blood to evaluate lead exposure, the metabolite mandelic acid is measured in urine for both styrene and ethyl benzene, and carboxyhaemoglobin is the intermediate measured in blood for both carbon monoxide and methylene chloride exposure. For exposure monitoring, the concentration of an ideal determinant will be highly correlated with intensity of exposure. For medical monitoring, the concentration of an ideal determinant will be highly correlated with target organ concentration.

The timing of specimen collection can impact the usefulness of the measurements; samples should be collected at times which most accurately reflect exposure. Timing is related to the excretion biological half-life of a chemical, which reflects how quickly a chemical is eliminated from the body; this can vary from hours to years. Target organ concentrations of chemicals with short biological half-lives closely follow the environmental concentration; target organ concentrations of chemicals with long biological half-lives fluctuate very little in response to environmental exposures. For chemicals with short biological half-lives, less than three hours, a sample is taken immediately at the end of the workday, before concentrations rapidly decline, to reflect exposure on that day. Samples may be taken at any time for chemicals with long half-lives, such as polychlorinated biphenyls and lead.

(7) Real-time monitors

Direct-reading instruments provide real-time quantification of contaminants; the sample is analysed within the equipment and does not require off-site laboratory analysis (Maslansky and Maslansky 1993). Compounds can be measured without first collecting them on separate media, then shipping, storing and analysing them. Concentration is read directly from a meter, display, strip chart recorder and data logger, or from a colour change. Direct-reading instruments are primarily used for gases and vapours; a few instruments are available for monitoring particulates. Instruments vary in cost, complexity, reliability, size, sensitivity and specificity. They include simple devices, such as colorimetric tubes, that use a colour change to indicate concentration; dedicated instruments that are specific for a chemical, such as carbon monoxide indicators, combustible gas indicators (explosimeters) and mercury vapour meters; and survey instruments, such as infrared spectrometers, that screen large groups of chemicals. Direct-reading instruments use a variety of physical and chemical methods to analyse gases and vapours, including conductivity, ionization, potentiometry, photometry, radioactive tracers and combustion. Commonly used portable direct-reading instruments include battery-powered gas chromatographs, organic vapour analysers and infrared spectrometers. Gas chromatographs and organic vapour monitors are primarily used for environmental monitoring at hazardous waste sites and for community ambient air monitoring. Gas chromatographs with appropriate detectors are specific and sensitive, and can quantify chemicals at very low concentrations. Organic vapour analysers are usually used to measure classes of compounds. Portable infrared spectrometers are primarily used for occupational monitoring and leak detection because they are sensitive and specific for a wide range of compounds. Small direct-reading personal monitors are available for a few common gases (chlorine, hydrogen cyanide, hydrogen sulphide, hydrazine, oxygen, phosgene, sulphur dioxide, nitrogen dioxide and carbon monoxide). They accumulate concentration measurements over the course of the day and can provide a direct readout of time-weighted-average concentration as well as provide a detailed contaminant profile for the day. Colorimetric tubes (detector tubes) are simple to use, cheap and available for a wide variety of chemicals. They can be used to quickly identify classes of air contaminants and provide ballpark estimates of concentrations that can be used when determining pump flow rates and volumes. Colorimetric tubes are glass tubes filled with solid granular material which has been impregnated with a chemical agent that can react with a contaminant and create a colour change. After the two sealed ends of a tube are broken open, one end of the tube is placed in a hand pump. The recommended volume of contaminated air is sampled through the tube by using a specified number of pump strokes for a particular chemical. A colour change or stain is produced on the tube, usually within two minutes, and the length of the stain is proportional to concentration. Some colorimetric tubes have been adapted for long duration sampling, and are used with battery−powered pumps that can run for at least eight hours. The colour change produced represents a time−weighted−average concentration. Colorimetric tubes are good for both qualitative and quantitative analysis; however, their specificity and accuracy is limited. The accuracy of colorimetric tubes is not as high as that of laboratory methods or many other real−time instruments. There are hundreds of tubes, many of which have cross−sensitivities and can detect more than one chemical.

This can result in interferences that modify the measured concentrations. Direct−reading aerosol monitors cannot distinguish between contaminants, are usually used for counting or sizing particles, and are primarily used for screening, not to determine TWA or acute exposures. Real−time instruments use optical or electrical properties to determine total and respirable mass, particle count and particle size. Light−scattering aerosol monitors, or aerosol photometers, detect the light scattered by particles as they pass through a volume in the equipment. As the number of particles increases, the amount of scattered light increases and is proportional to mass. Light−scattering aerosol monitors cannot be used to distinguish between particle types; however, if they are used in a workplace where there are a limited number of dusts present, the mass can be attributed to a particular material. Fibrous aerosol monitors are used to measure the airborne concentration of particles such as asbestos. Fibres are aligned in an oscillating electric field and are illuminated with a helium neon laser; the resulting pulses of light are detected by a photomultiplier tube. Light−attenuating photometers measure the extinction of light by particles; the ratio of incident light to measured light is proportional to concentration.

(8) Analytical techniques

There are many available methods for analysing laboratory samples for contaminants. Some of the more commonly used techniques for quantifying gases and vapours in air include gas chromatography, mass spectrometry, atomic absorption, infrared and UV spectroscopy and polarography.

1) Gas chromatography: A technique used to separate and concentrate chemicals in mixtures for subsequent quantitative analysis. There are three main components to the system: the sample injection system, a column and a detector. A liquid or gaseous sample is injected using a syringe, into an air stream that carries the sample through a column where the components are separated. The column is packed with materials that interact differently with different chemicals, and slows down the movement of the chemicals. The differential interaction causes each chemical to travel through the column at a different rate. After separation, the chemicals go directly into a detector, such as a flame ionization detector (FID), photo−ionization detector (PID) or electron capture detector (ECD); a signal proportional to concentration is registered on a chart recorder. The FID is used for almost all organics including: aromatics, straight chain hydrocarbons, ketones and some chlorinated hydrocarbons. Concentration is measured by the increase in the number of ions produced as a volatile hydrocarbon is burned by a hydrogen flame. The PID is used for organics and some inorganics; it is especially useful for aromatic compounds such as benzene, and it can detect aliphatic, aromatic and halogenated hydrocarbons. Concentration is measured by the increase in the number of ions produced when the sample is bombarded by ultraviolet radiation. The ECD is primarily used for halogen−containing chemicals; it gives a minimal response to hydrocarbons, alcohols and ketones. Concentration is measured by the current flow between two electrodes caused by ionization of the gas by radioactivity.

2) The mass spectrophotometer: To be used to analyse complex mixtures of chemicals present in trace amounts. It is often coupled with a gas chromatograph for the separation and quantification of different contaminants.

3) Atomic absorption spectroscopy: To be primarily used for the quantification of metals such as mercury. Atomic absorption is the absorption of light of a particular wavelength by a free, ground-state atom; the quantity of light absorbed is related to concentration. The technique is highly specific, sensitive and fast, and is directly applicable to approximately 68 elements. Detection limits are in the sub-ppb to low-ppm range.

4) Infrared analysis: A powerful, sensitive, specific and versatile technique. It uses the absorption of infrared energy to measure many inorganic and organic chemicals; the amount of light absorbed is proportional to concentration. The absorption spectrum of a compound provides information enabling its identification and quantification.

5) UV absorption spectroscopy: To be used for analysis of aromatic hydrocarbons when interferences are known to be low. The amount of absorption of UV light is directly proportional to concentration.

6) Polarographic methods: To be based upon the electrolysis of a sample solution using an easily polarized electrode and a nonpolarizable electrode. They are used for qualitative and quantitative analysis of aldehydes, chlorinated hydrocarbons and metals.

15.3　Control of exposures through interventions

After a hazard has been recognized and evaluated, the most appropriate interventions (methods of control) for a particular hazard must be determined. Control methods usually fall into three categories: engineering controls; administrative controls; personal protective equipment. As with any change in work processes, training must be provided to ensure the success of the changes.

15.3.1　Engineering control

Engineering controls are changes to the process or equipment that reduce or eliminate exposures to an agent. For example, substituting a less toxic chemical in a process or installing exhaust ventilation to remove vapours generated during a process step, are examples of engineering controls. In the case of noise control, installing sound-absorbing materials, building enclosures and installing mufflers on air exhaust outlets are examples of engineering controls. Another type of engineering control might be changing the process itself. An example of this type of control would be removal of one or more degreasing steps in a process that originally required three degreasing steps. By removing the need for the task that produced the exposure, the overall exposure for the worker has been controlled. The advantage of engineering controls is the relatively small involvement of the worker, who can go about the job in a more controlled environment when, for instance, contaminants are automatically removed from the air. Contrast this to the situation where the selected method of control is a respirator to be worn by the worker while performing the task in an "uncontrolled" workplace. In addition to the employer actively installing engineering controls on existing equipment, new equipment can be purchased that contains the controls or other more effective controls. A combination approach has often been effective.

Some common examples of engineering controls are: ventilation (both general and local exhaust ventilation); isolation (place a barrier between the worker and the agent); substitution (substitute less toxic, less flammable material, etc.); change the process (eliminate hazardous steps).

The occupational hygienist must be sensitive to the worker's job tasks and must solicit worker participation when designing or selecting engineering controls. Placing barriers in the workplace, for example, could significantly impair a worker's ability to perform the job and may encourage "work arounds". Engineering controls are the most effective methods of reducing exposures. They are also, often, the most expensive. Since engineering controls are effective and expensive, it is important to maximize the involvement of the workers in the selection and design of the controls. This should result in a greater likelihood that the controls will reduce exposures.

15.3.2   Administrative controls

Administrative controls involve changes in how a worker accomplishes the necessary job tasks—for example, how long they work in an area where exposures occur, or changes in work practices, such as improvements in body positioning to reduce exposures.

Administrative controls can add to the effectiveness of an intervention, but have several drawbacks:

(1) Rotation of workers may reduce overall average exposure for the workday, but it provides periods of high short—term exposure for a larger number of workers. As more becomes known about toxicants and their modes of action, short—term peak exposures may represent a greater risk than would be calculated based on their contribution to average exposure.

(2) Changing work practices of workers can present a significant enforcement and monitoring challenge. How work practices are enforced and monitored determines whether or not they will be effective. This constant management attention is a significant cost of administrative controls.

15.3.3   Personal protective equipment

Personal protective equipment consists of devices provided to the worker and required to be worn while performing certain (or all) job tasks. Examples include respirators, chemical goggles, protective gloves and faceshields. Personal protective equipment is commonly used in cases where engineering controls have not been effective in controlling the exposure to acceptable levels or where engineering controls have not been found to be feasible (for cost or operational reasons). Personal protective equipment can provide significant protection to workers if worn and used correctly. In the case of respiratory protection, protection factors (ratio of concentration outside there spirator to that inside) can be 1,000 or more for positive—pressure supplied air respirators or ten for half—face air—purifying respirators. Gloves (if selected appropriately) can protect hands for hours from solvents. Goggles can provide effective protection from chemical splashes.

15.3.4   Occupational health surveillance

The surveillance of workers' health entails medical examinations of workers to ensure that their state of health is compatible with their job assignment and that their occupational exposure to hazards does not have any detrimental effects on their health. Health examinations also help to identify conditions which may make a worker more susceptible to the effects of hazardous agents and to detect early signs of health impairment caused by them. Their main purpose is primary prevention of work—related injuries and diseases.

Surveillance should be carried out in consultation with the workers or their representatives, and should not result in any loss of earnings for them. Furthermore, medical examinations should be free of charge and, as far as possible, should take place during working hours. Workers' health surveillance at national, industry and enterprise levels should be organized so as to take into account several factors, including:

- The need for a thorough investigation of all work—related factors.
- The nature of occupational hazards and risks in the workplace which may affect workers' health.
- The health requirements of the working population.
- The relevant laws and regulations and the available resources.

● The awareness of workers and employers of the functions and purposes of such surveillance; and the fact that surveillance is not a substitute for monitoring and control of the working environment.

15.3.4.1　Medical examinations, health assessments and biological tests

Workers who are or have been exposed to occupational hazards, such as asbestos, should be provided with such medical examinations as are necessary to supervise their health in relation to those occupational hazards, and to diagnose occupational diseases caused by exposure to them.

Surveillance of workers' health in the form of medical screening or periodic medical examinations often leads to the identification of occupational hazards or diseases. It has been shown that special prescriptive surveys to detect ill health among the working population generally prove more rewarding in terms of avoiding or controlling hazards than a series of medical tests performed at a later stage to identify or confirm suspected occupational disease. Cases of occupational disease often remain "latent" (silent) among the labor force. As a condition slowly develops, workers adapt to it, and are often unwilling to report illness that may result in the loss of their jobs.

Health examinations of workers frequently reveal the existence of health hazards in the workplace, and in such cases, the necessary environmental evaluation and control measures must be implemented.

Surveillance of the workers' health should include, in the cases and under the conditions specified by the competent authority, all assessments necessary to protect the health of the workers, which may include:

● Health assessment of workers before their assignment to specific tasks which may involve a danger to their health or that of others.

● Health assessment at periodic intervals during employment which involves exposure to a particular hazard to health.

● Health assessment on resumption of work after a prolonged absence for health reasons for the purpose of determining its possible occupational causes, of recommending appropriate action to protect the workers and of determining the worker's suitability for the job and needs for reassignment and rehabilitation.

● Health assessment on and after the termination of assignments involving hazards which might cause or contribute to future health impairment.

Pre-assignment medical examinations: Pre-assignment medical examinations are carried out before the placement of workers in jobs or their assignment to specific tasks which may involve a danger to their health or that of others. The purpose of such an examination is to determine in what capacity the prospective employee can be utilized most efficiently without detriment to himself or herself or to fellow workers. The scope of pre-assignment medical examination is influenced by such factors as the nature and location of the industry, as well as by the availability of the services of physicians and nurses. Regardless of the size of the enterprise, it is advisable to conduct such examinations for all prospective employees. In the case of young people, such pre-assignment medical examinations are prescribed by specific ILO Conventions. The pre-assignment medical examination provides clinical information and laboratory data on the worker's health status at the moment of entering employment. It is also important with regard to the worker's subsequent occupational history, as it provides a baseline for the evaluation of any changes in health status that may occur later on. The results of pre-assignment medical examinations should be used to help place workers in jobs which are compatible with the status of their health, and not to screen out workers. In some cases, prospective employees who are found to be HIV-positive may be refused employment on the basis of their health status, or those already in employment may be summarily dismissed. These practices should not be condoned.

Periodic health evaluations: Periodic health evaluations are performed at appropriate intervals during employment to determine whether the worker's health remains compatible with his or her job assignment and to detect any evidence of ill health attributed to employment. Their objectives include identifying as early as possible any adverse health effects caused by work practices or exposure to hazards and detecting possible hazards. Changes in the body organs and systems affected by harmful agents can be detected during the periodic medical examination, usually performed after the worker has been employed long enough to have been exposed to any such hazards in the workplace. The worker may be physically fit, showing no signs of impairment and unaware of the fact that the substances he or she works with daily are slowly poisoning his or her system. The nature of the exposure and the expected biological response will determine the frequency with which the periodical medical examination is conducted. It could be as frequent as every one to three months, or it could be carried out at yearly intervals.

A return-to-work health assessment: A return-to-work health assessment is required to determine whether a worker is fit to resume his or her duties after a prolonged absence for health reasons. Such an assessment might recommend appropriate actions to protect the worker against future exposure, or may identify a need for reassignment or special rehabilitation. A similar assessment is performed on a worker who changes job, with a view to certifying him or her fit for the new duties.

Post-assignment health examinations: Post-assignment health examinations are conducted after the termination of assignments involving hazards which could cause or contribute to future health impairment. The purpose is to make a final evaluation of workers' health and compare it with the results of previous medical examinations to see whether the job assignments have affected their health.

In certain hazardous occupations, the competent authority should ensure that provision is made, in accordance with national law and practice, for appropriate medical examinations to continue to be available to workers after the termination of their assignment.

At the conclusion of a prescribed health assessment, workers should be informed in a clear and appropriate manner, by the attending physician, of the results of their medical examinations and receive individual advice concerning their health in relation to their work. When such reports are communicated to the employer, they should not contain any information of a medical nature.

They should simply contain a conclusion about the fitness of the examined person for the proposed or held assignment and specify the kinds of jobs and conditions of work which he or she should not undertake, for medical reasons, either temporarily or permanently.

When continued assignment to work involving exposure to hazardous substances is found to be medically inadvisable, every effort, consistent with national conditions and practice, should be made to provide the workers concerned with other means of maintaining an income. Furthermore, national laws or regulations should provide for the compensation of workers who contract a disease or develop a functional impairment related to occupational exposure, in accordance with the Employment Injury Benefits Convention. It must be mentioned that there are limitations to medical examinations, especially in developing countries, where generally the provision and coverage of health services is poor and there are relatively very few doctors. In these conditions, the heavy workload and other limitations often inhibit the thoroughness of medical examinations.

Where workers are exposed to specific occupational hazards, special tests are needed. These should be carried out in addition to the health assessments described above. The surveillance of workers' health should thus include, where appropriate, any other examinations and investigations which may be necessary to detect exposure levels and early biological effects and responses.

The analysis of biological samples obtained from the exposed workers is one of the most useful means of assessing occupational exposure to a harmful material. This analysis may provide an indication of the amount of substance that has accumulated or is stored in the body, the amount circulating in the blood, or the amount being excreted. There are several valid and generally accepted methods of biological monitoring which allow for the early detection of the effects on workers' health of exposure to specific occupational hazards.

These can be used to identify workers who need a detailed medical examination, subject to the individual worker's consent. Urine, blood and saliva are the usual body fluids examined for evidence of past exposure to toxic (harmful) agents. Lead concentrations in the urine or blood have long been used as indices of lead exposure.

Most biological monitoring measures are invasive procedures which may be undertaken only with legal permission. Moreover, many countries lack the laboratory facilities and other resources necessary to carry out such tests.

Consequently, priority should be given to environmental criteria over biological criteria in setting exposure limits, even though biological monitoring has certain advantages over environmental sampling. Biological monitoring takes account of substances absorbed through the skin and gastrointestinal tract (stomach), and the effects of added stress (such as increased workload resulting in a higher respiration rate with increased intake of the air contaminant) will also be reflected in the analytical results. Furthermore, the total exposure (both on and off the job) to harmful materials will be accounted for. Biological monitoring should not, however, be a substitute for surveillance of the working environment and the assessment of individual exposures. In assessing the significance of the results of biological monitoring, values commonly found in the general public should be taken into account.

15.3.4.2 Sickness absence monitoring

The importance of keeping a record of absence from work because of sickness is well recognized in various countries. Monitoring sickness absence can help identify whether there is any relation between the reasons for ill health or absence and any health hazards which may be present at the workplace. Occupational health professionals should not, however, be required by the employer to verify the reasons for absence from work. Their role is rather to provide advice on the health status of the workforce in the enterprise and on medical problems which affect attendance and fitness forwork. Occupational health professionals should not become involved in the administrative management and control of sickness absence, but it is acceptable for them to provide advice on medical aspects of sickness cases, provided that medical confidentiality is respected.

15.3.4.3 Reporting of occupational accidents, injuries and diseases

One of the tasks of the competent authority is to ensure the establishment and application of procedures for the notification of occupational accidents and diseases by employers and, when appropriate, insurance institutions and others directly concerned, as well as the production of annual statistics on occupational accidents and diseases. Consequently, national laws or regulations in many countries provide for:

• The reporting of occupational accidents and diseases to the competent authority within a prescribed time.

• Standard procedures for reporting and investigating fatal and serious accidents, as well as dangerous occurrences.

• The compilation and publication of statistics on accidents, occupational diseases and dangerous occurrences.

This compulsory reporting is usually carried out within the framework of programs for the prevention of occupational disease and injury or for the provision of compensation or benefits. In other countries there are voluntary systems for reporting occupational injury and disease. In either case, the competent authority is responsible for developing a system of notification of occupational diseases, in the case of asbestos for example. It must be acknowledged that occupational diseases are usually less well recorded than occupational accidents since the factors of recognition set out in the list of notifiable diseases differ from one country to another. Countries could use the ILO code of practice Recording and notification of occupational accidents and diseases as a basis for developing their own systems.

Whatever the system developed, it is the responsibility of the employer to present a detailed report to the competent authority within a fixed period of any accident or disease outbreak that results in a specified amount of lost working time (in many countries, three or four days). After a major accident, for example, the employer must submit a report containing an analysis of the causes of the accident and describing its immediate on-site consequences, as well as indicating any action taken to mitigate its effects. It is equally the responsibility of the employer to keep records of relevant occupational accidents and diseases. In this respect, it is worth pointing out that good record-keeping is beneficial to the company in many ways.

In many countries, lists of notifiable occupational diseases have been established by statute. The records of notified diseases give administrators some idea of the extent and types of occupational pathology. This presupposes that medical practitioners are sufficiently well informed to make such diagnoses accurately and are prepared to cooperate with the authorities, which unfortunately is not always the case: some doctors may try to cover for employers for fear of losing their own jobs. Workers' compensation schemes operated by ministries of labor also have lists covering occupational injuries for which compensation may be claimed.

Where an occupational disease has been detected through the surveillance of the worker's health, it should be notified to the competent authority, in accordance with national law and practice. The employer, workers and workers' representatives should be informed that this notification has been carried out. Specifically, the labor inspectorate, where it exists, should be notified of industrial accidents and occupational diseases in the cases and in the manner prescribed by national laws and regulations.

15.3.5 Health promotion, education and training

A healthy, motivated and contented workforce is fundamental to the social and economic well-being of any nation. To achieve such a workforce, it is not enough just to prevent occupational hazards or to protect workers against them. It is also necessary to take positive measures to improve health and to promote a safety and health-oriented culture. Such measures include health promotion, education and training.

15.3.5.1 Promotion of occupational safety and health

The promotion of occupational safety and health is an organizational investment for the future: enterprises will benefit from promoting health in the workplace in the form of lower sickness-related costs and higher productivity.

Consequently, OSH promotion in the workplace could be regarded as a modern corporate strategy which aims at preventing ill health at work (including work-related diseases, accidents, injuries, occupational diseases and stress) and enhancing the potential and well-being of the workforce.

As part of national OSH promotional activities, some countries organize annual awards based on certain criteria, including the number of accidents submitted for compensation claims, and continuous inspection and monitoring of hazards by the individual workplace. Companies that have kept good safety records are given awards in recognition of their efforts and to encourage others to emulate them. However, mechanisms for ensuring honesty and preventing under-reporting or inaccurate declaration should be put in place and enforced. In other instances, health promotion items, including hazard-monitoring equipment, safety devices, training manuals, and information packages on occupational safety and health are displayed at big annual events such as international trade fairs. Similar activities can be organized at the enterprise level to promote awareness about safety and health.

Such activities could include an annual safety festival. Workers' lifestyles, including diet, exercise, and smoking and drinking habits, are the key factors in health. Health education designed to promote good lifestyles and discourage those detrimental to health should be introduced into the workplace as part of the program of OSH activities.

OSH promotion covers a wide range of measures aimed at increasing interest in a safe and healthy working life. It includes:

- A comprehensive system of information dissemination.
- Targeted campaigns for the different sectors of occupational safety and health.
- Safety promotion activities, for example an annual safety week all over the country, featuring events centred on safety themes and culminating in a safety awards ceremony.

The OSH program should include strategies to promote wider awareness of the social and economic importance of improving working conditions and the environment.

An OSH awareness campaign is aimed at acquainting both management and workers with hazards in their workplaces and their role and obligations in the prevention of occupational accidents, injuries and diseases. It fosters improved communication and work relationships at all levels of the business enterprise, including top management, supervisors and workers on the shop floor. It helps a company to achieve the key objective of a good safety and health record.

Education in the context of occupational safety and health is designed to communicate a combination of knowledge, understanding and skills that will enable managers and workers in an enterprise to recognize risk factors contributing to occupational accidents, injuries and diseases, and be ready and able to prevent these factors occurring in their own work environment. OSH education is thus intended to foster the awareness and positive attitudes which are conducive to safety and health at work.

Education includes training, which is a process of helping others to acquire skills necessary for good performance in a given job. Training is therefore a narrower concept than education. Training, as opposed to full education, may be the only option where workers have limited academic background (and hence their comprehension is likely to be limited), or time is scarce.

Education and training provide individuals with the basic theoretical and practical knowledge required for the successful exercise of their chosen occupation or trade. Education and training must therefore also cover the prevention of accidents and injury to health arising out of or linked with or occurring in the course of work. There should be special emphasis on training, including necessary further training. In addition, attention should be paid to the qualifications and motivations of individuals involved, in one capacity or another, in the achievement of adequate levels of safety and health.

Where there are health hazards associated with hazardous materials, the competent authority should make appropriate arrangements, in consultation and collaboration with the most representative organizations of employers and workers concerned:

- To promote the dissemination of information on hazards and on methods of prevention and control.
- To educate all concerned about the hazards and about methods of prevention and control.

15.3.5.2 Training and information at the national level

The competent authority or authorities in each country should provide information and advice, in an appropriate manner, to employers and workers, and should promote or facilitate cooperation between them and their organizations, with a view to eliminating hazards or reducing them as far as practicable. Where appropriate, a special training program for migrant workers in their mother tongues should be provided.

Training at all levels should be emphasized as a means of improving working conditions and the work environment. OSH institutes and laboratories, labor institutes and other institutions concerned with training, technical support or research in occupational safety and health should be established. Workers' organizations as well as employers should take positive action to carry out training and information programs with a view to preventing potential occupational hazards in the working environment, and controlling and protecting against existing risks. In their own training, employers should also learn how to gain the confidence of their workers and motivate them; this aspect is as important as the technical content of the training.

The training of labor inspectors, OSH specialists and others directly concerned with the improvement of working conditions and the work environment should take into account the increasing complexity of work processes. In particular, with the introduction of new or advanced technology there is a need for training in methods of analysis to identify and measure the hazards, as well as in ways to protect workers against these hazards.

The OSH program should place particular emphasis on activities related to the collection, analysis and dissemination of information and take into consideration the differing needs of government agencies, employers and workers and their organizations, research institutions and others concerned with the improvement of working conditions and the work environment.

Priority should be given to the collection and dissemination of practical information, such as information on the provisions of legislation and collective agreements, training activities, research in progress and the content of technical publications.

Information should be easily accessible through a variety of means, including the internet, computerized databases, audiovisual materials, serial publications, information sheets and monographs. A special effort should be made to provide information at low cost or free of charge to trade unions and other interested organizations and audiences which might otherwise not be able to afford them.

The establishment of regional, subregional or national information systems on working conditions and on occupational safety and health should be encouraged. This could be achieved through the establishment of technical advisory services such as the ILO International Occupational Safety and Health Information Centre (CIS) national centers, as well as the organization of national and regional workshops and the inclusion of information activities in technical cooperation projects. Information systems should be examined to ensure that there is no overlap with the activities of other institutions providing information in the field of occupational safety and health, and that the most appropriate and cost-effective techniques are used.

15.3.5.3　Training and information at the enterprise level

The need to give appropriate training in occupational safety and health to workers and their representatives in the enterprise cannot be overemphasized. Training at all levels should be seen as a means of improving working conditions and the work environment. Employers should provide necessary instructions and training, taking account of the functions and capacities of different categories of workers. Furthermore, workers and their representatives should have reasonable time, during paid working hours, to exercise their safety and health functions and to receive training related to them. Employers' and workers' organizations should take positive action to carry out training and information programs with respect to existing and potential occupational hazards in the work environment. These programs should focus on prevention, control and protection.

Workers should be provided with the type of knowledge commensurate with the technical level of their activity and the nature of their responsibilities.

Representatives of workers in the enterprise should also be given adequate information on measures taken by the employer to secure occupational safety and health. They should be able to consult their representative organizations about such information provided that they do not disclose commercial secrets.

At an individual level, each worker should be informed in an adequate and appropriate manner of the health hazards involved in his or her work, of the results of the health examinations he or she has undergone and of the assessment of his or her health.

Information activities are a key means of support for OSH programs. These activities should emphasize practical materials targeted at specific groups. Special priority should be given to information that can be put to immediate use in enterprises. Policy—makers, labor inspectors and the staff of institutions carrying out research and technical support activities should also be provided with information relevant to their priorities. The participation of such institutions in information networks, both national and international, should be encouraged and developed.

Workers and their safety and health representatives should have access to appropriate information, which might include:

- Notice of any forthcoming visits to workplaces by the competent authority in relation to safety or health.

- Reports of inspections conducted by the competent authority or the employer, including inspections of machinery or equipment.

- Copies of orders or instructions issued by the competent authority in respect of safety and health matters.

- Reports prepared by the competent authority or the employer on accidents, injuries, instances of ill health and other occurrences affecting safety and health.

- Information and notices on all hazards at work, including hazardous, toxic or harmful materials, agents or substances used at the workplace.

- Any other documentation concerning safety and health that the employer is required to maintain.

- Immediate notification of accidents and dangerous occurrences.

- Any health studies conducted in respect of hazards present in the workplace.

15.3.5.4 Training methods and materials

The importance of training lies in the fact that regulations and warning signs will not prevent risky behavior unless workers understand dangers and believe that safety measures are worthwhile. Workers, in particular new recruits, need to be instructed in the safety aspects of their work and kept under close supervision to ensure that they have fully understood the dangers and how to avoid them. This instruction must be supported by effective materials and practical training methods. Specific training materials should be developed to assist action in poorly protected sectors, and emphasis should be placed on the training of trainers.

Developing countries have special needs to which training materials and methods will need to be adapted. In some cases, entirely new materials and methods will be required. This work should utilize research on sectors with particularly high safety risks and pilot experiments identifying the cost effectiveness and appropriateness of measures. Whenever possible, work on developing training methods and materials should be done in consultation with workers' and employers' representatives.

Given the fact that many workers in developing countries are either illiterate or semi—literate, great care must be taken in choosing an appropriate means of communication. Information on safety and health should be presented in a manner that is easily understood by all workers regardless of their level of education. Language should be kept simple. Everyday language, i. e. , the vernacular or local dialect, should be used whenever possible.

Information should be conveyed using a medium that doesn't rely heavily on the written word. Discussions or lectures in the vernacular, along with demonstrations, vivid posters or films, are often more effective than written material in putting across safety and health messages. Other techniques include on the – job demonstrations, role – playing, and audiovisual presentations accompanied by explanatory discussions.

Any new techniques implemented must be periodically evaluated. If communication is effective, it will produce the desired effects: a reduction in the number of accidents and diseases, or their elimination; savings in medical bills and compensation payments; and improved productivity and worker morale.

15.3.6 Legislation, enforcement and collective agreements

Appropriate legislation and regulations, together with adequate means of enforcement, are essential for the protection of workers' safety and health. Legislation is the very foundation of social order and justice; without it, or where it is not enforced, the door is wide open to all forms of abuse. Each country should therefore take such measures as may be necessary to protect workers' safety and health. This may be done by enacting laws or regulations, or by any other method consistent with national conditions and practice, undertaken in consultation with the representative organizations of employers and workers concerned. The law directly regulates certain components of working conditions and the work environment, including hours of work and occupational safety and health. There are also provisions relating to trade unions and collective bargaining machinery, which establish conditions for negotiations between employers and workers.

15.3.6.1 Occupation exposure limit

Over the past 50 years, many organizations in numerous countries have proposed occupational exposure limits (OELs) for airborne contaminants. The limits or guidelines that have gradually become the most widely accepted both in the United States and in most other countries are those issued annually by the American Conference of Governmental Industrial Hygienists (ACGIH), which are termed threshold limit values (TLVs).

The usefulness of establishing OELs for potentially harmful agents in the working environment has been demonstrated repeatedly since their inception. The contribution of OELs to the prevention or minimization of disease is now widely accepted, but many years ago, such limits did not exist, and even when they did, they were often not observed.

Simple observation of the working conditions and the illness and deaths of the workers readily proved that harmful exposures existed. Soon however, the need for determining standards for safe exposure became obvious.

The earliest efforts to set an OEL were directed to carbon monoxide, the toxic gas to which more persons are occupationally exposed than to any other (for a chronology of the development of OELs. The earliest and most extensive series of animal experiments on exposure limits were those conducted by K. B. Lehmann and others under his direction. In a series of publications spanning 50 years, they reported studies on ammonia and hydrogen chloride gas, chlorinated hydrocarbons and a large number of other chemical substances.

The first lists of standards for chemical exposures in industry, called maximum allowable concentrations (MACs), were prepared in 1939 and 1940. They represented a consensus of opinion of the American Standard Association and a number of industrial hygienists who had formed the ACGIH in 1938. A committee of the ACGIH met in early 1940 to begin the task of identifying safe levels of exposure to workplace chemicals, by assembling all the data which would relate the degree of exposure to a toxicant to the likelihood of producing an adverse effect.

In 1945 a list of 132 industrial atmospheric contaminants with maximum allowable concentrations was published by Cook, including the current values for six states, as well as values presented as a guide for occupational disease control by federal agencies and maximum allowable concentrations that appeared best supported by the references on original investigations.

15.3.6.2 Intended use of OELs

The ACGIH TLVs and most other OELs used in the United States and some other countries are limits which refer to airborne concentrations of substances and represent conditions under which "it is believed that nearly all workers may be repeatedly exposed day after day without adverse health effects" (ACGIH 1994). In some countries the OEL is set at a concentration which will protect virtually everyone. It is important to recognize that unlike some exposure limits for ambient air pollutants, contaminated water, or food additives set by other professional groups or regulatory agencies, exposure to the TLV will not necessarily prevent discomfort or injury for everyone who is exposed. The ACGIH recognized long ago that because of the wide range in individual susceptibility, a small percentage of workers may experience discomfort from some substances at concentrations at or below the threshold limit and that a smaller percentage may be affected more seriously by aggravation of a pre-existing condition or by development of an occupational illness. This is clearly stated in the introduction to the ACGIH's annual booklet Threshold Limit Values for Chemical Substances and Physical Agents and Biological Exposure Indices.

This limitation, although perhaps less than ideal, has been considered as practical one since airborne concentrations so low as to protect hypersusceptibles have traditionally been judged infeasible due to either engineering or economic limitations. Until about 1990, this shortcoming in the TLVs was not considered as serious one. In light of the dramatic improvements since the mid-1980s in our analytical capabilities, personal monitoring/sampling devices, biological monitoring techniques and the use of robots as a plausible engineering control, we are now technologically able to consider more stringent occupational exposure limits.

The background information and rationale for each TLV are published periodically in the Documentation of the Threshold Limit Values (ACGIH 1995). Some type of documentation is occasionally available for OELs set in other countries. The rationale or documentation for a particular OEL should always be consulted before interpreting or adjusting an exposure limit, as well as the specific data that were considered in establishing it.

TLVs are based on the best available information from industrial experience and human and animal experimental studies—when possible, from a combination of these sources. The rationale for choosing limiting values differs from substance to substance. For example, protection against impairment of health may be a guiding factor for some, whereas reasonable freedom from irritation, narcosis, nuisance or other forms of stress may form the basis for others. The age and completeness of the information available for establishing occupational exposure limits also varies from substance to substance; consequently, the precision of each TLV is different. The most recent TLV and its documentation (or its equivalent) should always be consulted in order to evaluate the quality of the data upon which that value was set. Even though all of the publications which contain OELs emphasize that they were intended for use only in establishing safe levels of exposure for persons in the workplace, they have been used at times in other situations. It is for this reason that all exposure limits should be interpreted and applied only by someone knowledgeable of industrial hygiene and toxicology.

The TLV Committee (ACGIH 1994) did not intend that they be used, or modified for use:
- As a relative index of hazard or toxicity.
- In the evaluation of community air pollution.

- For estimating the hazards of continuous, uninterrupted exposures or other extended work periods.
- As proof or disproof of an existing disease or physical condition.
- For adoption by countries whose working conditions differ from those of the United States.

The TLV Committee and other groups which set OELs warn that these values should not be "directly used" or extrapolated to predict safe levels of exposure for other exposure settings. However, if one understands the scientific rationale for the guideline and the appropriate approaches for extrapolating data, they can be used to predict acceptable levels of exposure for many different kinds of exposure scenarios and work schedules.

15.3.6.3   Philosophy and approaches in setting exposure limits

Exposure limits for workplace air contaminants are based on the premise that, although all chemical substances are toxic at some concentration when experienced for a period of time, a concentration (e.g., dose) does exist for all substances at which no injurious effect should result no matter how often the exposure is repeated. A similar premise applies to substances whose effects are limited to irritation, narcosis, nuisance or other forms of stress.

This philosophy thus differs from that applied to physical agents such as ionizing radiation, and for some chemical carcinogens, since it is possible that there may be no threshold or no dose at which zero risk would be expected. The issue of threshold effects is controversial, with reputable scientists arguing both for and against threshold theories. With this in mind, some occupational exposure limits proposed by regulatory agencies in the early 1980s were set at levels which, although not completely without risk, posed risks that were no greater than classic occupational hazards such as electrocution, falls, and so on. Even in those settings which do not use industrial chemicals, the overall workplace risks of fatal injury are about one in one thousand. This is the rationale that has been used to justify selecting this theoretical cancer risk criterion for setting TLVs for chemical carcinogens.

Several approaches for deriving OELs from animal data have been proposed and put into use over the past 50 years. The approach used by the TLV Committee and others is not markedly different from that which has been used by the US Food and Drug Administration (FDA) in establishing acceptable daily intakes (ADI) for food additives. An understanding of the FDA approach to setting exposure limits for food additives and contaminants can provide good insight to industrial hygienists who are involved in interpreting OELs.

Discussions of methodological approaches which can be used to establish workplace exposure limits based exclusively on animal data have also been presented. Although these approaches have some degree of uncertainty, they seem to be much better than a qualitative extrapolation of animal test results to humans.

Of those TLVs based on human data, most are derived from effects observed in workers who were exposed to the substance for many years. Consequently, most of the existing TLVs have been based on the results of workplace monitoring, compiled with qualitative and quantitative observations of the human response.

15.3.6.4   Limits for irritants

Prior to 1975, OELs designed to prevent irritation were largely based on human experiments. Since then, several experimental animal models have been developed. Another model based on chemical properties has been used to set preliminary OELs for organic acids and bases.

15.3.6.5   Limits for carcinogens

In 1972, the ACGIH Committee began to distinguish between human and animal carcinogens in its

TLV list. Do the TLVs Protect Enough Workers? The key question raised was, what percentage of the working population is truly protected from adverse health effects when exposed to the TLV?

A follow-up study attempted to quantify the safety margin and scientific validity of the TLVs. They concluded that there were serious inconsistencies between the scientific data available and the interpretation.

The degree of reduction in TLVs or other OELs that will undoubtedly occur in the coming years will vary depending on the type of adverse health effect to be prevented (central nervous system depression, acute toxicity, odour, irritation, developmental effects, or others). It is unclear to what degree the TLV committee will rely on various predictive toxicity models, or what risk criteria they will adopt, as we enter the next century.

15.3.6.6　Standards and nontraditional work schedules

The degree to which shift work affects a worker's capabilities, longevity, mortality, and overall well-being is still not well understood. So-called non-traditional work shifts and work schedules have been implemented in a number of industries in an attempt to eliminate, or at least reduce, some of the problems caused by normal shift work, which consists of three eight-hour work shifts per day. One kind of work schedule which is classified as nontraditional is the type involving work periods longer than 8 hours and varying (compressing) the number of days worked per week (e. g. , a 12-hours-per-day, 3-day workweek). Another type of non-traditional work schedule involves a series of brief exposures to a chemical or physical agent during a given work schedule (e. g. , a schedule where a person is exposed to a chemical for 30 minutes, 5 times per day with 1 hour between exposures). The last category of nontraditional schedule is that involving the "critical case" wherein persons are continuously exposed to an air contaminant (e. g. , spacecraft, submarine).

Compressed workweeks are a type of non-traditional work schedule that has been used primarily in non-manufacturing settings. It refers to full-time employment (virtually 40 hours per week) which is accomplished in less than five days per week. Many compressed schedules are currently in use, but the most common are: ①4-day workweeks with 10-hour days; ②3-day workweeks with 12-hour days; ③4-1/2-day workweeks with four nine-hour days and one four-hour day (usually Friday); ④the 5/4, 9 plan of alternating 5-day and 4-day workweeks of 9-hour days.

Of all workers, those on nontraditional schedules represent only about 5% of the working population. Of this number, only about 50,000-200,000 Americans who work nontraditional schedules are employed in industries where there is routine exposure to significant levels of airborne chemicals. In Canada, the percentage of chemical workers on nontraditional schedules is thought to be greater.

There are in practice only minor differences in the way OELs are set in the various countries that develop them. It should, therefore, be relatively easy to agree upon the format of a standardized criteria document containing the key information. From this point, the decision as to the size of the margin of safety that is incorporated in the limit would then be a matter of national policy.

15.3.7　Factors to consider for intervention

Often a combination of controls is used to reduce the exposures to acceptable levels. Whatever methods are selected, the intervention must reduce the exposure and resulting hazard to an acceptable level. There are, however, many other factors that need to be considered when selecting an intervention.

15.3.7.1　Effectiveness of controls

Effectiveness of controls is obviously a prime consideration when taking action to reduce exposures.

When comparing one type of intervention to another, the level of protection required must be appropriate for the challenge; too much control is a waste of resources. Those resources could be used to reduce other exposures or exposures of other employees. On the other hand, too little control leaves the worker exposed to unhealthy conditions. A useful first step is to rank the interventions according to their effectiveness, then use this ranking to evaluate the significance of the other factors.

15.3.7.2　Ease of use

For any control to be effective, the worker must be able to perform his or her job tasks with the control in place. For example, if the control method selected is substitution, then the worker must know the hazards of the new chemical, be trained in safe handling procedures, understand proper disposal procedures, and so on. If the control is isolation—placing an enclosure around the substance or the worker—the enclosure must allow the worker to do his or her job. If the control measures interfere with the tasks of the job, the worker will be reluctant to use them and may find ways to accomplish the tasks that could result in increased, not decreased exposures.

15.3.7.3　Cost

Every organization has limits on resources. The challenge is to maximize the use of those resources. When hazardous exposures are identified and an intervention strategy is being developed, cost must be a factor. The "best buy" many times will not be the lowest—or highest—cost solutions. Cost becomes a factor only after several viable methods of control have been identified. Cost of the controls can then be used to select the controls that will work best in that particular situation. If cost is the determining factor at the outset, poor or ineffective controls may be selected, or controls that interfere with the process in which the employee is working. It would be unwise to select an inexpensive set of controls that interfere with and slow down a manufacturing process. The process then would have a lower throughput and higher cost. In very short time the "real" costs of these "low cost" controls would become enormous. Industrial engineers understand the layout and overall process; production engineers understand the manufacturing steps and processes; the financial analysts understand the resource allocation problems. Occupational hygienists can provide a unique insight into these discussions due to their understanding of the specific employee's job tasks, the employee's interaction with the manufacturing equipment as well as how the controls will work in a particular setting. This team approach increases the likelihood of selecting the most appropriate (from a variety of perspectives) control.

15.3.7.4　Adequacy of warning properties

When protecting a worker against an occupational health hazard, the warning properties of the material, such as odour or irritation, must be considered. For example, if a semiconductor worker is working in an area where arsine gas is used, the extreme toxicity of the gas poses a significant potential hazard. The situation is compounded by arsine's very poor warning properties—the workers cannot detect the arsine gas by sight or smell until it is well above acceptable levels. In this case, controls that are marginally effective at keeping exposures below acceptable levels should not be considered because excursions above acceptable levels cannot be detected by the workers. In this case, engineering controls should be installed to isolate the worker from the material. In addition, a continuous arsine gas monitor should be installed to warn workers of the failure of the engineering controls. In situations involving high toxicity and poor warning properties, preventive occupational hygiene is practised. The occupational hygienist must be flexible and thoughtful when approaching an exposure problem.

15.3.7.5　Acceptable level of exposure

If controls are being considered to protect a worker from a substance such as acetone, where the acceptable level of exposure may be in the range of 800 ppm, controlling to a level of 400 ppm or less may be achieved relatively easily. Contrast the example of acetone control to control of 2-ethoxyethanol, where the acceptable level of exposure may be in the range of 0.5 ppm. To obtain the same per cent reduction (0.5 ppm-0.25 ppm) would probably require different controls. In fact, at these low levels of exposure, isolation of the material may become the primary means of control. At high levels of exposure, ventilation may provide the necessary reduction. Therefore, the acceptable level determined (by the government, company, etc.) for a substance can limit the selection of controls.

15.3.7.6　Frequency of exposure

When assessing toxicity, the classic model uses the following relationship:

Time×Concentration=Dose

Dose, in this case, is the amount of material being made available for absorption. The previous discussion focused on minimizing (lowering) the concentration portion of this relationship. One might also reduce the time spent being exposed (the underlying reason for administrative controls). This would similarly reduce the dose. The issue here is not the employee spending time in a room, but how often an operation (task) is performed. The distinction is important. In the first example, the exposure is controlled by removing the workers when they are exposed to a selected amount of toxicant; the intervention effort is not directed at controlling the amount of toxicant (in many situations there may be a combination approach). In the second case, the frequency of the operation is being used to provide the appropriate controls, not to determine a work schedule. For example, if an operation such as degreasing is performed routinely by an employee, the controls may include ventilation, substitution of a less toxic solvent or even automation of the process. If the operation is performed rarely (e. g. , once per quarter), personal protective equipment may be an option (depending on many of the factors described in this section). As these two examples illustrate, the frequency with which an operation is performed can directly affect the selection of controls. Whatever the exposure situation, the frequency with which a worker performs the tasks must be considered and factored into the control selection.

Route of exposure obviously is going to affect the method of control. If a respiratory irritant is presented, ventilation, respirators, and so on, would be considered. The challenge for the occupational hygienist is identifying all routes of exposure. For example, glycol ethers are used as a carrier solvent in printing operations. Breathing-zone air concentrations can be measured and controls are implemented. Glycol ethers, however, are rapidly absorbed through intact skin. The skin represents a significant route of exposure and must be considered. In fact, if the wrong gloves are chosen, the skin exposure may continue long after the air exposures have decreased (due to the employee continuing to use gloves that have experienced breakthrough). The hygienist must evaluate the substance – its physical properties, chemical and toxicological properties, and so on-to determine what routes of exposure are possible and plausible (based on the tasks performed by the employee).

In any discussion of controls, one of the factors that must be considered is the regulatory requirements for controls. There may well be codes of practice, regulations, and so on, that require a specific set of controls. The occupational hygienist has flexibility above and beyond the regulatory requirements, but the minimum mandated controls must be installed. Another aspect of the regulatory requirements is that the mandated controls may not work as well or may conflict with the best judgement of the occupational hygienist. The hygienist must be creative in these situations and find solutions that satisfy the regulatory as well as best practice goals of the organization.

15.3.7.7   Training and labeling

Regardless of what form of intervention is eventually selected, training and other forms of notification must be provided to ensure that the workers understand the interventions, why they were selected, what reductions in exposure are expected, and the role of the workers in achieving those reductions. Without the participation and understanding of the workforce, the interventions will likely fail or at least operate at reduced efficiency. Training builds hazard awareness in the workforce. This new awareness can be invaluable to the occupational hygienist in identifying and reducing previously unrecognized exposures or new exposures.

Training, labelling and related activities may be part of a regulatory compliance scheme. It would be prudent to check the local regulations to ensure that whatever type of training or labelling is undertaken satisfies the regulatory as well as operational requirements.

▶▶ *Summary*

The measurements to prevent and control occupational hazards include recognition, evaluation, forecast and control. All steps should follow the tertiary prevention principle.

Practice questions:

(1) How to recognize, evaluate, forecast and control occupational hazards?

(2) How many kinds of medical surveillance?

(3) What is the role of occupational legislation in the occupational hazards control?

Yao Sanqiao

References

[1]NING H,ZHOU Y,ZHOU Z. et al. Challenges to improving occupational health in China[J]. Occup Environ Med,2017,74(12):924-925.

[2]SEPULVEDA M J. From worker health to citizen health: moving upstream[J]. J Occup Environ Med, 2013,55(12):S52-S57.

[3]DING Q,SCHENK L,HANSSON S O. Occupational diseases in the people's Republic of China between 2000 and 2010[J]. Am J Ind Med,2013,56(12):1423-1432.

[4]MOREIRA S,VASCONCELOS L,SILVA SANTOS C. Sustainability of green jobs in Portugal: a methodological approach using occupational health indicators [J]. J Occup Health,2017,59(5):374-384.

[5]ZHANG X,WANG Z,LI T. The current status of occupational health in China[J]. Environ Health Prev Med,2010,15(5):263-270.

[6]MADSENI E H,NYBERG S T,MAGNUSSON L L,et al. Job strain as a risk factor for clinical depression: systematic review and meta-analysis with additional individual participant data[J]. Psychological Medicine,2017,47: 1342-1356.

[7]FRANCESCO C. Job stress models for predicting burnout syndrome: a review[J]. Ann Ist Super Sanità,2016,52(3): 443-456.

[8]MERITA T C,FERID K,MIRZA B,et al. Occupational overuse syndrome (technological diseases): carpal tunnel syndrome,a mouse shoulder,cervical pain syndrome[J]. Acta Inform Med,2014,22(5): 333-340.

[9]NAILYA N,MAZITOV A,SIMONOVA N I,et al. Current Status and Prospects of Occupational Medicine in the Russian Federation[J]. Annals of Global Health,2015,81(4) :576-586.

[10]CAROLINA E,MIQUEL P,JOACHIM S,et al. Environmental and Occupational Interventions for Primary Prevention of Cancer: A Cross-Sectorial Policy Framework [J]. Environ Health Perspect,2013, 121(4): 420-426.

[11]YUANAN H,HEFA C,SHU T. Environmental and human health challenges of industrial livestock and poultry farming in China and their mitigation [J]. Environment International,2017,107: 111-130.

[12]MOLLER D W. Environmental Health [M]. American:Harvard University Press,2011.

[13]ZHANG X,ZHONG T,LIU L,et al. Impact of soil heavy metal pollution on food safety in China [J]. PLoS ONE,2015,10(8): e0135182.

[14]TENG Y,WU J,LU S,et al. Soil and soil environmental quality monitoring in China: a review [J]. Environment International,2014,69:177-199.

[15]PAN L,WANG Y,MA J,et al. A review of heavy metal pollution levels and health risk assessment of urban soils in Chinese cities [J]. Environmental Science and Pollution Research,2018,25(2):1055-1069.

[16]YOU M,HUANG Y,LU J,et al. Environmental implications of heavy metals in soil from Huainan, China [J]. Analytical Letters,2015,48(11):1802-1814.

[17]WU S,PENG S,ZHANG X,et al. Levels and health risk assessments of heavy metals in urban soils in Dongguan,China [J]. Journal of Geochemical Exploration,2015,148(148):71-78.